general practice nursing

general
practice
nursing

Lynne Walker

Elizabeth Patterson

William Wong

Doris Young

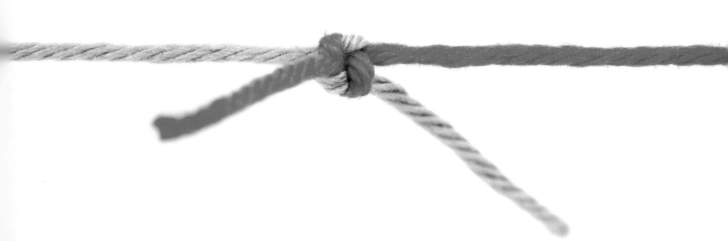

The **McGraw·Hill** Companies

Sydney New York San Francisco Auckland
Bangkok Bogotá Caracas Hong Kong
Kuala Lumpur Lisbon London Madrid
Mexico City Milan New Delhi San Juan
Seoul Singapore Taipei Toronto

Foreword

Primary health care is the frontline of our health system.

A stronger, multidisciplinary primary care system with a greater focus on preventative health is essential in delivering good health care to Australians in the 21st century. Since 2001 the number of nurses working in general practice has increased dramatically and more than half of all general practices now employ at least one practice nurse. This is a major and very positive step towards an improved primary health care system, to better meet the needs of Australian communities. In the course of using their considerable skills and expertise, practice nurses promote teamwork, improve patient access to health care, contribute to better health outcomes and assist general practitioners in many ways. Practice nurses will continue to play a vital role in our health system—not just in helping to manage existing health problems, but also in keeping people of all ages healthy and at reduced risk of hospitalisation. The Australian Government is delighted to see this workforce grow so that it may service communities' changing needs into the future, and is working to ensure that general practice nursing becomes a sought after career choice for the next generation of nursing graduates.

General Practice Nursing, the first book of its kind in Australia, will assist nurses entering the general practice workforce to gain the skills and understanding that will be required of them in this complex environment. It will reinforce and expand the knowledge of those currently working in this area, and hopefully inspire them to become leaders in the field while igniting interest generally. Skilled practitioners and leadership are essential in developing the specialty of general practice nursing, and will contribute to the reform process initiated by the Australian Government.

As Federal Minister for Health and Ageing, I wish to congratulate all nurses and students of nursing on their choice of career path. For those seeking to specialise in general practice nursing, or hone their skills, I wish you all the best in your future learning and in helping Australians live healthier lives.

Nicola Roxon MP
Minister for Health and Ageing

Contents

Part one   *Professional issues*
Edited by Lynne Walker

Part two   *Fundamentals of practice nursing*
Edited by William Wong

Part three · *Clinical skills and management in practice nursing*
Edited by Doris Young

Part four · *The way forward in practice nursing*
Edited by Elizabeth Patterson

About the authors

Lynne Walker Lynne was one of the first nurses to graduate from nursing education delivered through the higher education sector in 1977. Since then further education has been a focus with courses in midwifery, diabetes education, Pap testing and health counselling, and Lynne is currently undertaking a Master of Nursing Leadership. She was a founding member and former president (2001–2007) of the Australian Practice Nurses Association, and is currently Quality Care Project Manager at the Royal Australian College of General Practitioners and practice nurse consultant for the Department of General Practice at the University of Melbourne. In addition to this, Lynne is co-director of **walker-evans**, a small consultancy delivering education to practice nurses.

Elizabeth Patterson Elizabeth has been a Registered Nurse since 1979, undertaking her initial training at Royal Prince Alfred Hospital in Sydney, and subsequent postgraduate education at the University of New England, Queensland University of Technology and finally Griffith University, where she attained a PhD with a focus on the role of practice nurses in primary health care. Since 1991 Elizabeth has been employed at Griffith University where she is now Professor of Nursing and Head of School. She has developed and taught postgraduate education programs and facilitated continuing education sessions and workshops about practice nursing for the Royal College of Nursing, Australia and Divisions of General Practice in Queensland. Elizabeth has also been a keynote speaker at several national conferences on practice nursing.

William Wong William was Associate Professor and Director of General Practice and Primary Care Education at the University of Melbourne (2007–2009), during which time he was in charge of the distance-learning postgraduate diploma and masters programs in general practice nursing, and coordinator of the risk management in general practice module. He has previously worked in the UK, Hong Kong, China and Australia and his main research interests are sexual health, infectious diseases and health inequality. He has been the recipient of many grants and published over 70 manuscripts in such internationally peer-reviewed journals as *British Medical Journal* and *Social Science & Medicine*. Among other editing credits, he is Associate Editor of the journal *Sexually Transmitted Infections*.

Doris Young Doris is Professor and Chair of General Practice, and Associate Dean, Academic, in the Faculty of Medicine, Dentistry and Health Sciences at the University of Melbourne. As an academic general practitioner for over 25 years, she has extensive teaching, clinical and research experience in general practice, adolescent and community health, and communication skills. She has long been actively involved in undergraduate, vocational and postgraduate general practice education in Australia. For over 20 years she has worked as a part-time general practitioner in a multidisciplinary team based in a community health centre serving a multicultural and disadvantaged community, and currently leads the chronic disease research group in the Primary Care Research Unit located in the Department of General Practice.

Preface

General practice nursing has existed as a profession in Australia for many years, but the number of nurses in this field, and their scope of practice, has been limited. Recent government initiatives have, however, helped to boost employment and development. Never has there been a greater opportunity for the nursing profession to engage with patients on a widespread community level and work collaboratively with general practitioners and other health care providers at the primary health care level. With the proposed introduction of further health care reforms, it is likely that practice nurses will become embedded in the general practice setting in a manner that fully acknowledges and utilises their expertise, skills and experience to the benefit of patients and their medical and allied health colleagues. This brings with it the need for increased educational resources to support the development of this role, from novice through to expert practice nurse.

General Practice Nursing is the first book of its kind to be published in Australia. The breadth of general practice is extensive and this text provides practice nurses with the fundamentals and—hopefully—the impetus to develop their knowledge and skills to an advanced degree. Expanding the specialty of general practice nursing and the capacity of these nurses to be clinical leaders, innovators and critical thinkers has been uppermost in the minds of the editors of this text. In order for practice nurses to achieve specialisation status, become essential members of the primary health care team and contribute to patient care at an advanced level, certain commitments are called for. These involve continuing professional development, clinical leadership, expert clinical skills and undertaking responsibility to plan, implement and evaluate services provided in general practice. Fundamental to these aspirations will be the practice nurse's requirement to seek out, critique and apply the best available evidence to underpin and evolve their practice.

The first three parts of this text feature chapters on professional issues, fundamentals and clinical skills and management in practice nursing. The final section presents ideas on how practice nurses can contribute to the strengthening of primary health care provision in Australia by building capacity in leadership, education and research. The great variety of interest and expertise in Australian general practice nursing—professional, clinical and academic—is captured by 29 contributing authors across 21 chapters. The inclusion of real-life case studies and testimonials enhances the practical context of the array of topics covered. Importantly, *General Practice Nursing* provides a stimulus for practice nurses to question the way in which they and their colleagues provide care for their patients. By understanding the working relationships that practice nurses form with each other and their patients, better care can be delivered to the communities of which we are all a part.

The collaboration between nursing and medical professionals in the joint editing of this book has been demonstrative of how well health professionals can work together for the benefit of their professions, patients and the community.

Lynne Walker, Elizabeth Patterson, William Wong, Doris Young

Acknowledgment

Thank you to practice nurses, who provide nursing care, face the challenges, and tie it all together.

Contributing authors

Julianne Bryce

Judy Evans

Elizabeth Foley

Dr Kim Forrester

Dr Stephanie Fox-Young

Dr Marie Gerdtz

Dr Elizabeth Halcomb

Dr Kelsey Hegarty

Peter Larter

Dr Anne McMurray

Katrina McNalty

Rosemary Mahomed

Dr Elizabeth Manias

Christine Mathieson

Dr Lucio Naccarella

Dr Cate Nagle

Dr Rhian Parker

Dr Elizabeth Patterson

Julie Porritt

Jan Rice

Dr Natisha Sands

Gerry Silk

Dr Christine Walker

Lynne Walker

Dr Donna Waters

Michelle Wills

Dr William Wong

Rachel Yates

Dr Doris Young

Part one

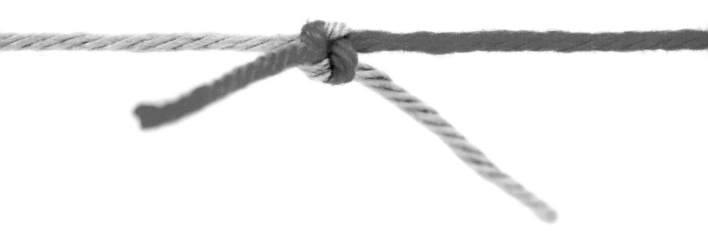

Professional issues

Edited by Lynne Walker

Chapter one

Practice nursing

by Lynne Walker

Overview

Australian general practice is experiencing an era of change which includes an increase in the number of nurses working in this area. This recent growth in nursing has been attributed to several factors, which include the shortage of general practitioners, changing health care needs of consumers, and the availability of significant funding and incentives for the employment of nurses in this role. The growth and development of the practice nurse role has been influenced by both opportunities and challenges. This chapter will examine the context of nursing in general practice and some of the many influences on this role.

Objectives

At the completion of this chapter you should be able to:

- identify and value the unique contribution of nursing to general practice;

- differentiate between acute and general practice nursing;

- recognise the changing influences on the development of the practice nurse role; and

- reflect on your own role and what it might be like in the future.

Introduction

Primary care has traditionally been seen as the provision of medical care to patients at their initial entry into the health system, and one component of primary care is general practice. There is no universally accepted definition of general practice but it is generally accepted that there is a trend to think more broadly of a general practice as an entity rather than focusing on individual general practitioners. The role of general practice has been described by Powell-Davies and Fry (2005) as:

- **providing the first point of contact for individuals seeking help from the health system**. Depending on the diagnosis made, the point of contact may end after an initial consultation.

- **creating a gateway to the rest of the system**. The next step may be a prescription or a referral for an investigation or to another health provider. It is here that the general practitioner (GP) is seen as the gatekeeper to the broader health system.

- **providing ongoing or coordination of care**. This is particularly true for patients with chronic and complex care needs, and staff often advocate and interpret the maze of services available for patients.

- **introducing and implementing disease prevention and health promotion activities**. Most people will visit a general practice in any given year, and this makes it an ideal environment to offer disease prevention and screening.

With the recent recommendations from the National Health and Hospitals Reform Commission (2009) and the development of the National Preventive Health Agency, it is likely that there will be a greater emphasis on disease prevention. The coordination role of general practice is expected to expand because of an ageing population and increasing numbers of patients with chronic illnesses. This coordination will provide opportunities to integrate and increase the services of other health professionals, including nurses, into primary care health team models of care. With their ability to triage, educate, refer, coordinate, manage disease, prevent complications and promote health to individuals and communities, nurses can play an integral role in fulfilling the requirements expected of an effective primary health system.

Nursing

Because of its nature, it is often difficult for patients and other disciplines to understand the complexities of nursing and this is even more pronounced in the general practice context. The Royal College of Nursing (2003, p. 3) has described nursing as:

The use of clinical judgement in the provision of care to enable people to improve, maintain, or recover health, to cope with health problems, and to achieve the best possible quality of life, whatever their disease or disability, until death.

The defining characteristics of nursing have been described by The Royal College of Nursing as having:

1. a particular **purpose**—to promote health, healing, growth and development, to minimise stress and suffering and to enable people to understand and cope with their disease, its treatment and its consequences. When faced with death, nursing maintains the best quality of life until its end.

2. a particular **mode of intervention**—to empower people and help them achieve independence. Nursing is a physical, intellectual, emotional and moral process which includes the identification of nursing needs and the provision of education, advice and advocacy as well as physical, emotional and spiritual support. Nursing practice also includes management, teaching, and policy and knowledge development.

3. a particular **domain**—the specific domain of nursing is people's unique responses to and experiences of health, illness, frailty, disability and health-related life events. The term 'people' includes individuals of all ages, families and communities, throughout their entire life span.

4. a particular **focus**—the whole person.

5. a particular **value base**—nursing is based on ethical values which respect the dignity, autonomy and uniqueness of human beings. The nurse has acceptance of and accountability for decisions and actions. This is supported by a code of ethics, a code of conduct and a regulatory process.

6. a **commitment to partnership**—with patients, carers, relatives and members of a multidisciplinary team. Where appropriate, nurses will lead the team, and at times work under the leadership of others. At all times, however, they remain personally and professionally accountable for their own decisions and actions.

General practice nursing

Over the years nursing has been described as a vocation, a practice, an occupation, an industry, an art, a science, a craft and a profession (Gray & Pratt 1991). Perhaps it can be described as a combination of all of these things, and general practice is an environment where all of these descriptors have meaning in the work undertaken by practice nurses.

A practice nurse is defined as 'a registered nurse or an enrolled nurse who is employed by, or whose services are otherwise retained by, a general practice' (Department of Health and Ageing 2009).

Very often practice nurses describe their work in general practice as a culmination of the various roles and previous employment opportunities that they have undertaken prior to commencement in general practice. Time has seen nursing progress from simple tasks to a complex knowledge-based practice undertaken in a variety of rapidly changing health care organisations, in this case general practice.

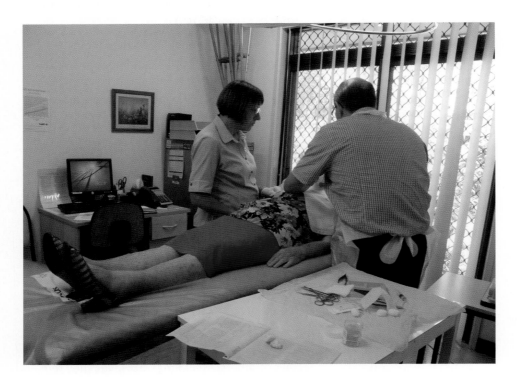

Testimonial

Why am I a practice nurse? Why am I still practice nursing after 18 years? Why do I still enjoy my job and go home feeling I've made a difference each day? Sometimes I ask myself these questions and the answer is—I'm part of a family that cares and we pull together and not apart to support each other, our clients and our community. I know the answer when I take a BP on an 80-year-old who really wants to tell me about her dog that got run over, and I want to give her the acknowledgment of her loss. I know the answer when I'm there for the 32-year-old mother of six who has just found out that she has a brain tumour, and just hopes I'm on duty so that she can share her shock and disbelief with me. It's when I can make a quick cuppa for a doctor who has been up all night and hasn't had time for a break, and his quiet 'thank you' lets me know he appreciates the thought behind the gesture. I know that through being able to make time for people, in all the different roles I play in my capacity as a practice nurse, I can make a difference to the wellbeing of the inhabitants of the town I love. That's why I enjoy being a practice nurse. (Cathy, rural practice nurse)

Based on the characteristics described above, practice nurses should be involved in health promotion, disease prevention, palliative care, advocating for patients, research, policy planning and development, and education both for the profession and the health consumer. As well as caring for individuals, their families and the community, practice nurses can be involved in the development of appropriate systems for the management of patients, information and quality improvements.

As an evolving profession, nurses have been given the responsibility of developing an appropriate scope of practice. Never has this been truer than in the area of general practice, where the development of practice nursing is moving towards the status of a legitimate specialty of nursing. The perceived traditional role of nurses has been determined by the context which has the most meaning for most patients; usually the acute or tertiary environment of a hospital. The general public's perception of nurses and their view of what happens in general practice is often influenced by their individual hospital experiences (Hegney et al. 2004), albeit that the views formed about general practice are inaccurate at times. Practice nurses have yet to develop a professional profile akin to that of acute nursing specialties (Patterson 2000); however, the need to do so is important to the future perception, role, education and career path of practice nurses in Australia.

As nursing in general practice is a new and evolving context for nursing, most practice nurses have a background of employment within the acute or hospital sector. Working in general practice brings contextual challenges which differentiate the roles of practice nurses from those of their colleagues in the acute sector. For nurses contemplating working in general practice, identifying these differences will assist them in adapting to the unique working environment of general practice and in recognising the impact on their nursing practice. Differences described by Keleher and St John (2007) between the institutional setting and community setting are described in Table 1.1 overleaf.

Reflections

Can you describe other differences between hospital-based nurses and those working in general practice?

Table 1.1 Impact on nursing practice of institutional/hospital setting versus a community setting

	Hospital/institutional setting	Community setting
Focus of care	– Individual focus, family as context	– Individual, family, group, aggregate, community as unit of care
Aim of care	– Secondary and tertiary prevention, discharge from institution	– Primary, secondary and tertiary prevention, self-care
Duration of care	– Episodic	– Continuous
Power	– Nurse in charge, patient on health professionals' turf	– Client in charge, nurse on patients' turf
Patient/client	– Sick role, called a patient	– Well role, called a client
Responsibility	– Treatment and care provision is nurses' responsibility	– Self-care, responsibility for treatment and care is shared between client and nurse
Resources	– Structures, well resourced, quick access to resources	– Unstructured, less access to resources, community as a resource
Nurse/patient relationship	– Nurse as expert care provider, patient dependant	– Collaborative, nurse as consultant or advisor
Change	– Responds to political and organisational change	– Responds to political and community change
Professional support	– Quick access to health teams, interdependent	– Sole practitioner, independent access to partnerships and networks
Philosophies of practice	– Illness focus, treatment and therapy – Individual holistic care	– Health and rehabilitation focus – Family and community holistic care – Primary health care

Source: Keleher & St John 2007, p. 10

Prior to the availability of financial incentives to employ more nurses in general practice, very little data was available to ascertain practice nurse demographics. Since 2003, the Australian General Practice Network (AGPN) has compiled a biannual compilation of national information and statistics regarding practice nurses. This survey is conducted via the Divisions of General Practice Network and is the only survey of its type to offer such comprehensive information. The key findings from the National Practice Nurse Workforce Survey Report 2007 include the following:

- The estimated number of practice nurses has increased from 4924 in 2005 to 7824 in 2007.

- An estimated 58% of general practices employ one or more practice nurses, an increase of 1% from 2005.

- About 79% of all practice nurses are registered nurses, with 15.3% reporting that they are enrolled nurses.

- Forty-one per cent of the practice nurse population is aged between 40 and 49 years, with 78% over 40 years of age.

- General practice nursing is still a predominantly part-time workforce. However, the percentage of nurses working part-time in general practice has decreased consistently, falling from 87% in 2003 to 82% in 2005 and 75% in 2007. This equates to 25% of the practice nurse workforce now working full-time.

- Rural and remote areas have the highest rate of practice nurse employment at 60%.

- Sixty-two per cent of practice nurses have additional graduate nursing qualifications, for example, accredited nurse immuniser, midwifery, women's health nurse or asthma education.

Currently, the eastern states have higher numbers of nurses employed in general practice but this may reflect the larger population in these states. As the number of nurses employed in general practice increases, it is likely the role will continue to change. Supported by evidence, increasing familiarity with the practice nurse role by general practitioners, the nursing profession and consumers will help promote and expand practice nursing.

The overseas experience

Nurses in the United Kingdom have been documented as having worked in general practice from as far back as 1913 (Hampson 2000). As a result of government initiatives, the numbers have increased since the 1960s and continue to grow. Historically, however, the relationship between employing bodies and practice nurses has been a 'troubled liaison' since early times (Hampson 2000, p. 7).

Similar to their Australian colleagues, practice nurses and general practitioners in the UK have experienced frustrations with limitations, such as 'hierarchical relationships, interprofessional disputes, skill mix and inappropriate utilization of the skills of team members' (Galvin et al. 1999, p. 239). However, this has changed since significant health reforms based on quality and outcome were introduced in 2000 and practice nurses have consistently expanded their roles to take on some activities traditionally fulfilled by the GP (Parker & Keleher 2008). Although the funding mechanism is different from that in Australia, an understanding remains that patient care is delivered for quality not volume and the focus is the 'right care in the right place at the right time' (National Health Service UK 2002, p. 34).

Components of the practice nurse role

'Role' has been described by Williams (2000) as a 'slippery concept' signifying function or a part to play. It is an expected outcome of behaviours of members occupying a particular position within an organisational structure. Importantly though, it also takes into consideration the way nurses perceive their own situation (Goffman 1969, cited in Hampson 2000). In its early developmental stage, practice nursing in the UK was described as flexible, generic and somewhat ill-defined (Aitken & Lunt 1996; Hampson 2002). This has also been noted in the Australian context with only 66.2% of practice nurses having a clear job description (Halcomb, Patterson & Davidson 2006). General practice is an area where medicine and nursing meet at an elementary level and the potential for overlap of roles and responsibilities of nurses and medical practitioners is high.

Although the Future Directions in Practice Nursing Workshop in 2001 articulated an expectation of general practice to 'enhance the quality and delivery of health care by providing nursing services' (DoHA 2001, p. 3), none of the five objectives of the nursing in general practice initiative emphasised the contribution from a nursing perspective. These objectives related to access, cost, integration and relieving workforce pressure, presumably of the general practitioners (Healthcare Management Advisors 2005).

In the most comprehensive study of the practice nurse role, Watts et al. (2004) identified four dimensions of responsibility:

- **clinical care**—which may include injections, wound management, applying casts, performing Pap tests, assessment of patients and first aid;
- **clinical organisation**—which requires management and coordination of clinical activities, such as infection control, recalls and reminders, population health, research and quality assurance;
- **practice administration**—which provides support to the business aspect of general practice and may include staff orientation, education and rostering; and
- **integration**—which includes patient advocacy, liaising with other professionals and developing effective communication channels.

The interaction and overlap of these role components are perhaps best illustrated by Figure 1.1 below.

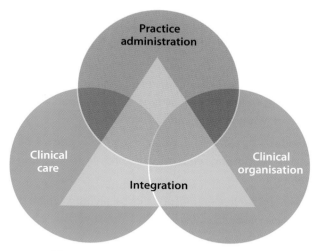

Figure 1.1 Components of the practice nurse role

Interestingly, none of the identified dimensions include a professional nursing perspective, such as leadership, research, education, professional development or development of the specialty. This may be explained partly by the intent of government policy in this area to support medical workforce issues, with little thought given to the effect it would have on the individual nurse or nursing profession as a whole. The role of the practice nurse has similarly but more broadly been described in the *Competency Standards for Registered and Enrolled Nurses in General Practice* (Australian Nurses Federation 2006). These standards attempt to address this lack of professional perspective by describing the role in more comprehensive dimensions, such as:

- **professional practice**—including contributing to review and modification of nursing and general practice standards, codes and guidelines, establishing networks, and educating nurses and students of general practice health care;

- provision of **clinical care**—including the operation of health care clinics while considering the ethical implications in decision making about allocation of health care resources;

- management of **clinical systems**—including quality improvement; and

- **collaborative practice**—including referral of patients, contribution to practice meetings, communication of research evidence and monitoring of population health.

In more recent research, Phillips et al. (2009), through observational visits to practices, identified six roles that practice nurses fulfil:

1. **carer**—seen as a core function of the practice nurse, with participation in clinical care, advocacy and nurturing the patient–nurse relationship. This study demonstrated that 43.5% of nurse time was spent in clinical activities;

2. **organiser**—recognised by practice staff as a key function, both in terms of clinical organisation of recalls, reminders and triage, and in management organisation of stock, cleaning of instruments, maintenance of a safe working environment, and writing policies and procedures;

3. **quality controller**—by establishing processes and systems for practice accreditation and supporting regulatory requirements including occupational health and safety;

4. **problem solver**—proactive and responsive behaviours which indicate that nurses are strategic problem solvers, often innovative, thinking, reflecting and acting as agents of change;

5. **educator**—educating predominantly in an informal manner to patients, other nurses, GPs, registrars and other practice staff; and

6. **agent of connectivity**—both within the practice and externally to community resources.

It can be seen from most studies that the practice nurse has been identified as not only playing an important part in patient care but also in contributing to practice infrastructure, building the capacity of the practice, maintaining quality, contributing to sustainability of general practice and generally tying together the complex elements of general practice.

Testimonial

When you've have had an exceptionally gruelling day and feel like throwing in the towel, being an emergency nurse, coronary care nurse, immuniser, Pap smear provider, asthma and diabetes educator, counsellor, health promoter, liaison nurse and support person, as well as being pulled from pillar to post by doctors and reception staff, it all makes it worthwhile when one of your favourite patients whispers in your ear, 'I don't know what I would do without you', and gives you a bag of chocolate éclairs. (Christine, rural nurse)

Reflections

How do you perceive your role and is it the same as your job description?
How does your role compare to the dimensions described above?

> **Testimonial**
>
> The practice nursing role is constantly developing. It is all about change, utilising and expanding your skill set and being adaptable. Many practices have never worked with a nurse and simply employing a PN brings enormous change to the workings and culture of the GP surgery. The nurse may not realise it when taking the job but the nurse is the catalyst for change. (Karen, metropolitan practice)

Influences on the role of the practice nurse

The role of the practice nurse has been described as a 'slippery concept' (see p. 10). Therefore, it is no surprise that when asked to describe their role, practice nurses will give an individual account of the work they do, which will often differ from those of their colleagues, even within the same workplace. The factors which determine what each practice nurse does on a daily basis are varied and arise from global and local initiatives and the nurse's background. The more global factors which impact on the practice nurse role are described in Table 1.2 overleaf and include national health priorities and government policy, professional issues, consumer needs, legislative requirements, educational opportunities, and workforce supply and demand.

Local factors will vary according to the state or territory, the geographical location of the practice, the demographics of the community, the building and space available for the nurse to use, and the owners of the practice and their ethics and philosophies. For example, rural nurses have been shown to enjoy slightly more extended care roles with increased autonomy and extended skill sets (Phillips et al. 2009) and have benefited from earlier introduction of Medicare Benefits Schedule (MBS) item numbers.

The nurse's individual characteristics are important and are related to their educational qualifications, personal and professional experiences, attitudes, general knowledge, skills, goals and expectations (Watts et al. 2004; Phillips et al. 2009). Moreover, the practice nurse role is influenced by how the individual nurse perceives it and how he or she works towards fulfilling that expectation.

The predominantly small-business structure of Australian general practice has been described as a major impediment to the development of the role of the practice nurse (Halcomb et al. 2005; Halcomb, Patterson & Davidson 2006). Limited understanding by employers of the abilities and education of practice nurses further restricts the ability of nurses to work to their full capacity. The constant focus on the nurse as a strategy for increasing practice income rather than for the provision of nursing care is one that limits the role and reduces it to a task-oriented service rather than part of a holistic approach to patient care.

Practice nurses are in a unique situation whereby they are employed by another professional group. The professional relationship between the general practitioner and the practice nurse is entrenched with issues that affect the role

Table 1.2 Factors that enhance and constrain development of the practice nurse role in Australia

	Enhancing	Constraining
Health system	– Global shift from secondary to primary care – Trend towards group rather than solo general practices – Publicly funded practice – National and international health priority areas of chronic and complex diseases	– Predominantly episodic illness management—no national primary health care policy – Narrow interpretation of primary health care – Biomedical domination of primary and secondary health service – Complex interface between secondary and primary care – Trend to highly corporate centre with high turnover
Legislation	– Introduction of nurse practice legislation	– Current Medicare benefits largely restricted to medical practitioners, optometrists and some dentists – State registration boards have variable requirements and regulations – Issues regarding professional liability and malpractice are poorly defined for nurses in the general practice setting
Financial	– Practice and division of general practice grants for specific projects – Commonwealth Government incentives to employ practice nurses, such as the practice incentive program and enhanced primary care – MedicarePlus item numbers for immunisation, wound care and Pap smear services	– Limited subsidy/financial incentive to employ practice nurses (particularly from urban practices) – Economic rationalism – Decreased profit margin of general practice – Short-term nature of project funding and the need to incorporate self-sustainability into project development – Lack of a specific industrial award to define appropriate conditions of employment and remuneration packages

	Enhancing	Constraining
Social	– Nurses viewed as approachable, ethical and trustworthy by the community	– Negative power relationship between nurses and GPs relating to employee–employer status, gender, socioeconomic status, nurses generally passive nature – Historical development of the professions – Cure more valued than care by consumers in primary care – Lifestyle benefits of practice nurses role valued more highly than career opportunities
Professional issues	– Nurse practitioner movement – Growth of the Australian Practice Nurse Association – Development of Australian practice nurse research – Development of competency standards for both registered and enrolled nurses – Conduct of accredited practice nurse specific education – Practice nurse specific professional development opportunities (e.g. annual conference)	– Fragmented nursing organisations – Limited understanding of the role of the practice nurse by other nurses and health professionals – Medical control of the scope of practice in primary care – Use of nurses for general administrative and cleaning duties in addition to clinical nursing practice – Appropriation of nursing work to receptionists and unskilled employees – Lack of clearly defined career path, thus reducing the recruitment/retention of career-oriented workforce
Knowledge development	– Tertiary nursing education – Curriculum underpinned by primary health care – Availability of focused educational opportunities through divisions of General Practice and Royal College of Nursing, Australia	– Limited orientation to practice nursing or post-basic practice nurse qualifications – Segregated medical and nurse education – General paucity of health promotion and primary health care training among current practice nurses – Poor access to appropriate, graded education, training and accreditation for both registered and enrolled nurses
Workforce supply	– Shortage of GPs in rural and remote areas – Dissatisfaction of nurses in the public health system – Employment conditions could be more suitable to nurses lifestyle needs	– Disproportionate representation of GPs in metropolitan areas – Global shortage of educated and experienced nurses

Continued >

Table 1.2 *continued*

	Enhancing	Constraining
Public demand	– Increased demand for, and public awareness of, alternative health practitioners – Increased GP visits nationally – Increased numbers of consumers, particularly with chronic disease, requiring health education, lifestyle modification and psychosocial support	– High demand for low-cost/bulk-billed services

Source: Patterson 2000

that practice nurses are able to fulfil. These include implicit power differences, economic power wielded through the employer–employee relationship and gender differences (Halcomb, Patterson & Davidson 2006; Phillips et al. 2009). Medical training has traditionally been concerned with diagnosis and treatment, with little time left for management and issues relating to human resources (Hampson 2002), which creates tension between practice nurses as employees and practice nurses as accountable health professionals. Ideally the relationship between two health professionals should be an equal one. Furthermore, despite having a clear scope of practice, many practice nurses are impeded in fulfilling their potential due to the direction given by their employers. The desire to work to full capacity in terms of their scope of practice has been expressed as a priority for practice nurses (Australian Practice Nurses Association 2009). Conversely, the pressure from practice nurses to work outside this scope of practice is also an issue of significance. Respect, recognition of skills and trust are essential components of teamwork and these can be a challenge to achieve in some workplaces.

Substitution of work of general practitioners

Practice nurses have traditionally been associated with delegated work supervised by medical practitioners but in recent times much has been written about their role as substitutes for providing certain elements of care that have previously been delivered by general practitioners. Sibbald (2008) argues that efficiency gains are possible if general practitioners stop providing services that nurses are competent to undertake, such as immunisation, wound management, cervical screening, lifestyle counselling and suturing, to name a few, and focus on the tasks that they alone are licensed to perform. Although the concept of substitution creates debate between the medical and nursing professions, it is a debate that needs to happen and be resolved if the future health system is going to be able to manage the growing number of patients with the limited resources available. Avoiding the duplication of services, which can accompany substitution, will increase efficiencies in general practice and allow better access for more patients.

Delegation of work by general practitioners to practice nurses

The delegation of work by general practitioners to practice nurses is reflected and reinforced by the Australian Government in its MBS criteria. Funding via MBS practice nurse item numbers, which supports employment of practice nurses, is limited primarily to those services that have been directly supervised by the GP. Nursing work done 'for and on behalf of the GP' undermines nursing responsibility and accountability as determined by the Nursing Code of Ethics and Code of Conduct. Currently, only 21% of clinical activities performed by practice nurses are funded by the MBS (Phillips et al. 2009), so this is not a true indication of the contribution that nurses can make to general practice, despite the argument for employment of nurses often being based on the business model. Furthermore, it restricts or expands the nurse role at the discretion of the employing GP and allows payment only for those holding a provider number, rather than those doing the work. Conversely, a UK study found that most practice nurses felt they had considerable autonomy in organising their work (Aitken & Lunt 1996). The most likely explanation for this variation in practice nurse autonomy between Australia and the UK is how they are funded.

Evidence of benefits of practice nurses

Keleher et al. (2009, p. 16) has concluded 'that there is modest international evidence that nurses in primary care settings can provide effective care and achieve positive health outcomes for patients similar to that provided by doctors'. Although limited to date, research is now seeking to confirm these findings in the Australian context. Information about some of this research can be found in Chapter 18.

International studies have identified health promotion, chronic disease management and illness prevention as particularly significant roles for practice nurses. Furthermore, primary care nurses, including those in general practice, have been shown to deliver care of as high a quality as that of general

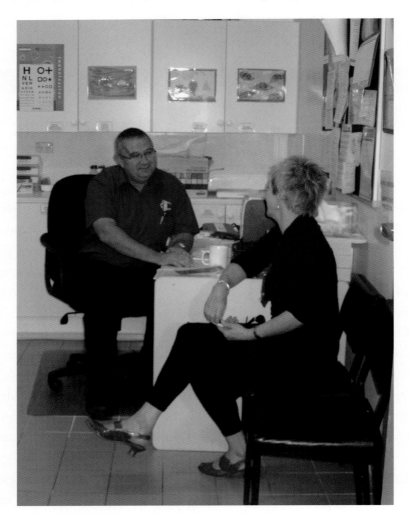

Testimonial

At the end of a two-week clinical placement at a local medical centre, I was offered a job there. The past two years have been a wonderful experience. Exposure to all kinds of different wounds and dressings has broadened my experience and skills. The vaccination programs for cervical cancer, H1N1 and childhood immunisation have finetuned my vaccination skills. And my professional relationships with some of our long-term as well as drop-in patients have really made me feel like a part of the local community. (Greg, metropolitan practice)

practitioners in the areas of preventive health care, routine follow-up of patients with long-term conditions and first contact care for people with minor illness (Laurant et al. 2008). Indeed, a review of research completed by Richardson (1999) suggested that 25–70% of the work undertaken by doctors might be moved to nurses. A decade later, nurses in Australia were shown to contribute to appropriate, responsive, continuous, safe and sustainable care with an often unrecognised contribution to quality and safety in general practice (Phillips et al. 2009). Although consumers have indicated that they expect practice nurses to work within their professional boundaries, they have also indicated that they enhance the services available to them (Cheek et al. 2002).

Future role of practice nurses

Favourable opportunities often follow as a result of conjecture, occurring unplanned and providing the prospect of experiencing something new, suggest Wilson, Averis and Walsh (2004). These writers argue that the development of nurses' positions through augmenting nursing activities has created chances for nurses to extend their boundaries and explore new areas, especially in the realm of private practice. Such expansion requires practice nurses to be educated at an advanced level and undertake regular professional development to maintain and grow their competencies. This will be discussed further in Chapter 3.

Suggestions for vocational development include:

- further expansion of multidisciplinary care;
- identification of core skills of team members which could be shared;
- clarification of specialist skills;
- accessibility of affordable and accredited formal education;
- provision of quality education and career framework;

- education of GPs regarding clinical skills and scope;
- standardisation of systems which would enable evaluation of patient outcomes;
- collection of primary care activity data by provider type;
- creation of formal and informal models of clinical supervision and mentorship of practice of nurses;
- specification of national training standards for practice nursing;
- sustainable remuneration commensurate with the level of practice;
- availability of career pathways; and
- identification of organisational changes and a support systems for change.

(Galvin et al. 1999; Palm Consulting Group 2005; Halcomb & Davidson 2007; Keleher et al. 2007; Parker & Keleher 2008; Parker et al. 2009; Nelson et al. 2009.)

Until certain issues, such as a funding model which supports nursing skills and rewards an expanded scope of practice, are resolved, difficulties will remain for general practice nurses.

Conclusion

Although practice nursing is in the early stages of its evolution, health reforms, workforce shortages and consumer expectations have provided endless opportunities for nurses working in the unique context of general practice. Nurses have demonstrated infinite ability in solving the problems and challenges they face in their workplaces and fulfilling the aim of enhancing the quality and delivery of health care. As further prospects arise, today's practice nurses will lead tomorrow's graduates into a recognised and rewarding career.

Key messages

The role of the practice nurse is varied and influenced by national, local and personal factors.

Appropriately trained practice nurses can make a significant and cost effective contribution to primary health care and good health outcomes for patients.

Practice nurse numbers and scope of practice are expanding.

Useful resources

Australian Practice Nurses Association
http://www.apna.asn.au

Department of Health and Ageing Nursing in General Practice program
http://health.gov.au

Nursing in General Practice Business Models
http://generalpracticenursing.com.au

Nursing in General Practice Recruitment and Orientation Resource
http://generalpracticenursing.com.au

Nursing in General Practice: A Guide for the General Practice Team
http://generalpracticenursing.com.au

References

1. Aiken, K & Lunt, N 1996, 'Negotiating the role of the practice nurse in general practice', *Journal of Advanced Nursing*, vol. 24, pp. 498–505.

2. Australian General Practice Network (AGPN) 2007, *National Practice Nurse Workforce Survey report 2007*, Canberra, viewed November 2009, <http://generalpracticenursing.com.au/__data/assets/pdf_file/0006/15378/National-Practice-Nurse-Workforce-Survey-2003.pdf>.

3. Australian Nurses Federation 2006, *Competency standards for nurses in general practice*, viewed October 2009, <http://www.anf.org.au/nurses_gp/resource_03.pdf>.

4. Australian Practice Nurses Association 2009, *Salary and conditions survey*, unpublished report.

5. Cheek, J, Price, K, Dawson, A, Mott, K, Beilby, J & Wilkinson, D 2002, 'Consumer Perceptions of Nursing and Nurses in General Practice', Centre for Research into Nursing and Health Care (CRNHC), Adelaide, viewed November 2009, <http://www.health.gov.au/internet/main/publishing.nsf/Content/work-pr-nigp-res-cons-rept>.

6. Department of Health and Ageing (DoHA) 2009, *Nursing in General Practice—education and training*, viewed October 2009, <http://health.gov.au/>.

7. Galvin, K, Andrews, C, Jackson, D, Cheesman, S, Fudge, T, Ferris, R & Graham, I 1999, 'Investigating and implementing change within the primary care health nursing team', *Journal of Advanced Nursing*, vol. 30, no. 1, pp. 238–47.

8. Gray, G & Pratt, G 1991, *Towards a discipline of nursing*, Churchill Livingstone, Marrackville, NSW.

9. Halcomb, E & Davidson, P 2007, 'Strategic directions for developing the Australian general practice nurse role in cardiovascular disease management', *Contemporary Nurse*, vol. 26, Issue 1, pp. 125–35.

10. Halcomb, E, Davidson, P, Daly, J, Griffiths, R, Yallop, J & Tofler, G 2005, 'Nursing in Australian general practice: directions and perspectives', *Australian Health Review*, vol. 29, no. 2, pp. 156–66.

11. Halcomb, E, Patterson, E & Davidson, P 2006, 'Evolution of practice nursing in Australia', *Journal of Advanced Nursing*, vol. 55, no. 3, pp. 376–90.

12. Hampson, G 2002, *Practice Nurse Handbook*, 4th edn, Blackwell, Oxford.

13. Healthcare Management Advisors 2005, *Evaluation of the 2001 Nursing in General Practice Initiative: Final Report*, Adelaide, viewed October 2009, <http://www.health.gov.au/>.

14. Hegney, D, Price, K, Patterson, E, Martin-McDonald, K & Rees, S 2004, 'Australian consumers' expectations for expanded nursing roles in general practice—choice not gatekeeping', *Australian Family Physician*, vol. 33, no. 10, pp. 845–9, viewed November 2009, <http://www.racgp.org.au/>.

15. Keleher, H, Joyce, C, Parker, R & Piterman, L 2007, 'Practice Nurses in Australia: current issues and future directions', *Medical Journal of Australia*, vol. 187, no. 2, pp. 108–10.

16. Keleher, H, Parker, R, Abdulwadud, O & Francis, K 2009, 'Systematic review of the effectiveness of primary care nursing', *International Journal of Nursing Practice*, 15, pp. 16–24.

17. Keleher, H & St John, W 2007, *Community Nursing Practice Theory, Skills and Issues*, Allen & Unwin, Sydney.

18. Laurent, M, Reeves, D, Hermens, J, Braspenning, J, Grol, R & Sibbald, B 2008, 'Substitution of doctors by nurses in primary care', *Cochrane Database of Systematic Reviews*, 2008, issue 4.

19. National Health and Hospitals Reform Commission (NH&HRC) 2009, 'A Healthier Future for All Australians', <http://www.health.gov.au/>.

20. National Health Service (NHS) 2002, *Delivering the NHS plan: next steps on investment, next steps on reform*, <http://www.dh.gov.uk/>.

21. Nelson, K, Wright, T, Connor, M, Buckley, S & Cumming, J 2009, 'Lessons from eleven primary health care nursing innovations', *New Zealand International Journal of Nursing Review*, vol. 56, pp. 291-8.

22. Palm Consulting Group 2005, 'Nursing in General Practice Training and Support Workshop; Summary Report', viewed November 2009, <http://www6.health.gov.au/>.

23. Parker, R & Keleher, H November 2008, 'Preparing nurses for primary health care reforms', Faculty of Health, University of Canberra and Department of Health Science, Monash University, viewed March 2010, <http://www.anu.edu.au/aphcri/Spokes_Research_Program/Stream_Ten/S10_ParkerKeleher_25.pdf>.

24. Parker, R, Keleher, H, Francis, K & Abdulwadud, O 2009, 'Practice nursing in Australia: a review of education and career pathways', *BMC Nursing*, 8:5, viewed November 2009, <http://www.biomedcentral.com/content/pdf/1472-6955-8-5.pdf>.

25. Patterson, E 2000, Primary health care nursing: a case study of practice nurses (PhD thesis), Griffith University, Australia as cited in Halcomb, E, Davidson, P, Daly, J, Griffiths, R, Yallop, J & Tofler, G 2005, 'Nursing in Australian general practice: directions and perspectives', *Australian Health Review*, vol. 29, no. 2, p. 159.

26. Phillips, C, Pearce, C, Hall, S, Klijakovic, M, Sibbald, B, Dawn, K, Porritt, J & Yates, R 2009, 'Enhancing care, improving quality: the six roles of the general practice nurse', *Medical Journal of Australia*, vol. 191, no. 2, pp. 92–7.

27. Powell-Davies, G & Fry, D 2005, 'General Practice in the Health System', chapter in *General Practice in Australia: 2004*, Commonwealth of Australia.

28. Richardson, M 1999, 'Identifying, evaluating and implementing cost effective skill mix', *Journal of Nurse Management*, 5, pp. 265–70, cited by Laurant, M, Reeves, D, Hermens, J, Braspenning, J, Grol, R & Sibbald, B 2004, 'Substitution of doctors by nurses in primary care', *Cochrane Database of Systematic Reviews*, issue 4.

29. Royal College of Nursing 2003, *Defining Nursing*, London, <http://www.rcn.org.uk/>.

30. Sibbald, B 2008, 'Should primary care be nurse led?', *British Medical Journal*, vol. 337, p. 658.

31. Watts, I, Foley, E, Hutchison, R, Pascoe, T, Whitecross, L & Snowdon, T 2004, *General Practice Nursing in Australia*, RACGP and RCNA, Melbourne, viewed October 2009, <http://www.racgp.org.au/>.

32. Williams, A 2000, *Nursing, Medicine and Primary Care*, Open University Press, Buckingham.

33. Wilson, A, Averis, A & Walsh, K 2004, 'The scope of private practice nursing in an Australian sample', *Public Health Nursing*, vol. 21, no. 5, pp. 488–94.

Chapter two

The Australian health care system

by Lucio Naccarella, Julie Porritt and Rachel Yates

Overview

This chapter provides an overview of the current Australian health care system. Discussed in detail is the development of policy and how it relates to the primary health care system, general practice and practice nurses. Information provided in this chapter is essential for practice nurses to understand the complex environment in which they work, and the funding implications for both the workplace and the patient. It demonstrates how national and state policies directly influence the role of practice nurses and why nurses need to be aware of and participate in formulation of policy.

Objectives

At the completion of this chapter you should be able to:

- have an understanding of the Australian health care system;

- have an understanding of funding arrangements for primary care providers;

- have knowledge about the current primary health care policy reform directions; and

- recognise the role of divisions of general practice.

Introduction

Currently, Australians enjoy one of the highest life expectancies in the world, at 81.4 years, second only to Japan. Death rates are falling for many of our leading health concerns, such as cancer, heart disease, strokes, injury and asthma (AIH&W 2008). Despite the good health that Australians enjoy in comparison to other countries, concerns about quality of care, workforce shortages, and the increasing burden of complex and chronic diseases demand discussion and reform of the health care system. Emphasis is being placed on the central role and contribution of the primary health care system to address these concerns.

Nursing in general practice, despite its recent introduction into the primary health debate, is of paramount importance in seeking to maintain and improve life expectancy by preventive health care and monitoring of chronic illness.

The Australian health care system

Australia has a complex, multilayered health care system that can be confusing for both patients and practitioners alike. The complexity arises due to the system's many elements and interactions. Major elements in the system include:

- levels of care (primary, secondary and tertiary)
- settings and facilities (hospitals, consulting rooms, aged-care homes, community clinics)
- sectors and funders (private/public, state/federal)
- services and providers (pharmaceutical/medical/allied health agencies and Home And Community Care (HACC) program).

A useful way to understand the national health care system is to consider how the different elements of the system sit within the different tiers of care. A simplified view is provided in Table 2.1 opposite.

Reflections

In which parts of the system do nurses have a role to play? How will the activities pertaining to work vary from one part of the system to another?

Sources of funding

A further complexity in the Australian health care system is that each of the elements can have different mechanisms for obtaining funding. There are currently four main contributors, each providing funds to enable the provision of health care delivery to all Australians.

These are:

- **Commonwealth Government**—funds most, but not all, primary care, general practice and public hospitals through the Medicare Benefits Schedule (MBS) and the Pharmaceutical Benefits Schedule (PBS).
- **State governments**—fund public hospital and community health services by finance determined through the Australian health care agreements and state/territory taxes. Recent policy initiatives, such as GP Plus in South Australia, HealthOne in New South Wales and the Australian Better Health Initiative (ABHI)

Table 2.1 Australian health system elements

Level of care	What it is	Setting	Provider	Funder
Primary care	Frontline care that can be accessed directly by individuals without referral	– General practices – Community/private clinics – Hospital emergency departments – Various government and non-government agencies	– Medical practitioners (mainly GPs) – Nurses (PNs, NPs and community nurses) – Community-based (public and private) allied health professionals	– Commonwealth (general practice) – State health (community clinics and other state-based health services) Private health insurance
Secondary care	More specialised care that can only be accessed by referral from other primary care providers (usually GPs and in some cases, nurse practitioners)	Area health services – Local/district hospitals – Residential aged care facilities	– Specialist medical practitioners – Hospital-based nurses and allied health professionals	– Commonwealth (private medical practitioner services) – State (public hospital services, personnel and facilities) – Private health insurance private hospital services, facilities and non-medical personnel)
Tertiary care	Care provided by highly trained specialists on referral from primary or secondary medical care personnel Such care also often involves advanced technology	– Specialist/teaching hospitals and units (e.g. burns, cancer, plastic and neurosurgery units) – Residential aged-care facilities	'Super specialists'; highly trained doctors and nurses and some allied health professionals	– Commonwealth (private medical practitioner services) – State (public hospital services, personnel and facilities) – Private health insurance private hospital services, facilities and non-medical personnel

have led to states funding an extended range of primary care services, including a number of general practice clinics. The emphasis on general practice by the state governments is seen as a cost-effective approach to health, especially in relation to chronic disease.

- **Private health insurance (PHI)**—financed through individual consumer payments for specific health insurance policies. These policies fund services from a variety of health professionals (except GPs) for the services they provide in private practices in the community and in private hospitals.

The fourth contributor to health funding is *the individual*, who often contributes to funding health care by direct payment for services not subsidised or funded by any of the means described above. Co-payments are made by patients in addition to subsidised services funded through the MBS, PBS or PHI.

Reflections

How does the funding of the Australian health care system affect access to health care for some groups in the community?

Methods of funding

The Commonwealth Government's major contributions to health funding include Medicare and the Pharmaceutical Benefit Scheme.

Medicare is a universal medical insurance scheme that was introduced in 1975 as Medibank and renamed to Medicare in 1984. Medicare was introduced to provide eligible Australian residents with affordable, accessible and high-quality health care. Payments are subsidised for services provided by doctors and optometrists, and allied health professionals such as clinical psychologists (Mediguide 2007). Medicare is financed through a tax levy on income and this is currently set at 1.5% with an additional 1.0% surcharge for those on high incomes who do not have private health insurance. The schedule fees for items are uniform across Australia and are determined by the Department of Health and Ageing in consultation with professional bodies.

Medicare is also responsible for administering government health programs such as:

- General Practice Immunisation Incentives Scheme (GPII)
- Practice Incentives Program (PIP)
- **Australian Childhood Immunisation Register** (ACIR)

The WHO definition includes three main parts:

1. a holistic understanding of health as overall wellbeing, rather than just as the absence of disease
2. a set of strategies aimed at creating health care consistent with this underlying holistic philosophy
3. a view of PHC as the first level of health care, which individuals and communities can directly access without referral from anyone else.

The combination of all these elements is sometimes referred to as *comprehensive primary health care.*

Selective PHC and primary (medical) care

Within the broader literature, several other recognised conceptualisations and meanings of primary health care also exist. The first of these is sometimes called *primary medical care* or just *primary care* (Fry & Furler 2000). It is a narrow definition which focuses solely on the provision of medical services and medical treatment of individuals by doctors, to those with acute medical conditions who can access frontline care.

Others have suggested that primary health care, as defined in the Alma-Ata Declaration, is idealised and difficult to achieve in practice. This is because it relies on a multidimensional approach to health which goes against the segmented way that most countries, including Australia, organise their public service portfolios. At the same time, they recognise that primary health care is much more than just medical (that is, doctor only) interventions and care, involving many other health professionals and services such as nurses and allied health. This has resulted in what is known as *selective primary health care* (Wass 1995; Baum 1998). The differences between these definitions are summarised in Table 2.3 overleaf.

Variations on the selective PHC theme have also arisen, with some authors incorporating aspects of non-medical intervention into PHC, but not reaching the full-blown comprehensive PHC defined by WHO.

In general, the way that PHC is seen in Australia and referred to in this chapter is largely based on selective PHC. However, if the suggested future health policy reforms go ahead (National Health and Hospitals Reform Commission (NHHRC) 2009; Preventative Health Taskforce (PHT) 2009), such as workplace interventions for preventative health, town planning to support healthy lifestyles and substantial taxation increases on substances that increase health risk (for example, alcohol, junk food and cigarettes), then a more comprehensive, intersectoral approach to PHC may emerge in Australia.

Table 2.3 Differences between comprehensive and selective PHC

	Comprehensive PHC	Selective PHC	Medical model (primary medical care)
View of health	Positive wellbeing	Absence of disease	Absence of disease
Locus of control over health	Communities and individuals	Health professionals	Medical practitioners
Major focus	Health through equity and community empowerment	Health through medical interventions	Disease eradication through medical interventions
Health care providers	Multidisciplinary teams	Doctors plus other health professionals	Doctors
Strategies for health	Multisectoral collaboration	Medical interventions	Medical interventions

Source: Rogers & Veale 2000

Policy reforms proposed in this area are likely to affect primary care nurses, including practice nurses, as more preventive activities and screening are introduced and funded in general practice.

Why PHC is important

There is growing evidence that PHC, more than other parts of the health system, can enable fairer access to care, make best use of health resources, improve overall population health outcomes and tackle inequities in health, especially for impoverished and marginalised groups.

It is widely recognised that health care systems with strong primary health care orientations are associated with improved equity, increased access and appropriate services at lower costs, and improved population health (WHO 1978; WHO 2008; Starfield 1994).

This is important in Australia where we still face significant health inequalities in certain population subgroups, such as Indigenous Australians, those in rural and remote areas and those in lower socioeconomic groups. A reorientation of the system towards PHC is important for other reasons too. Like many other parts of the world, Australia has seen a significant rise in the ageing population as well as in chronic disease over the last few decades. People are living longer but with more ailments. The result is that more people are making demands on the health budget but fewer are adding to Australia's overall economy. Without a more cost-effective system, health budgets will not be able to keep pace with the growing demand for services.

A further consideration is that much of the chronic (and other) disease that is adding to these costs is potentially preventable. The setting best suited to the primary and secondary prevention of illness is PHC. Comprehensive PHC can help tackle the social determinants that contribute to disease while selective PHC can provide the health workforce that is best suited to promoting health, aiding disease prevention and reducing costly avoidable hospital admissions, often through better patient education and self-management.

The workforce required for such approaches includes a team of health professionals who can provide comprehensive, multidisciplinary approaches to illness prevention, as well as to the treatment and management of disease. This is particularly important in chronic disease management (CDM) where multidisciplinary team approaches have been shown to improve outcomes. No single profession can meet all the aims of primary health care. In many instances this multidisciplinary PHC workforce is not only better suited to delivering preventative care but is also often a more cost-effective option than one based on using doctors alone.

The need to reorient health systems towards better performance to meet these growing challenges has been recognised internationally (WHO 2008). Australia has also recently recognised the need for a return to primary health care and undertaken some significant work in health reform to achieve this (NHHRC 2009; PHT 2009). This will be discussed in more detail later in the chapter.

Primary health care in Australia

As outlined in Figure 2.1 (p. 32), the primary health care sector in Australia, similar to the health system overall, is a complex mix of public and private services and of Commonwealth and state government funded programs. Its main components include:

- general medical practice provided by GPs in private practice who operate through a fee-for-service framework where patients are eligible for Medicare rebates which are largely Commonwealth funded;
- community health services which are staffed by salaried GPs, nurses and multidisciplinary care teams of salaried non-medical allied health professionals, largely funded by state/territory governments;
- community health programs that support the frail, aged and disabled people, and are funded through both Commonwealth and state governments; and

- child and maternity services that are a combination of Commonwealth, state, local and private providers.

Although complex, the current PHC system does have has several strengths. These include:

- universal access to rebates against the cost of medical visits and pharmaceutical coverage via the MBS and the PBS;
- a robust general practice and community health sector, including maternal and child health;
- strong education and training in medical, nursing and allied health; and
- innovative initiatives in rural, remote and Aboriginal and Torres Strait Islander (ATSI) communities.

Although part of primary health care, practice nurses mainly work in the general practice context, which is a Commonwealth responsibility. The remainder of this chapter will focus on this area.

General practice

Further reforms to general practice introduced over the last 10 years include a range of alternative initiatives for blended and targeted payments to improve access to primary health care and address ongoing use of limited resources. These reforms are designed to provide incentives for a range of quality focused activities in general practice and have had a direct impact on practices and in particular, the role of nurses working in general practice. The reforms have included:

- **Divisions of General Practice**—see page 44.
- **Nursing in General Practice Initiative**—see page 37.
- **Practice Incentive Program (PIP)**—provides incentives that encourage general practices to improve the quality of care provided to patients. PIP payments are part of a blended approach to payment for general practice. Practices can register and receive payments over and above the MBS for after-hours access, employment of a practice nurse, quality prescribing of medicines, teaching of undergraduate medical students and acting as a referral point for people experiencing domestic violence.
- **Service Incentive Payments (SIP)**—additional payments provided to GPs to improve care. For example, payments can be accessed for: cervical screening of under-screened women; diabetic patients on completion of a diabetes cycle of care; patients with moderate to severe asthma on completion of an asthma cycle of care; operation of a secure messaging capability; and access to electronic evidence-based resources.

- **Outcome Payments (OP)**—paid once practices reach certain targets, for example, when 50% of eligible women have a Pap test taken or 20% of patients with diabetes mellitus have a completed cycle of care.

- **A Rural Incentives Program**—provides payments for GPs to relocate to rural and remote communities and outer urban areas.

More recent policy reforms have introduced some limited access under Medicare to PHC services provided by nurses and allied health professionals. In rural areas and outer metropolitan areas where there are workforce shortages, general practices can apply for grants which enable them to employ practice nurses on a sessional basis, particularly to assist GPs with chronic disease management and prevention programs.

Nursing in General Practice Initiative

In 2001–2002, the Australian Government provided funding for the Nursing in General Practice Initiative (NiGP Initiative), to be administered over four years (Jolly 2007). The three components of this initiative were:

1. **Practice Incentive Payment (PIP)**—to support the employment of a practice nurse in eligible practices. This incentive was extended to additional practices in urban areas of GP workforce shortage in 2003. The incentive, which is still available to eligible practices today, is based on a patient activity indictor and is capped at a maximum of $35 000 per annum in rural and remote practices and $40 000 in urban practices.

2. **Training and Support Component**—to develop the practice nurse role and provide support via the following:

   a. Informing consumers, nurses and GPs about practice nursing

   b. Increasing the capacity of the Divisions of General Practice

   c. Providing accessible and affordable training for practice nurses

   d. Encouraging nursing networks and mentoring

   e. Evaluating the initiative.

3. **Rural and Remote Nurse Re-entry and Upskilling Scholarship Scheme**—to encourage nurses within rural and remote areas to return to the nursing workforce.

From a nursing perspective perhaps the most significant of all the initiatives was the seed funding provided by the Commonwealth Government to establish the Australian Practice Nurses Association (APNA). This funding saw the support of the newly formed organisation run by nurses, for nurses and the administration of scholarships supporting practice nurses to undertake additional education.

An evaluation of the NiGP Initiative in 2005 showed that:

- 71% of practices had accessed the funding to employ a nurse;
- the throughput of patients had increased in practices which employed a nurse;
- there were reduced patient waiting times in practices that employed a nurse;
- GPs had more time and reduced workforce pressures;
- GPs could liaise more effectively with other health professionals about care of patients; and
- increased awareness by patients of the role of the practice nurse raised the nursing profile and encouraged the idea of specific practice nurse education (Healthcare Management Advisors 2005).

Additional MBS items have also been added to support multidisciplinary team care. For example, Enhanced Primary Care Items (RACGP 2000) have encouraged Care Planning, Case Conferencing, and Team Care Arrangements (TCAs) as part of the National Chronic Disease Strategy. Furthermore, the MBS primary care items have grown in complexity.

However, due to the reasons outlined previously, as well as for other reasons (such as the dwindling health care workforce and rising consumer expectations), Australia's health system still faces some significant challenges, some of which arise from its complex structure. To further address this situation, Australia is about to undergo significant health policy reform.

Australian government health policy

Before expanding the detail about recent health policy and its relevance to PHC and nursing, it is useful to understand more about policy in general and how it is developed.

What is policy?

Policy can be formulated in virtually any organisational setting. For example, schools may have internal policies about student conduct and workplaces may have their own policies about staff leave. The type of policy referred to in this section, however, is government policy—that is, the group of principles and ideals that those in government (or aspiring to be in government) set as the direction that the country should take in a given area such as education, health, employment and so forth. This package of ideals, principles and aspirations that formulate government policy are influenced by several factors including:

- identified need
- evidence of what works or has a good chance of working to overcome the need
- the ideologies of different political parties
- cost effectiveness and available public funds
- consideration of the public good
- consideration of public acceptability.

Each political party has its own policy platform which can include policy statements on key areas of public interest. Governments are elected on the basis of these (Irvine et al. 2006). Over recent years, health has become an increasingly important policy platform for both major Australian political parties.

Policy development

Ideally, good policy is well-informed, concise, rigorous and able to be implemented. Its purpose is to act as an instrument of change which impacts positively on the population as a whole or on selected population groups that have been identified as having specific needs. Where possible, policy development should undergo a cycle of progression that begins with a presentation of the evidence (academic and otherwise) pertaining to the issue to be addressed, and possible solutions. This often takes the form of an initial discussion paper. Consultation with relevant stakeholders follows to gain feedback. The feedback is then incorporated into a revised policy proposal (such as policy recommendations or a draft position statement) and 'road tested' again on stakeholders after which final revisions are made.

Reflections

How does this process relate to the development of policy in your practice?

National primary care policies

Over the last 10 years, policy reforms have occurred within primary care in response to the challenges previously discussed. These polices have, to some extent, helped alleviate certain health system issues by: assisting with cost containment; improving the public/private funding balance; improving efficiency and effectiveness; and measuring how well the health system is functioning.

A number of these have impacted on nursing especially the increased employment of nurses within general practice. Major policies include:

- establishment of Divisions of General Practice
- various workforce policies—Rural Incentives Program to provide payments for GPs to relocate to rural and remote communities, Rural Locum Relief Program (RLRP), overseas trained doctors (OTD) policies, establishment of the Rural Workforce Agencies (RWAs)
- Access programs—Allied Psychological Services (ATAPS), More Allied Health Services (MAHS), Round the Clock Medicare, after hours programs
- Quality initiatives—Practice Incentive Program (PIP) to improve quality and accountability of GP services, the National Primary Care Collaboratives (NPCC), National Commission on Quality and Safety in Healthcare, national performance measures
- Chronic disease initiatives—Better Access, Australian Better Health Initiative (ABHI)
- Health training and education—registration/GPET, national registration for health care professionals
- E-health—National E-Health Transition Authority (NEHTA)
- Targeted subgroups—Indigenous policies, Council of Australian Government (COAG), Aged Care GP panels, early child health (immunisation)
- Research—Primary Health Care Research Evaluation & Development (PHCRED), Australian Primary Health Care Research Institute (APHCRI).

Health reform 2009

In June 2009 the Commonwealth Government released both *A Healthier Future For All Australians – Final Report of the National Health and Hospitals Reform Commission'* and *Building a 21st Century Primary Health Care System: A Draft of Australia's First National Primary Health Care Strategy* (NHHRC 2009; PHT 2009). The NHHRC report makes 123 recommendations. With regard to primary health care, the NHHRC report makes several statements relevant to nursing in general practice including:

- Primary health care should be established as the cornerstone of a future person-centred health system.
- The Australian Government should take responsibility for funding and policy for primary health care and provide national leadership. This includes becoming responsible for services currently funded by state, territory and local governments, such as community health services, family and child

health services, community nursing, allied health, and alcohol and drug treatment services. States may continue to operate public primary health care services.

- The Commonwealth Government should encourage the establishment of Comprehensive Primary Health Care Centres, supported by government through initial fixed capital grants. The centres would be a 'one-stop shop' so that patients could get access to an expanded range of services (such as pathology, imaging, community nursing or allied health), with extended opening hours at more convenient times for patients.

- Young families and complex care patients should have the option of enrolling voluntarily with a single primary health care service of their choice, which would provide an ongoing point of contact for patients. This is designed to provide continuity of care, particularly in the early years of life, and assist shared-care arrangements between primary health care practitioners and specialists— especially for people with chronic, complex conditions.

- The establishment of performance payments for prevention, timeliness and quality of care will help embed a strong focus on quality and health outcomes and complement fee for service payments.

- The establishment of Primary Health Care Organisations (evolving from or replacing Divisions of General Practice) will provide future service coordination and population health planning within local communities.

- In the medium to longer term, investment should be made in strengthened primary care to reduce growth in projected health expenditure.

Alongside both the NHHRC and the Draft National PHC Strategy, the federal government also introduced several other key reform processes in 2008–09, a number of which are relevant to nursing in general practice. These include:

- the Preventative Health Taskforce (PHT);
- review of Maternity Services;
- review of MBS items;
- development of a National E-Health Strategy;
- review of rural health programs; and
- development of the fourth National Mental Health Plan.

At the time of writing, decisions about the exact direction that health policy will take as a result of these reforms is still unclear. However, it is likely that significant reform will be introduced into the health system—and especially primary health care.

Practice nurse MBS changes

Since 2004 the Australian Government has introduced a number of items to the MBS specifically for a practice nurse to provide a patient service on behalf of a general practitioner. This has been a significant policy initiative and has been extended to provide the opportunity for GPs to claim payment for a service provided by a nurse on their behalf. Although important, these fee-for-service items have been criticised by both nursing and medical professions due to their task focus (Phillips et al. 2008) and inadequate dollar value.

The practice nurse MBS item numbers have had the effect of determining the type of care delivered in general practice by nurses. Table 2.4 below outlines these item numbers.

Table 2.4 MBS practice nurse item numbers

MBS Item Number	Description
10993	Immunisation
10994	Pap test and preventative check
10995	Pap test and preventive check (no Pap in the last 4 years)
10996	Wound management
10997	Service provided to a person with a chronic disease (GPMP or TCA in place)
10998	Pap test only
10999	Pap test only (no Pap in the last 4 years)
16400	Antenatal service
10986	4-year-old check with immunisation

Other Australian Government initiatives

There has also been a range of other Australian Government health care initiatives introduced, which have included provision for the practice nurse to undertake a specific role in supporting the GP (see Table 2.5 opposite).

The first of these was the Enhanced Primary Care Package in the 1999 budget. Many of these MBS changes signalled support to practice to involve practice nurses in chronic disease management, although the exact role and was unclear and services were still provided on behalf of the general practitioner. The focus of the package was to improve the health of older Australians and

Table 2.5 Other relevant practice incentives and initiatives

Introduced	Initiative	Description
1999	Enhanced Primary Care package	Provision for a practice nurse to support a GP with some aspects of health assessments and care plans
2001	More Allied Health Service Program	Specialist nurses in areas such as asthma, diabetes and mental health can be employed to support general practice in caring for patients needing allied health support
2001	Chronic Disease Management Program	GPs can delegate some aspects of care for diabetes and asthma and maintenance of cervical screening registers to a practice nurse
2005	Lifescripts Program	Lifestyle information package can be used by practices nurses to support patient education
2006	45-year-old health check	GPs are able to delegate some aspects of the health check to a practice nurse
2006	Aboriginal & Torres Strait Islander Child Health Check	Provision for a nurse to assist the GP with the information collection components of the health assessment
2006	Health Assessment for Refugees and other Humanitarian Entrants	Provision for a nurse to assist the GP with the information collection components of the health assessment
2008	Type 2 Diabetes Risk Evaluation	The nurse can assist the patient to complete the Diabetes Risk Assessment tool
2008	Lifestyle Modification Programs	Practice nurses can undertake training to provide lifestyle modification programs

those with chronic and complex conditions (Royal Australian College of General Practitioners 2000).

Practice nurses and policy

In order to progress the nursing profession and improve the access and safety of health care for patients, nurses need to contribute to and influence policy at a national, state, local and practice level. There are numerous ways of achieving this. The following list provides some avenues to consider:

- becoming a member and participating in nursing professional groups such as the Australian Practice Nurses Association (APNA) the Royal College of Nursing

Australia (RCNA), or the Australian Nurses Federation (ANF). The strategic direction and representation of practice nurses in the development of national policy is directly influenced by professional nursing organisations such as the APNA.

- participation in planning committees or reference groups through your local division of general practice
- contributing to health planning committees in your local community, through local government or your state health bodies
- making personal representation to your local state or federal member of parliament
- responding to requests by government for community comment on draft policy documents.

Government decisions can be influenced by professional organisations or individual representation so it is important to contribute and express your views and opinions. Governments also routinely seek input from the peak organisations, such as the Australian Practice Nurses Association, the Royal College of Nursing Australia and the Australian General Practice Network, to develop, draft and implement new policy. These organisations rely on feedback from their members in order to respond to government policy, so through these groups you can keep abreast of current initiatives and have input into government policy. It is important to recognise that the policies subsequently developed can directly influence the way nurses work and the care provided to patients.

Reflections

How can you contribute to policy at a national, state, local and practice level?

Divisions of General Practice

Divisions of General Practice is an Australian national primary health care network established in response to the emerging burden of disease and health imperatives for our population (Scott & Coote 2007). Other countries, including England and New Zealand, have also established models of network-based primary health care organisations; however, divisions were established and have evolved to meet the specific needs and circumstances for Australia (Naccarella et al. 2006).

The Australian General Practice Network (AGPN), which receives core funding from the Australian Government Department of Health and Ageing, is a national network comprising a national peak body, eight state-based organisations (SBO) and 111 divisions of general practice.[2] AGPN is the primary interface for the network with the Australian Government and is responsible for the development of national policy and the provision of program expertise in primary care service delivery and support of the network as a whole. Although members of Divisions of General Practice are predominantly from the medical profession, small numbers of practice nurses, practice staff and allied health professionals are members (Hordacre et al. 2008).

By delivering local solutions through general practice, the network aims to improve health outcomes by ensuring all Australians can access a high-quality health system (Hordacre et al. 2008). The eight SBOs work at a state and territory level to interface with state and territory governments.

At a local level, the 111 divisions play a major role in implementing health policy and supporting change through general practice, providing a range of support programs and managing health programs. Divisions provide 'grassroots' knowledge and experience of primary health care delivery and innovation. Divisions of General Practice have been responsible for progressing many of the current developments in Australian general practice (PHCRIS 2008).

Key roles for the Divisions of General Practice network include:

- engaging the consumer and community in the health care system
- delivering services for the Indigenous population
- implementing strategies to alleviate primary health care workforce shortages
- providing support activities to general practitioners, practice nurses and other practice staff
- engaging in prevention and early intervention activities
- contributing to primary health care research.

(Hordacre et al. 2008)

The Divisions of General Practice acknowledge that multidisciplinary teams play an important role and that essential members of those teams include general practitioners, practice nurses and practice managers (ADGP 2005a). The Divisons of General Practice have been at the forefront of the transition of general practice to include a significantly larger proportion of practice nurses and a much more multidisciplinary team approach to primary health care. Despite the broadening of membership of the Divisions of General Practice and the influence that they have on development of policy for primary care, in 2006–07 only 12% of board members were not

GPs (Hordacre et al. 2008). Effectively this means that nurses have very little input into the strategic direction and policy of the primary care organisation which has capacity to influence the current and future role of a rapidly expanding area of the nursing workforce.

> **? Reflections**
>
> *What is your role in the division and how are you able to influence policy development?*

Divisions' support for practice nurses

Many divisions have been providing support to practice nurses since as early as 1992 (Hall 2007), although support formally began in 2002 with funding to appoint a Principal Advisor for Nursing in General Practice to provide national coordination, leadership and policy advice. Today all Divisions of General Practice provide some level of support to nurses in general practice, including professional development, facilitation of networks for management of chronic disease, support for use of Medicare items, involving practice nurses in division activities, induction/orientation into general practice, provision of clinical support, provision of mentoring, and contracting nurses on behalf of general practices (Hordacre et al. 2008).

For practice nurses some of the benefits derived from the support provided through divisions have been reported as (ADGP 2005b):

- increased recognition and promotion of the general practice nurse workforce
- professional development opportunities
- overcoming the isolation experienced by practice nurses
- clarification of issues relating to supervision and mentoring
- increased satisfaction and pride in their work
- greater rapport and interaction among local nurses
- opportunities for nurses to vent frustrations and problems and to seek solutions among their peers and with division representatives
- networking and opportunities to share experiences and knowledge
- dissemination of information pertinent to the general practice
- assistance in the implementation of the various DoHA Nursing in General Practice initiatives

- stronger links with the community through participation in divisional programs
- increased capacity for practice nurses to undertake extended roles in chronic disease management and preventive/population health programs.

Reflections

What opportunities does your division provide to support your work in general practice?

Conclusion

This chapter has highlighted that nurses have a role in all parts of the health care system and at all levels of care, although the specific activities they perform may vary depending on which part of the system they are working in. Australia has a complex health care system with many differing elements, thus it is essential that nurses understand how these elements fit together both professionally as well as in understanding a patient's journey through it. To address the growing demands from patients with complex and chronic illness, the workforce required for primary health care approaches is not only medical but includes other health professionals. The Australian Government is currently reforming the health system, with the primary health care system being a cornerstone of policy reforms, and practice nurses have various ways to influence government policy. Primary health care will no doubt be the cornerstone of Australia's future health care system, with nursing having a key role and contribution within general practice.

C A S E   S T U D Y

THE AUSTRALIAN PRACTICE NURSES ASSOCIATION
Name of nurse

Belinda Caldwell, CEO of the Australian Practice Nurses Association

The Australian Practice Nurses Association (APNA) was incorporated in 2001 and born out of a need to support the expanding group of nurses working in general practice. Prior to this, as a small proportion of the nursing workforce, no nursing organisation was familiar with challenges confronting this group. Hence, a small group of practice nurses took on the challenge to develop the organisation known as APNA. Fortunately, APNA was able to capitalise on government policy by requesting and receiving seeding funding from the Nursing in General Practice Initiative. Historically, very few nursing organisations have been the recipient of money for this purpose and it remains one of the outstanding achievements of APNA to date.

Today, APNA has a membership of over 1600 and continues to grow. The mission of APNA, first formulated in 2001, remains relevant in 2009 'to support members to be *recognised, professional and empowered*'.

During its short but productive history, APNA has strived to influence policy, particularly at a national level. It was recognised very early on that as general practice was a Commonwealth responsibility, any professional organisation supporting nurses in this area needed to have a national perspective.

Over the ensuing years APNA has lobbied the Department of Health and Ageing in a variety of ways, and although it is difficult to claim total responsibility for policy changes, in combination with other factors, having input and representation at a national level has been fundamental to the success of APNA. As described in this chapter, the ability to identify a need, gather evidence and link into government policy has allowed APNA to lead, inform and be part of the consultation process which ultimately recognises and empowers its members. Major successes in this area have been:

· a standard of education (credentialing) attached to the MBS Pap smear item number
· introduction and expansion of scholarships for practice nurses to undertake relevant education
· input into the National Health and Hospitals Reform Commission, National Preventive Health Taskforce, and National Primary Health Care strategy, all part of a major government health reform process
· development of a roundtable consensus statement on the primary health care nursing advocating nursing's central role
· participation in reference and advisory groups such as the National Primary Health Care Partnerships, National Heart Foundation GP Advisory Group
· Membership of the Nurse Practitioner Advisory Group
· Consultation on all MBS item numbers affecting practice nurses.

Although by comparison a small professional organisation, APNA has demonstrated that through the power of numbers, partnering with other key organisations, consultation and lobbying, it has been able to influence formulation of government policy to achieve the objectives of its membership. Only by achieving a critical mass are practice nurses capable of determining their own role—albeit to a smaller degree than what it would like—but important progress nevertheless in becoming an influential organisation on a national level.

ONE NURSE'S CONTRIBUTION TO NATIONAL POLICY

Name of nurse

Cathy Pattullo

Practice

Well Women's Clinic, Mudgee, NSW

In 2003, Mudgee was faced with the prospect of having no access to female GPs. As a midwife and a general practice nurse I was well aware of the crisis we were facing. The female doctors were highly sought after to discuss personal female conditions that women often felt uncomfortable discussing with a male. As a midwife I had shared in the responsibility of providing women's health care and was the first port of call for many 'female' questions which I would then refer onto the female or male doctors.

I was aware of the vulnerability that the women of Mudgee were feeling and was fully aware that if there was no female doctor in town, women may choose not to have preventive health care at all.

In order to improve access to cervical screening and breast health, I successfully completed the Well Women's Screening Course. As there was no Medicare item available to support practice nurses to undertake cervical screening and the medico-legal issues were unclear, the practice was reluctant to allow me to expand my scope of practice and provide this service to women. Some thought this barrier insurmountable—not me! All I needed was a Medicare item number—easy! I can do that thought I, who had battled years of droughts and floods and plagues on the land.

In my first attempt at changing policy, I started by organising a petition. Signatures poured in to the front desk from the community eager to support my idea, with people appreciating that their plight was recognised. The local paper highlighted the need and local groups approached me to give me their support. A member of the Country Women's Association knocked on my door in the middle of one morning surgery to say Deputy Prime Minister John Anderson MP (leader of the National Party) was in town and I should meet with him immediately. Leaving a few startled faces behind, I bolted out of the surgery with urges to 'go get them' ringing in my ears. I managed to get a moment with John Anderson and explained the need in Mudgee and my idea to have practice nurses run Well Women's Clinics to address this need and an item number to support practices offering this service. John Anderson requested the petition be sent to him and he would support the idea in the election campaign. He identified the two-fold benefit of supporting GPs to provide more acute care and women having access to a female provider. Unknowingly, I was putting a human face to a need already identified by NSW Cervical Screening, Department of Health & Ageing and the Family Planning Association (FPA).

John Anderson was re-elected and subsequently a media release announced the introduction of the 10994 item number. I was now confident of providing a much needed nurse-led service but the practice remained reluctant make this happen due to the medico-legal issues and a resistance to handover what had been historically been a role for the GP.

Using existing guidelines from the FPA and Victorian Cytology, I compiled a policy which was endorsed by the practice. This complied with insurance requirements and the last hurdle was overcome—we had our Well Women's Clinic! The weekly article I wrote in the local paper to provide information on women's health was widely read and women came from outlying areas to utilise the clinic as a result.

In recognition of my achievements I received and APNA Award for Innovation & Commitment to the General Practice. This has allowed me to further my knowledge in the area of sexual health and I have found it invaluable in providing a comprehensive service that can identify relevant symptoms and refer to the appropriate provider. The GPs now refer women to me—I think that says it all!

Further to the Well Women's service which is now embedded into our practice, I have successfully applied to have two female GPs visit Mudgee/Gulgong as part of the Royal Flying Doctor's Rural Women's GP Service. These GPs have acted as mentors to me and I now realise this professional recognition is so imperative to providing an ongoing service of this level. I now feel supported and recognised by GPs for the service I am providing, and my service has now been extended to a fortnightly service in Rylstone.

This whole process has taught me many things—changing policy, especially at a government level, can be difficult and it is important not to give up. The impossible is possible: it just means you have to sometimes take the long way around. Success builds more opportunity and that none of this happens without the support of the wonderful people in the community who continue to inspire me to provide preventive health care for women in the rural community.

Key messages

Nurses need to understand the various elements of the health system in order to recognise the patient journey and the challenges that patients face.

The primary health care workforce requires a multidisciplinary approach to illness prevention as well as to management and treatment of disease.

Practice nurses can influence reform and government policy.

Notes

1. Australia is currently in the midst of significant health care reform in which the Commonwealth could eventually fund and oversee all primary health care. The results of the reform recommendations were still to be decided at the time of going to press.

2. At the time of going to press, several divisions were in the process of amalgamating prior to formation of primary health care organisations.

Useful resources

Australian Divisions of General Practice
http://www.agpn.com.au/

Department of Health and Aging Nursing in General Practice program
http://www.health.gov.au/

Australian Primary Health Care Research Institute
http://www.anu.edu.au/aphcri/

Medicare
http://www.medicareaustralia.gov.au/

Mediguide—A Guide to Medicare and other Medicare Australia health programs, 11th edn, Medicare Australia

The Australian Primary Care Collaboratives (APCC) Program
http://www.apcc.org.au/

Medicare Benefits Schedule (MBS)
http://www.health.gov.au/internet/mbsonline/publishing.nsf/Content/Medicare-Benefits-Schedule-MBS-1

References

1. Australian Divisions of General Practice (ADGP) 2005a, *Primary Health Care Position Statement*, ADGP, Canberra, viewed 7 January 2010, <http://www.agpn.com.au/__data/assets/pdf_file/0006/16269/20051026_pos_AGPN-Primary-Health-Care-Position-Statement-FINAL.pdf>.

2. Australian Divisions of General Practice (ADGP) 2005b, *Demonstration Divisions National Resource Kit*, ADGP, Canberra, viewed 31 December 2009, <http://www.agpn.com.au/>.

3. Australian Institute of Health and Welfare (AIHW) 2008, *Australia's health 2008*, cat. no. AUS 99, AIHW, Canberra.

4. Baum, F 1998, *The New Public Health: an Australian perspective*, Oxford University Press, Melbourne.

5. Department of Health and Ageing 2010, *The Changes to Medicare Primary Care Items: A Fact Sheet for General Practitioners*, viewed February 2010, <http://www.health.gov.au/internet/main/publishing.nsf/Content/mbsprimarycare-changes-to-medicare-primary-care-items-for-gps>.

6. Fry, D & Furler, J 2000, 'General practice, primary health care and population health interface', in *General Practice in Australia*, Department of Health and Aged Care, Canberra.

7. Hall, S 2007, 'Divisions of general practice and practice nurse development in Australia', *Contemporary Nurse*, Advances in Contemporary General Practice Nursing, Special Issue, vol. 26, issue 1, pp. 37–47.

8. Healthcare Management Advisors 2005, *Evaluation of the 2001 Nursing in General Practice Initiative: Final Report*, Adelaide, viewed October 2009, <http://www.health.gov.au/>.

9. Hordacre, A, Howard, S, Moretti, C & Kalucy, E 2008, *Moving ahead. Report of the 2006–07 Annual Survey of Divisions of General Practice*, Primary Health Care Research & Information Service, Department of General Practice, Flinders University, Adelaide, and Australian Government Department of Health and Ageing, viewed 7 January 2010, <http://www.phcris.org.au/>.

10. Irvine, L, Elliot, L, Wallace, H & Crombie, I 2006, 'A review of major influences on current public health policy in developed countries in the second half of the 20th century', *The Journal of the Royal Society for the Promotion of Health*, vol. 126, no. 2, pp. 73–8.

11. Jolly, R 2007, *Practice Nursing in Australia*, Parliamentary Library, <http://www.aph.gov.au/>.

12. Medicare Benefits Schedule (MBS) 2009, MBS online, viewed 29 December 2009, <http://www.health.gov.au/internet/mbsonline/publishing.nsf/Content/Medicare-Benefits-Schedule-MBS-1>.

13. *Mediguide 2007—A Guide to Medicare and other Medicare Australia health programs*, 11th edn, viewed 7 January 2010, <http://www.medicareaustralia.gov.au/provider/pubs/mediguide/index.jsp>.

14. Naccarella, L, Southern, D, Furler, J, Scott, A, Prosser, L & Young, D 2006, *Narrative Review of Innovative Models of Primary Care Delivery*, final report to APHCRI, Department of General Practice, University of Melbourne.

15. National Health and Hospitals Reform Commission (NHHRC) 2009, *A Healthier Future for All Australians*, viewed 7 January 2010, <http://www.health.gov.au/>.

16. Phillips, C, Pearce, C, Dwan, K, Hall, S, Porritt, J, Yates, R, Kljakovic, M & Sibbald, B 2008, *Charting New Roles for Australian General Practice Nurses: Abridged Report of the Australian General Practice Nurses Study*, Australian Primary Health Care Institute, Canberra.

17. Preventative Health Taskforce (PHT) 2009, *Australia: The healthiest country by 2020 National Preventative Health Strategy–Overview*, Department of Health and Ageing, Canberra, viewed 7 January 2010, <http://www.health.gov.au/>.

18. Primary Health Care Research Institute (PHCRIS), 2008, *What Divisions Do. A Snapshot of the General Practice Network 2006–07,* Australian General Practice Network, Canberra.

19. Rogers, W & Veale, B 2000, *Primary health care: a scoping report,* National Information Service, Department of General Practice, Flinders University, p. 18, viewed November 2009, <http://www.phcris.org.au/publications/catalogue.php?elibid=1150>.

20. The Royal Australian College of General Practice (RACGP) 2000, *Enhanced Primary Care: standards and guidelines for the enhanced primary care Medicare Benefits Schedule items,* Commonwealth Department of Health and Ageing, Canberra, pp. 51–69.

21. Scott, A & Coote, B 2007, *The value of the Divisions network: an evaluation of the effect of Divisions of General Practice on primary care performance,* Melbourne Institute Report No. 8, Melbourne Institute of Applied Economic and Social Research, University of Melbourne.

22. Starfield, B 1994, 'Is primary care essential?', *Lancet,* vol. 344, no. 8930, pp. 1129–33.

23. Wass, A 1995, *Promoting health: the primary health care approach,* WB Saunders, Bailliere Tindall, Harcourt Brace and Company, Sydney.

24. World Health Organisation (WHO) 1978, *Alma Ata Declaration on Primary Health Care,* viewed 7 January 2010, <http://www.who.int/hpr/NPH/docs/declaration_almaata.pdf>.

25. World Health Organisation (WHO) 2008, *The World Health Report 2008: Primary Health Care–Now More Than Ever,* viewed 7 January 2010, <http://www.who.int/mediacentre/news/releases/2008/pr38/en/index.html>.

Chapter three

Scope of practice

by Julianne Bryce and Elizabeth Foley

Overview

It is the intent of this chapter to outline the legislative, regulatory, educational and professional environment in which nurses and midwives practice within the general practice setting, in Australia. From a description of existing frameworks the reader will gain an understanding of the factors influencing nurses' and midwives' scope of practice; and be stimulated to examine their own practice for creatively meeting future community health needs, resulting in greater levels of personal, professional and interprofessional satisfaction.

Objectives

At the completion of this chapter you should be able to:

- describe the regulatory and professional frameworks which underpin nurses' and midwives' scope of practice;

- identify the factors which influence and shape the scope of practice of nurses and midwives;

- understand how these factors interact with professional scope of practice;

- recognise the importance of flexibility in scope of practice for nurses and midwives; and

- identify strategies for expanding scope of practice of nurses and midwives working in the general practice environment.

Introduction

If you don't know where you are going, any road will take you there.
(Alice in Wonderland *by Lewis Carroll*)

The Cat's advice to Alice when she found herself at a crossroad in Wonderland would seem to have little relevance to nursing and midwifery practice. However, without an understanding of their scope of practice, the 'roadmap' it provides, and the factors which shape and influence that practice, it is likely that nurses and midwives in the general practice setting will be no clearer than poor Alice as to the direction to take and the possibilities ahead for developing their role.

There are challenges for nurses (registered nurses and enrolled nurses) and midwives in considering their scope of practice within general practice. The environment in which they deliver primary care is often unpredictable and involves caring for a broad group of people from diverse backgrounds and at all stages of life (Australian Nursing Federation 2009). In addition to this recognition of a breadth of scope, there is a need for a flexible approach in pushing the boundaries of their practice and being cognisant of the impact of that on others in the general practice setting. For example, as nursing and midwifery expands their scope of practice to more advanced levels to include the nurse practitioner role, and to increase the numbers of people taking on this role, nurses and midwives need to be mindful that aspects of their current activities may need to be delegated to other workers within the general practice environment, such as practice managers. And, just as nurses and midwives want support and recognition from medical colleagues in their expansion of scope of practice, support structures must also be developed for those taking on roles that were previously the province of nursing and midwifery as the professions grow and expand.

The scope of practice for nurses and midwives is defined as practice for which nurses and midwives are educated, competent and authorised to perform (Australian Nursing Federation 2006). It is critical that all nurses and midwives employed in general practice have a clear role description with a scope of practice that is appropriate to the educational preparation of the nurse or midwife and consistent with the legislative framework of the state or territory in which the nurse or midwife is employed (Australian Nursing Federation 2008). This chapter outlines the regulatory and professional factors which shape and impact on the scope of practice for nurses and midwives in general practice.

The *National Practice Nurse Workforce Survey Report* (Australian General Practice Network 2007) states that 20% of nurses employed in general practice have postgraduate qualifications in midwifery, although it is not known how many of these practice nurses still practice in the area of midwifery. While the information contained in this chapter applies to both practice nurses and midwives, the following text will mostly refer only to nurses (Australian General Practice Network 2007).

International perspective

In its 2009 publication titled *Global standards for the initial education of professional nurses and midwives,* the World Health Organisation outlines a global standard for initial education for nurses and midwives which will prepare them for roles within the health workforce 'where they will be called upon to strengthen health systems to meet population needs and protect the public' (World Health Organisation 2009). The standards describe nursing and midwifery education program graduates as being able to demonstrate:

- use of evidence in practice;
- cultural competence;
- the ability to practise in the health care systems of their respective countries and meet population needs;
- critical and analytical thinking;
- the ability to manage resources and practise safely and effectively;
- the ability to be effective client advocates and professional partners with other disciplines in health care delivery;
- community service orientation; and
- leadership ability and continual professional development.

(World Health Organisation 2009, p. 21)

These attributes, in whole or in part, are reflected in the writings from many countries on scope of practice for nurses and midwives. The following commentary provides just a snapshot of views from the international nursing and midwifery community.

The International Council of Nurses' (ICN) *Position Statement: Scope of Practice* says that 'nursing is responsible for articulating and disseminating clear definitions of the roles nurses engage in, and the profession's scope of practice' (International Council of Nurses 2004). The ICN points out that in addition to essential input from professional, regulatory and industrial nursing and midwifery organisations to the development and evaluation of scope of practice, it is also important to seek the 'views of others in society in defining scope of practice'. In the general practice setting this would be other members of the general practice team and the local community.

So what elements does the ICN consider form the scope of practice? The council statement outlines the following:

- specific tasks, functions/responsibilities;
- direct care giving and evaluating of its impact;
- advocating for patients and for health;
- supervising and delegating to others;
- leading, managing, teaching, undertaking research; and
- developing health policy for health care systems.

(International Council of Nurses 2004)

In acknowledgement of the ever-changing nature of the broader context in which nurses and midwives practice, the ICN makes an important point that:

As the scope of practice is dynamic and responsive to health needs, development of knowledge, and technological advances, periodic review is required to ensure that it continues to be consistent with current health needs and supports improved health outcomes.

(International Council of Nurses 2004, p. 1)

As the ICN position statement highlights, and which will be discussed in this chapter, the practice and competence of an individual nurse within the legal scope of practice is influenced by a variety of factors, including education, experience, expertise and interests as well as the context of practice (International Council of Nurses 2004, p. 2).

The body responsible for the regulation of the practice of nursing and midwifery in Ireland, An Bord Altranais, developed a guiding framework in 2000, which says that

the role and scope of practice of nurses and midwives must respond to changes in a dynamic way ... [therefore] the framework ... aims to support nurses and midwives in determining their scope of practice and, in so doing, to practice with flexibility and innovation.

(An Bord Altranais 2000)

The Nursing Council of New Zealand developed four scopes of practice under the *Health Practitioners Competence Assurance Act 2003* (NZ) which encompass the scopes and practice of registered nurses, nurse practitioners, enrolled nurses and nurse assistants (Te Kaunihera Tapuhi o Aotearoa/Nursing Council of New Zealand 2004).

In relation to registered nurses it is acknowledged that their practice occurs in a range of settings and clinical contexts depending on their educational preparation and practice experience. Essentially they

> *... utilise nursing knowledge and complex nursing judgement to assess health needs and provide care, and to advise and support people to manage their health. They practise independently and in collaboration with other health professionals, perform general nursing functions and delegate to and direct Enrolled Nurses and Nurse Assistants. They provide comprehensive nursing assessments to develop, implement, and evaluate an integrated plan of health care, and provide nursing interventions that require substantial scientific and professional knowledge and skills.*

(Te Kaunihera Tapuhi o Aotearoa/Nursing Council of New Zealand 2004)

As in Australia, the enrolled nurse in New Zealand practices under the direction of a registered nurse or midwife to implement nursing care for people who have stable and predictable health outcomes in situations that do not call for complex nursing judgment (Te Kaunihera Tapuhi o Aotearoa/Nursing Council of New Zealand 2004).

Lanette Anderson (Anderson 2009) provides a succinct overview of the situation in the United States of America. Scope of practice is defined as the actions, procedures, etc. that are permitted by law based on specific experience and educational qualifications, as determined by the board of nursing in each state. Anderson stresses that it is just as important for nurses and midwives to know their own scope of practice as it is to know the scope of practice of others who form their team providing patient care. This is particularly important when a registered nurse is delegating aspects of care, as the registered nurse remains accountable for the care delegated to other health care workers. As Anderson (2009) says, 'our primary concern as nurses [and midwives] must always be safe and proficient nursing [and midwifery] care. Scopes of practice for the various levels of nursing [and midwifery] providers exist specifically for that reason'.

Reflections

What influence has your practice team had in determining the scope of your practice in the general practice context?

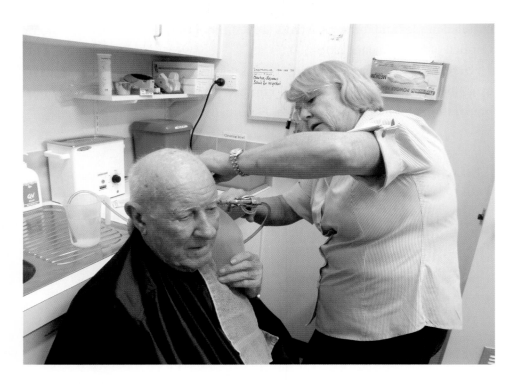

Australian frameworks

In Australia, regulatory bodies and professional organisations have worked extensively, particularly over the past decade, to establish frameworks to guide the professional practice of nurses, including practice nurses. The overriding aim is to promote safe and competent professional practice to ensure protection of the public. The standards required for practice as a nurse or midwife in Australia are that of:

- regulation;
- scope of practice;
- decision-making framework;
- code of ethics;
- code of professional conduct;
- competency standards; and
- other relevant legislation.

Regulation

Regulation (or licensure), the purpose of which is to protect the public, imposes an obligation on nurses, making them accountable to the community for providing quality care through safe, ethical and effective practice (see also Chapter 19, p. 442). This means maintaining the competence necessary for practice; and practicing within their scope of practice. The other standards or frameworks nurses and midwives must consider in their professional practice are the codes of ethics and professional conduct, competency standards, and other relevant legislation such as nursing Acts, poisons and controlled substances Acts and mental health Acts. Ongoing regulation or licensure as a nurse or midwife requires that the nurse practices within their scope, competently, in accordance with their code of ethics and code of professional conduct, and within a legislative framework. Currently nurses and midwives are registered under state and territory nursing Acts. As of 1 July 2010 a national legislative framework for nurses and midwives in Australia applies.

Scope of practice

The ICN position, referred to previously, states that the entire scope of practice for nurses and midwives should be within a legislative regulatory framework (International Council of Nurses 2004).

In Australia, some aspects of practice are covered by statutory regulation such as protection of the title of registered nurse/enrolled nurse/midwife/nurse practitioner; medication management under the drugs and controlled substances Acts; certain aspects of the nurse practitioner role (such as prescribing, referral, admitting rights and clinical privileging); and supervision of enrolled nurses by registered nurses. These areas of practice are rightly covered by legislation as they encompass elements which hold a greater degree of potential risk to the public than other aspects of care. Australian regulatory bodies take a more liberal approach than that described by the ICN, in that all other aspects of practice remain in the self-regulatory arena. The importance of this for the scope of practice for nurses and midwives is that it allows for the flexibility required to respond to changes in the environment, such as innovations in practice brought about by research or new technology, development of new or enhanced roles, and innovation to meet future challenges in health care.

The National Nursing and Nursing Education Taskforce (N[3]ET), established to implement recommendations of *Our Duty of Care*, the report of the National Review of Nursing Education, made the point in its 2005 *Scopes of Practice Commentary Paper* that:

There are ... risks for nurses and midwives from drawing tight boundaries around their practice. Their scopes of practice may be interpreted as the absolute limit to their capacity rather than as the threshold of opportunity. Nurses and midwives may appear rigid and inflexible when in reality their scopes of practice are fluid and constantly shifting.

(Australian Health Ministers' Advisory Council 2005, p. 46)

It could also be argued that the public interest is not being served when limits are placed on the scope of practice of nurses or midwives that unnecessarily restrict the provision of health or maternity services required by their community now, and in the future (Australian Health Ministers' Advisory Council 2005, p. 53). The factors which influence the scope of practice of individual nurses in general practice include:

- the context in which they practice;
- the health needs of the client and community;
- the level of competence, education and qualifications held by the nurse or midwife;
- the general practice facility's policies and protocols;
- relevant legislation, such as state/territory Acts relating to nursing and midwifery or to drugs and poisonous substances (Australian Nursing Federation 2006, p. 8); and
- government policy decisions and funding mechanisms.

Particularly relevant to practice nurses is the influence of government policy decisions and funding mechanisms. The growth in numbers of practice nurses and the introduction of Medicare Benefit Schedule (MBS) item numbers has directly and significantly determined the role and the scope of practice for many nurses working in general practice.

Reflections

How has your scope of practice changed since working in general practice? Has it extended or has it been limited?

Decision-making framework

In 2005 the Australian Nursing and Midwifery Council (ANMC) embarked on a two-year project to develop a national framework to assist nurses and midwives in decision making about their scope of practice (Australian Nursing and Midwifery Council 2007). The intention of the framework is not only to provide guidance to nurses and midwives in decision making about their practice but also to encourage them to think about ways to expand their scope of practice in responding to workforce supply issues and in meeting the health needs of their community. In its deliberations on developing a framework for nurses and midwives in Australia, the ANMC noted the principles which have been used in the United Kingdom to form the basis for making decisions on scope of practice for registered nurses, midwives and health visitors. These principles are reproduced here because of their perceived usefulness and applicability for nurses and midwives in general practice.

The registered nurse, midwife or health visitor must:

- Be satisfied that each aspect of practice is directed to meeting the needs and serving the interests of the patient.
- Endeavour always to achieve, maintain and develop knowledge, skill and competence to respond to those needs and interests.
- Honestly and openly acknowledge any limits or personal knowledge and skill and take steps to remedy any relevant deficits in order effectively and appropriately to meet the needs of patients and clients.
- Ensure that any enlargement or adjustment of the scope of personal professional practice must be achieved without compromising or fragmenting aspects of professional practice and care and that the requirements of the Council's code of professional conduct are satisfied through the whole area of practice.
- Recognise and honour the direct or indirect personal accountability borne for all aspects of professional practice.
- In serving the interests of patients and clients and the wider interests of society, avoid any inappropriate delegation to others which compromise those interests.

(Australian Nursing and Midwifery Council 2007, p. 8)

A decision-making framework gives practice nurses a support tool for analysing their scope of practice, whatever the context of that might be, within existing regulatory constraints. It therefore assists them to assess and manage risk in their practice, which is a requirement for obtaining professional indemnity cover either through their employer (as vicarious liability) or as an individual. A decision-making framework also promotes the use of the most appropriate health care worker for the care required and so supports flexible workforce practices.

The National Decision-making Framework (DMF) developed by the ANMC was subsequently endorsed by state/territory nursing and midwifery registration boards in 2008, for use across the country. The national framework provides a consistent approach to decisions on the scope of practice for nurses and midwives and allows for changes and expansion of practice as the health needs of the population evolve. The final national DMF includes decision-making template tools for nurses' and midwives' practice decisions (incorporating a guide for practice, a flowchart, a flowchart narrative and a summary guide diagram for each profession) and explanation of terms used in the template tools (Australian Nursing and Midwifery Council 2007, p. 1).

General practitioners and practice managers need to be familiar with the nursing professional framework to understand the role and scope of practice of the nurse and how the DMF can be used to determine and expand the nursing scope.

Codes of ethics and professional conduct

The Code of Ethics and Code of Professional Conduct for Nurses in Australia has been developed by the Australian Nursing and Midwifery Council, the Australian Nursing Federation, Royal College of Nursing, Australia, and the Australian College of Midwives. First published in the 1990s, these codes have been revised over time, with the latest versions being issued in August 2008. There are now four sets of codes:

- Code of Ethics for Nurses in Australia
- Code of Ethics for Midwives in Australia
- Code of Professional Conduct for Nurses in Australia
- Code of Professional Conduct for Midwives in Australia.

(Australian Nursing and Midwifery Council 2008)

The codes of ethics provide fundamental ethical guidance as well as a mechanism to assist decision making for nurses and midwives in situations where ethical boundaries or responsibilities are unclear. They help nurses and midwives identify the essential moral commitments of the profession; provide nurses and midwives with a basis for professional and self-reflection on ethical conduct; act as a guide to ethical practice; and indicate to the community the moral values which nurses and midwives can be expected to hold.

The codes of professional conduct outline how nurses and midwives are expected to conduct themselves personally and professionally in a way that will maintain public trust and confidence in the professions. These codes articulate the responsibility nurses and midwives have to the individual, society and to the professions to provide safe and competent nursing and midwifery care which is responsive to individual, group and community needs, and the professions; identify minimum requirements for conduct in the professions; and inform the community of those standards.

As stated previously, the scope of practice for any nurse or midwife is defined as that which the nurse is educated, competent and authorised to perform. A nurse may be taught to perform a particular scope of practice, but not be competent. A nurse might feel competent, but not be qualified. A practice nurse must be all three—educated, competent and authorised.

Reflections

What areas of the nursing role in general practice require reflection about ethical issues?

Education

In Australia, registered nurse and midwife preparatory education is universally, at the minimum level of entry to practice, an undergraduate degree. This level of education equips the nurse or midwife to critically analyse their clinical practice, make comprehensive assessments of care needs, undertake research and problem solve and initiate highly complex care regimes. The educational preparation also enables a nurse or midwife to function effectively in a broad range of health and aged care settings, in acute or community and primary health care environments. All graduating nurses and midwives must meet an agreed national set of minimum competency standards developed by the Australian Nursing and Midwifery Council to be able to register to practice (Australian Nursing and Midwifery Council 2002, 2006a, 2006b). The educational preparation of enrolled nurses varies between states and territories across Australia, with there being both diploma level and certificate IV level qualifications. Some of the differences in curricula relate to variations in the scope of practice of enrolled nurses—principally the extent to which enrolled nurses are permitted to administer medicines independently of the supervision of a registered nurse, as set down in regulations governing the type of medication enrolled nurses are allowed to administer.

In addition to nurses and midwives undertaking formal undergraduate and postgraduate education, it is imperative that they maintain and enhance their level of education to remain relevant to their context of practice. Lifelong learning is promoted aggressively by professional nursing and midwifery bodies along with the need for continuous self-assessment of practice performance and identification of professional development needs, to enable nurses and midwives to demonstrate accountability and autonomy as professionals, within their scope of practice. The link between professional development and professional accountability means that it is important that the promotion of professional development be included in scope of practice documents.

With the introduction of the National Health Professional Regulation Scheme in Australia in 2010, nursing and midwifery are moving towards a mandatory continuing competence framework which recognises the vital importance of recency of practice and continuing professional development to practice (see also Chapter 19).

Postgraduate courses are now available to specifically address the expansion of practice nurses' knowledge and their ability to contribute to primary health care. This education will assist practice nurses to expand their scope of practice and help build the specialty of general practice nursing.

Competence

Nurses and midwives, as regulated health care professionals, are required by law to be competent to perform nursing and midwifery care wherever they practice. Competence is defined as 'the ability to perform tasks and duties to the standard expected in employment'. Competency standards are 'industry-determined specifications of performance which set out the skills, knowledge and attitudes required to operate effectively in employment' (Australian Nursing Federation 2006, p. 11).

Nurses and midwives have for some years now used competency standards as their professional framework against which to measure performance and prepare a professional development plan so that competence is maintained and enhanced. These standards were developed by the ANMC, the peak national body responsible for nursing regulation, following considerable consultation and validation with nurses and midwives.

The ANMC competency standards are important in undergraduate education programs for nurses and midwives where they form the basis of course content and clinical assessment in both higher education and vocational education settings. Universities also use these standards to assess student and new graduate performance.

Nursing and midwifery regulatory authorities in each state and territory use the professions' competency standards to assess the competence of:

- people applying for a licence to enter practice as a nurse or midwife such as an undergraduate nurse or midwife;
- nurses and midwives as part of the annual renewal assessment for registration;
- overseas nurses and midwives seeking to work in Australia;
- nurses or midwives wishing to re-enter the register after a period of time out of practice; or
- a nurse or midwife involved in professional conduct breaches.

Employers use competency standards to develop position descriptions and also for performance appraisal processes.

The competency standards outlined above refer to the minimum standards for the nursing and midwifery professions. Since the 1990s advanced competencies have been developed for practising at advanced levels across practice settings, and for nurse practitioners; in addition to the creation of standards by a range of individual nursing specialty areas, such as critical care, mental health, gastroenterology and operating room nurses.

Of critical importance to nurses and midwives working in general practice are competency standards specifically for registered and enrolled nurses in general practice. These standards were developed in 2005 by the University of South Australia and Royal College of Nursing, Australia. The project was funded by the Department of Health and Ageing, managed by the Australian Nursing Federation (Australian Nursing Federation 2006) and overseen by a steering committee with broader nursing and general practice nursing representatives. The development of these standards heralded a significant acknowledgement of the unique environment in which nurses and midwives function in general practice. The standards recognise the role for both registered and enrolled nurses in general practice as well as highlighting the differences in responsibility level according to the legislative framework under which each practice.

Competency standards for nurses and midwives in general practice provide a useful framework within which to reflect on scope of practice in terms of individual professional development. In this regard it is worth noting an observation of the N³ET:

> ... *while pre-registration education and ANMC competencies shape the limits of a nurse's [or midwife's] scope of practice on entry to practice, they do not circumscribe or limit the nurse's [or midwife's] actual or potential scope of practice.*

Indeed, there is an implicit expectation that practitioners expand their repertoire of knowledge, skills and competence as they become immersed in professional practice.

> *As they become more experienced and exposed to a range of practice settings, there is an expectation that nurses [and midwives] become more capable, confident and competent in different areas of practice.*

(Australian Health Ministers' Advisory Council 2005)

Nurses and midwives in general practice should be familiar with the competency standards prepared specifically for their context of practice. In addition to using these standards to guide their current practice and to expand their practice to meet future health demands in primary care, feedback should be provided to the standard for future revisions to ensure these standards remain relevant to nurses and midwives in general practice.

Reflections

How does your job description relate to the Competency Standards for Nurses in General Practice? How has it changed?

Authorised or endorsed nurses

In addition to regulation for all nurses and midwives in Australia, there are specific aspects of practice for which authorisation or endorsement is granted by state/territory nursing and midwifery regulatory boards.

These authorisations and endorsements include:

- **Nurse practitioner** Authorisation or endorsement involves a rigorous process to meet educational and professional predetermined standards culminating in the right to: use the title 'nurse practitioner'; prescribe medicines; refer to other health professionals; order other diagnostic testing; and, in some jurisdictions, claim admitting rights and clinical privileges.

- **Enrolled nurses**   Medication management authorisation or endorsement is conferred after successful completion of an educational program for prescribed medication management. This extension of the scope of practice for enrolled nurses enables them to be able to administer Schedule 2, 3 and 4 medications—and in some jurisdictions such as Tasmania, Schedule 8 medications—under the supervision of a registered nurse. Amendments were made to the drugs and controlled substances Acts in each state and territory enabling these changes in the scope of practice of the enrolled nurse in medication management. This important expansion of the role of the enrolled nurse in Australia has meant that they can now more fully complement the role of the registered nurse, and together provide safe competent care to the community.

Collaboration

An essential component of the role of practice nurses, an indeed all staff in general practice, is that of collaboration with others in the general practice team. Collaborative practice is longstanding between health professionals and especially between nurses and their medical colleagues. The manner in which collaboration occurs between nurses and others in the general practice team can impact on their scope of practice.

In 2000 Way and colleagues reported on a research project undertaken with family doctors and nurse practitioners in Canada (Way, Jones & Busing 2000). They suggested that collaboration is a term that is often used with little understanding by health providers of its accurate meaning. Through their project on collaborative practice they developed the following definition:

> *Collaborative Practice is an inter-professional process for communication and decision making that enables the separate and shared knowledge and skills of care providers to synergistically influence the client/patient care provided.*

(Way, Jones & Busing 2000, p. 3)

The authors concluded that collaborative practice involves working relationships and ways of working that fully utilises and respects the contribution of all providers involved. Seven essential elements were identified through this research project as being integral to successful collaborative practice:

1. responsibility and accountability
2. coordination
3. communication
4. cooperation

5. assertiveness

6. autonomy

7. mutual trust and respect.

Reflections

How do team members in your general practice setting incorporate these seven elements of collaboration in their daily work?

It is worth noting the commentary on 'autonomy'.

Autonomy involves the authority of the individual providers to independently make decisions and carry out the treatment plan. Autonomy is not contrary to collaboration and serves as a complement to shared work. Without the ability to work independently, the provider team becomes inefficient and work becomes unmanageable. .... Both partners need to fully understand and support practice autonomy, as well as, shared decision making from a liability perspective.

(Way, Jones & Busing 2000, p. 5)

Collaboration means respecting each other's interest and professional responsibilities and does *not* mean one profession dominating or overseeing another. In the general practice setting, nurses, midwives and medical colleagues must have confidence that each will inform the other and discuss client needs at an appropriate time. It also means that each health professional will act in an ethical and professional manner at all times, and recognise the breadth/limits of one's scope of practice. Existing regulatory processes for each profession which underpin professional practice ensure quality, safety, accountability and responsibility in the public's interest.

While collaboration with other health professionals and with individuals and groups requiring care is inherent in nursing practice in any setting including general practice, registered nurses are autonomous health care professionals. Under law, they are required to be accountable and responsible for their own actions and must be able to identify the nursing care which they have the knowledge and skill to provide.

Legislation in most states and territories also requires that enrolled nurses are supervised by registered nurses. Supervision can be direct, where the registered nurse is present, observes, works with and directs the enrolled nurse, or indirect where the registered nurse is easily contactable but does not directly observe the activities. The level of supervision required depends on a number of factors including the skills and knowledge of the enrolled nurse, the acuity and stability of the person receiving the nursing care, and the complexity of the nursing care being provided.

Professional supervision of an enrolled nurse is solely the responsibility of the registered nurse. These professional supervisory arrangements must be in place irrespective of any other employer oversight including that provided by an employing general practitioner. In general practices employing enrolled nurses, arrangements for professional supervision should be developed and guidelines prepared to assist both the enrolled nurse and the supervising registered nurse (Australian Nursing Federation 2006, p. 9).

Reflections

What are the professional supervisory arrangements for enrolled nurses employed in your general practice?

Future scope of practice

The growth in the numbers of nurses and midwives working in general practice has altered the face of general practice. Through policy and funding introduced in recent years, and through their own initiative, practice nurses had been able to enhance their contribution to general practice with the establishment of nurse-led clinics for such health issues as asthma, diabetes, wound management, obesity/eating disorders and immunisation programs. Further developments such as the establishment of a professional body specifically for nurses and midwives in general practice—the Australian Practice Nurses Association—and the development of the competency standards for registered and enrolled nurses in general practice have meant the emergence of professional practice frameworks for this group of nurses. Sharing of experiences at conferences, forums and publications has helped influence and shape the evolution of scope of practice for nurses and midwives in general practice.

The current Australian Government's reform agenda offers the nursing and midwifery professions a unique opportunity to reflect on innovations to practice to meet future health and aged care challenges. The National Primary Health Care Strategy and the National Preventative Health Strategy are two areas which should challenge nurses and midwives in general practice to analyse their current scope of practice against the health profile and demographics of their local population. Questions to be asked include: is there a match in our general practice between nursing/midwifery practice and our clients' needs? Are there gaps in service provision? Are the nurses and midwives using all of their knowledge and expertise at present? Are there health promotion and health prevention strategies or chronic disease management issues which are not being met by the nurses and midwives in our facility? Are there additional skills and knowledge that the nurses and midwives in our general practice need to acquire?

The challenge for nurses and midwives in general practice is to be creative in assessing the fit between current scope of practice and possibilities for broadening that scope. Over the past 15 years nurses have consistently rated as the 'most favoured profession' by the public in terms of ethics and integrity (Roy Morgan Research 2009). The public trusts nurses and midwives, as health professionals, to deal with a wide range of health issues pertaining to themselves and their families. This is particularly pertinent in general practice environments as the nurses and midwives become well known to individuals and whole families who attend the practice. Practice nurses have a responsibility, as professionals, to ensure that their scope of practice not only fits within relevant regulatory and professional frameworks but also, and just as importantly, meets the needs of their communities. When there is a need to expand scope of practice and the practice nurse does not have requisite knowledge or skills to do so, continuing professional development activities, supervised practice, or formal education programs must be undertaken.

Practice nurses have great opportunity to show leadership and to model new thinking as the 19th century, militaristic 'orders' mentality in nursing (and medicine) moves into the modern health era of sciences grounded in knowledge, innovation and critical thinking (Villeneuve 2008).

Conclusion

The scope of practice of nurses and midwives in general practice is influenced by a range of factors. Essentially, while there are some limitations imposed by regulation, nurses and midwives can take the initiative in expanding their practice to meet the needs of the clients presenting to their facility. The focus on prevention, health promotion and chronic disease management in the current primary health care reforms provides an ideal opportunity for nurses and midwives in general practice. The challenge is to reflect on individual practice, ensure that their scope of practice is relevant for contemporary community health needs, and take necessary action to expand that scope to meet emerging health issues.

Key messages

Scope of practice is defined as practice for which nurses and midwives are authorised, educated and competent to perform.

Nurses and midwives are legally required to be accountable and responsible for their own actions and must be able to identify the nursing care which they have the knowledge and skill to provide.

Scope of practice changes depending on the skills, attitude and knowledge of the nurse.

It is the responsibility of individual nurses and midwives to identify and work within their own scope of practice.

The challenge to nurses and midwives is to seek opportunities to broaden their scope of practice to meet the needs of the community served by their general practice, in collaboration with the general practice team.

Useful resources

Codes of ethics and professional conduct

Competency standards for the registered nurse, enrolled nurse, midwife and
    nurse practitioner

National decision-making framework
    http://www.anmc.org.au/professional_standards/

Competency standards for the advanced registered nurse, advanced enrolled
    nurse and nurses in general practice
    http://www.anf.org.au/html/publications_compstandards.html

References

1. An Bord Altranais 2000, *Scope of Nursing and Midwifery Framework*, viewed 10 January 2010, <http://www.nursingboard.ie/en/about_us.aspx>.

2. Anderson, L 2009, *Nursing Scope of Practice. Nurse Together*, viewed 23 November 2009, <http://www.nursetogether.com/tabid/102/itemid/707/Nursing-Scope-of-Practice.aspx>.

3. Australian General Practice Network 2007, *National practice nurse workforce survey report 2007*, viewed 10 January 2010, <http://www.agpn.com.au/>.

4. Australian Health Ministers' Advisory Council 2005, *National Nursing and Nursing Education Taskforce (N³ET): Scopes of Practice Commentary Paper*, p. 46, viewed 7 January 2010, <http://www.nnnet.gov.au/>.

5. Australian Nursing Federation 2006, *Competency standards for nurses in general practice*, p. 8, viewed 10 January 2010, <http://www.anf.org.au/nurses_gp/>.

6. Australian Nursing Federation 2008, *ANF position statement: nursing in general medical practice*, viewed 10 January 2010, <http://www.anf.org.au/html/publications_policies.html>.

7. Australian Nursing Federation 2009, *Fact sheet: A snapshot of practice nurses in Australia*, viewed 10 January 2010, <http://www.anf.org.au/html/publications_factsheets.html>.

8. Australian Nursing and Midwifery Council 2002, *National Competency Standards for the Enrolled Nurse*, viewed 7 January 2010, <http://www.anmc.org.au/>.

9. Australian Nursing and Midwifery Council 2006a, *National Competency Standards for the Registered Nurse (2006)*, 4th edn, viewed 7 January 2010, <http://www.anmc.org.au/>.

10. Australian Nursing and Midwifery Council 2006b, *National Competency Standards for the Midwife (2006)*, viewed 7 January 2010, <http://www.anmc.org.au/>.

11. Australian Nursing and Midwifery Council 2007, *Report of the national framework for the development of decision-making tools for nursing and midwifery practice*, viewed 7 January 2010, <http://www.anmc.org.au/publications#dmf>.

12. Australian Nursing and Midwifery Council 2008, *Code of Ethics for Nurses in Australia; Code of Ethics for Midwives in Australia; Code of Professional Conduct for Nurses in Australia; Code of Professional Conduct for Midwives in Australia.* viewed 7 January 2010, <http://www.anmc.org.au/>.

13. International Council of Nurses 2004, *Position Statement: Scope of nursing practice*, viewed 10 January 2010, <http://www.icn.ch/>.

14. Roy Morgan Research Pty Ltd 2009, *Image of Professions survey*, viewed 7 January 2010, <http://www.roymorgan.com/news/polls/2009/4387/>.

15. Te Kaunihera Tapuhi o Aotearoa/Nursing Council of New Zealand 2004, *Scopes of practice*, viewed 7 January 2010, <http://www.nursingcouncil.org.nz/scopes.html>.

16. Way, D, Jones, L & Busing, N 2000, *Implementation Strategies: Collaboration in Primary Care—Family Doctors & Nurse Practitioners Delivering Shared Care*, discussion paper written for the Ontario College of Family Physicians, 18 May 2000, viewed 7 January 2010, <http://www.cfpc.ca/>.

17. Villeneuve, M 2008, 'Yes we can! Eliminating health disparities as part of the core business of nursing on a global level', *Policy, Politics & Nursing Practice*, vol. 9, no. 4, pp. 334–41.

18. World Health Organisation 2009, *Nursing & Midwifery Human Resources for Health: Global standards for the initial education of professional nurse and midwives*, viewed 10 January 2010, <http://www.who.int/hrh/nursing_midwifery/en/>.

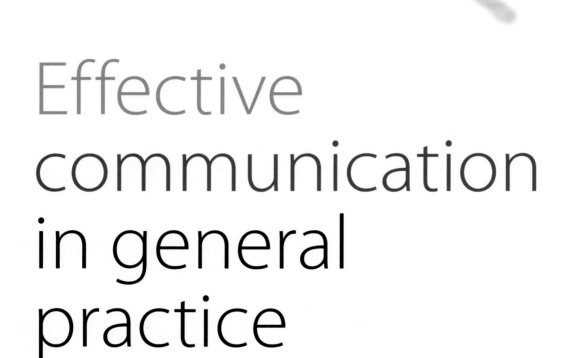

Chapter four

Effective communication in general practice

by Kelsey Hegarty and Lynne Walker

Overview

This chapter outlines the skills needed to communicate effectively with patients and colleagues to enhance patient health outcomes and reduce risk. Ways in which nurses can demonstrate assertiveness and the language that they can use to successfully convey their expectations to colleagues and employers will also be discussed. Reflective practice and teamwork, which enable successful working relationships, are also described.

Objectives

At the completion of this chapter you should be able to:

- understand the principles and skills of effective communication with patients, including the patient-centred approach;

- describe psychological therapies available to patients, including **cognitive behaviour therapy** and problem solving; and

- understand the value of relationship-centred care, teamwork, assertiveness skills and reflective skills to enhance practice.

Introduction

Assessment of medico-legal claims shows that communication has been identified as a medico-legal risk (Avant Mutual Group 2007). As general practices become larger and multidisciplinary, the continuity of patient care relies heavily on effective communication by all members of the practice team. The provision of safe, continuous, systematic and effective care by a variety of medical, nursing, administrative and management staff relies on the ability of all staff to communicate with patients from a variety of ages, experiences, cultures and educational backgrounds. Furthermore, staff need to be able communicate with each other.

Communicating with patients

The Code of Ethics for Nurses in Australia states that 'nurses value respect and kindness for self and others' (Australian Nursing and Midwifery Council 2008, p. 5). It further states that 'respect for people who are health consumers recognises their capacity for active and informed participation in their healthcare'. The aim of nurse communication is not just to understand the details of a person's illness or a colleague's work role, but to understand the reactions of the individuals involved; the significance and meaning of the situation to them; and to foster the relationship through the process of communication. There is a need for nurses to both learn and practice communication skills that enhance the nurse patient relationship (McCabe 2007) as well as teamwork (Talia et al. 2006). Central to this in primary care are empathy, ensuring respect and dignity, interview and negotiation skills, and reflecting on practice and roles (Sully & Dallas 2005).

Benefits of effective communication

Charlton and colleagues (2008) reviewed the evidence for the impact of communication styles on patient outcomes. They show that bio-psycho-social or patient-centred communication styles can make a difference to outcomes of patient care. Here are some examples of the outcomes of effective communication:

- improved patient satisfaction
- patients more likely to comply with the medication or advice they are given
- improved patient health
- resolution of symptoms in some cases relates to the ability to discuss their issues and problems fully
- better control of some chronic diseases, e.g. hypertension
- fewer legal issues—poor communication is a critical factor in malpractice suits.

Kurz, Silverman and Draper (1998) identified that the longer the health practitioner takes before they interrupt the more likely they are to find out more of the issues that the patient is attending with. They also found that the use of open questions leads to greater disclosure of issues.

Having clinical knowledge and skills, systems and effective communication are thought to contribute to good risk management (Avant Mutual Group

2007). Methods of reducing risk to the medical profession in the area of communication include:

- building a patient–provider relationship built on trust and honesty
- listening to patients and showing empathy
- minimising interruptions during consultations
- managing unrealistic patient expectations
- communicating with practice staff
- encouraging an environment in the practice where patients feel welcome and staff are skilled in all aspects of managing patients
- fostering strong relationships with colleagues and other health professionals
- keeping open channels of communication with other health facilities
- managing complaints in a way that does not leave the patient feeling abandoned or that their concerns were ignored
- ensuring the consent process is robust.

The reasons outlined above suggest that effective communication is an essential element for not just the medical profession but for all staff employed in general practice. Having effective communication skills has advantages to the patient, the staff and the employer.

Reflections

To what extent is communication reflected in risk management within your practice?

The role of empathy

Nurse–patient studies have mainly focused on the use of empathy, rather than style of communication and the effects on patient outcomes (Barry 2009). Empathy is identification with and understanding of another's situation, feelings and emotions. Empathetic people have the skill to be able to:

- attend to what is said;
- retain objectivity and distance;
- recognise non-verbal cues;
- understand both the content and the feelings in the message; and
- communicate their understanding to others.

(Dwyer 2002)

Empathy and empathetic statements are the basis of supportive communication in primary care.

The context of communication

The clinical encounter between practice nurses and patients is influenced by many factors including culture, experience and understanding of health. For example, practice nurses have knowledge and skills in their field and patients have their own understanding of their health and illness (Chant et al. 2002). In addition, age and gender can impact on the way nurses communicate with patients. There is an inherent power imbalance in the health care environment between the patient and the nurse (Kettunen, Poskiparta & Gerlander 2002). The power imbalance between a patient and a nurse can be significant, particularly where the person has limited knowledge; experiences pain, illness and fear; needs assistance with care; or experiences an unfamiliar loss of self-determination (Australian Nursing and Midwifery Council 2008). This imbalance can arise from disparities in knowledge, social status and loss of control over health. There is an additional gender power imbalance as the

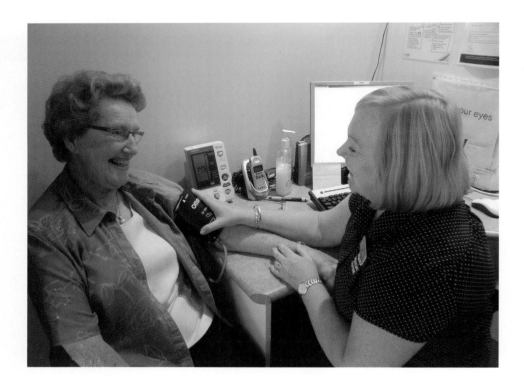

majority of doctors are male. However, as the majority of nurses are women, this power imbalance is not so overt. A patient with a different cultural background, for example an Indigenous person, requires a nurse to develop a cultural awareness and understanding to be able to communicate better to meet the needs of the patient and their family.

Skills of effective communication

Communicating with both patients and colleagues is fundamental to working in health care. Basic communication requires skills which can be learned and practiced (Robertson 2006). They include the following categories of skills.

Active listening

Listening is a core skill which involves more than merely hearing. It is an interactive, engaging process in which the listener attempts to understand and interpret the non-verbal and verbal messages of the speaker. With active listening, the listener then uses verbal and non-verbal techniques to convey that they have heard and understood the message. The following behaviours (Robbins et al. 2001) are associated with active listening skills:

- making eye contact
- affirmative head nods and facial expressions
- avoiding distracting actions or gestures
- asking questions
- paraphrasing
- avoiding interrupting the speaker
- don't overtalk.

Questions

Verbal questions can be classified into four types:

1. **Open-ended questions**   Open-ended questions elicit more information and often start interactions and then, depending on the answers, move to focused or closed questions.

    For example, *'How are you feeling?'*

2. **Focused questions**   Well-focused questions are precise and should be phrased to elicit facts and meaningful information from the patient.

    For example, *'Where is your pain?'*

3. **Closed questions**   Closed questions are designed to limit the response. They invite a brief response from the patient.

   For example, *'How long have you had…?'*

4. **Leading and compound questions**   Leading and compound questions are used less as they usually elicit insufficient or inaccurate information.

   For example, *'Tell me, have you decided on who you want to go see and whether you want to take the medication?'*

   Or *'You agree that seeing a counsellor is the only way you're going to feel better, don't you?'*

The choice of the type of question to be used will be influenced by the person to whom you are speaking. For example, with a very talkative, rambling speaker, questions need to be more focused and direct. However, for shy or reticent speakers the frequent use of open-ended questions may elicit maximum information.

Following skills

Being a good listener means following what the speaker is trying to communicate without interrupting unnecessarily, leading or taking control of the conversation.

Interpreting and following non-verbal cues

The listener receives a great deal of information about the speaker's emotions from visual cues such as facial expression, gesture, posture and eye contact. Auditory cues such as speed, pitch and volume of speech, tone of voice, number and length of pauses and hesitations, and silence are all non-verbal cues. People often send non-verbal clues that they want to talk about something.

A listener may be able to interpret these non-verbal clues and offer a 'door opener' which typically includes the following four elements:

1. **An acknowledgement of the speaker's body language**   The way the speaker is sitting in the chair, or if they are fiddling with personal items, such as rings or clothing, can let the listener know that the speaker might need to talk.

   For example, *'You look as though you're upset about something…'*

2. **An invitation to talk or continue talking**   When the speaker seems hesitant or reluctant to continue, they may need to be encouraged.

   For example, *'Tell me more…'*

3. **Silence**   Silence gives the speaker time to decide whether they want to talk and to decide what to say.

4.   **Attending behaviour**   When the listener gives the speaker physical attention it indicates that they are listening.

For example, non-verbal clues, such as head nodding, smiling or eye contact, and verbal clues such as 'mm-mm', 'yes', 'I see', 'uh-huh'.

Attentive silence

This is one of the hardest skills to master, as people often feel uncomfortable with silence and cannot resist the temptation to jump in and fill the silence. However, there are times during an interaction when silence is the most appropriate response, for example, when the person is obviously distressed.

Other skills that are useful to show you are attending include:

- **Clarifying skills** For example, *'Sounds to me like you're saying…'*

- **Confirmation or validation skills** For example, *'It can be very hard to talk about these sensitive issues. Abuse is common in relationships and talking about what the problems are sometimes helps.'*

- **Probing skills** For example, *'Let's talk about …'* rather than 'how', 'what', 'when', 'where', or 'who' questions.

Not all interactions with patients are the same and hence nurses require a variety of communication skills to be able to interact with patients in the most appropriate manner.

Reflective listening skills

Further to hearing, the listener also attempts to communicate their ability to help, accept and support the speaker.

- **Confronting** involves the listener giving honest feedback to the speaker. Confrontation is based on an observation about the speaker's behaviour, appearance or story. Confronting responses typically focus on discrepancy. For example, *'You say this doesn't bother you, yet you looked upset when we were talking about it'*.

- **Reflecting feelings (empathetic responses)** facilitate and deepen communication by focusing on the speaker's feelings rather than content details. Many people find it difficult to master this skill as they counter long experience of responding primarily to the content. This can be done by asking yourself. *'What one word describes the speaker's feelings when they made that statement?'* Empathetic responses may be introduced by phrases such as, *'It sounds as though you felt…'*. Remember, when you make an empathetic statement, you withhold judgment and the offering of a solution.

Other skills that show you are reflectively listening may include:

- **paraphrasing,** where synonyms are used to paraphrase what the speaker has said but in a briefer form
- **restating** to echo a proportion of the speaker's last statement
- **summarising**, where the listener provides an overview of the content when the speaker concludes a lengthy and confusing account, when they are rambling or to conclude a section.

Finally, some authors suggest that simply allowing patients to tell their stories is a therapy within itself (Dowrick 2008) and use of the above techniques will allow and enable people to tell their story.

Barriers to effective communication

There are many barriers to effective communication in the clinical setting. There are structural barriers such as lack of appropriate room, excessive noise and lack of privacy. There are also interaction barriers. As practitioners, we are often guilty of excessive questioning or advising, or avoiding the patient's concerns by reassuring them. Patients may have been subjected to this type of communication from their partners, friends and families and so are disappointed further when they receive it from their practitioner. What they are seeking is for someone to really listen to them.

Bolton (1987) outlines some of the communication responses that cause barriers. These include:

- **Judging**
  - Criticising—'You've got no one else to blame but yourself.'
  - Diagnosing—'You are just doing that to irritate me.'
  - Praising evaluatively—'You are always such a good girl.'
- **Sending solutions**
  - Moralising—'You ought to tell him you are sorry.'
  - Excessive, inappropriate questioning—usually closed ended—'When did it happen?'
  - Advising—'If I were you, I'd sure tell him off.'
- **Avoiding the other's concerns**
  - Diverting—'Don't dwell on it. Let's think about something more pleasant.'
  - Logical argument—'Look at the facts: if you hadn't bought the new car we could afford the house.'
  - Reassuring—'It will all work out in the end.'

Patient-centred communication

One model that provides a framework to understand different aspects of a holistic approach to health care is the patient-centred model (Stewart et al. 1995). Current evidence shows that patients prefer a patient-centred approach to their care. A United Kingdom study (Little et al. 2001a; Little et al. 2001b) reports that patients are less satisfied, less enabled and may suffer greater symptom burden if they do not receive a patient-centred response.

The six related concepts of the model are:

1. Exploring both the experience and impact of disease and illness, and the patient's feelings and how the problem impacts on their life
2. Understanding the patient as a whole person
3. Finding common ground
4. Incorporating prevention and health promotion
5. Enhancing the care provider–patient relationship
6. Being realistic.

The following list of questions can be incorporated into a patient-centred model of care (Gunn 2006).

Questions exploring both the experience and impact of care issues

'How do you feel about ...?'
'How are you feeling in yourself?'
'What for you is the most important thing to talk about today?'
'What changes has ... had on your life?'

Questions understanding the patient as a whole person

'How has your ... affected your family and friends?'
'Apart from ... what other things are going on in your life?'
'What information would you like about looking after yourself at the moment?'

Questions assisting in finding common ground regarding care

'What do you know about...?'
'What would help you make a decision?'
'What have you tried?'

Questions incorporating prevention and health promotion

'How is your health in general?'
'What do you do to keep you healthy?'

How do you tell if a consultation is patient centred?

For some health care professionals it may be the extent to which:

- decisions about care are shared;
- a person has been treated as an individual with individual preferences reflective of their social context; or
- the focus is on the individual needs of a person rather than on clinical aspects of care.

There is extremely limited research on primary care nurse or nurse practitioner–patient communication styles (Barry 2009). Often it is assumed that nursing care will be patient centred. Barry (2009) calls for more research in this area including the barriers and possible solutions, as in her small study of nurse practitioners' consultations (N = 53) this hypothesis was not borne out. Only a minority (30.2%) of nurse practitioners used a patient-centred communication style with the majority using a provider-centred communication style.

To provide holistic and comprehensive patient care, nurses need to incorporate skills and behaviour that will encourage a patient-centred approach to consultations, however, this maybe difficult at times.

Barriers to patient-centred care in primary care

There are many barriers to conducting patient-centred care in the primary care setting. Myerscough (1996) outlines the following:

- Time
- Physical setting
- Presence of a third party
- Knowing the patient outside the primary care setting
- Nature of the issues, for example, impending death, sexuality problems
- Cultural barriers
- Health professional's personal anxieties, for example, anxious about failing, introducing sensitive issues, unresolved personal problems.

Many of these barriers can be overcome: the practice of patient-centred care can be a rewarding experience for primary care nurses (Greenhalgh 2007).

Reflections

How can you overcome the barriers to patient-centred care in your practice?

Psychological therapies

In addition to the generic skills of active listening and supportive counselling, there are several other specific skills that primary care practitioners may find useful, with additional training. These include:

- Cognitive behaviour therapy
- Problem-solving therapy
- Motivational interviewing.

Cognitive behaviour therapy

When people get depressed or anxious they often think negatively about themselves, what will happen in the future and about what is going on in their lives. Negative thinking makes people more vulnerable to depression. Cognitive behaviour therapy (CBT) is a structured psychological therapy that is based on the idea that the way we think affects the way we feel (Burns 1980). CBT teaches people to think rationally about life's common difficulties. It is often used in association with medication following treatment of an acute episode of stress and depression. The framework for CBT is represented in Figure 4.1 below.

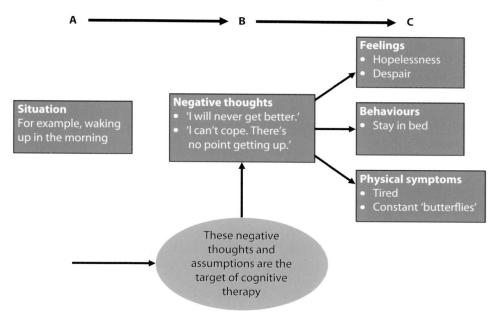

Figure 4.1 Cognitive behaviour therapy: the ABC of thinking
Source: Burns 1980

Features of CBT include asking a patient to keep a diary of their thoughts and feelings to enable them to recognise and challenge negative thoughts. Some people have had negative thoughts all their life and require more extensive cognitive treatment by their doctor or another mental health professional.

Problem solving

Problem solving assists individuals in using their own skills and resources to function better. When used by doctors and nurses trained in problem-solving techniques, non-directive problem solving in primary care has been effective in the treatment of depression (Mynors-Wallis, Gath & Baker 2000).

Problem solving occurs in the following stages:

- Clarification and definition of problems
- Choice of achievable goals
- Generation of solutions
- Implementation of preferred solutions
- Evaluation.

(Gath & Mynors-Wallis 1997)

When used by practice nurses, problem solving engages the patient as an active partner in their care. It creates a framework for individuals to refocus on practical approaches to perceived problems and learn new cognitive skills. Whether the solution chosen by the patient is successful is not as important as what the patient learns during the process and can apply in other situations. A structured approach as described by Hickie (2000) may be useful in helping patients to solve problems. The steps are:

Step 1: Identify the problems that are worrying or distressing you and write them down.

Step 2: Work out what options are available to deal with the problem and write them down.

Step 3: List the advantages and disadvantages of each option, taking into account the resources available to you.

Step 4: Identify the best option to deal with the problem.

Step 5: List the steps required to carry out this option.

Step 6: Carry out the best option and check its effectiveness.

Motivational interviewing

Motivational interviewing is a counselling style for helping people explore and resolve ambivalence about whether they want to change their behaviour. It is an approach designed to help patients build on their own motivation and reach a decision to change (Miller & Rollnick 2002). Specific responses are given depending on which stage the person is at. It has been used successfully for many lifestyle issues in primary care, for example, smoking and alcohol abuse and is discussed further in Chapter 16.

Relationship-centred care

Relationship-centred care can be defined as care in which all participants appreciate the importance of their relationships with one another. It is founded upon four principles:

1. Relationships in health care ought to include the personhood of the participants

2. Affect and emotion are important components of these relationships

3. All health care relationships occur in the context of reciprocal influence

4. The formation and maintenance of genuine relationships in health care is morally valuable.

In this framework of care, relationships between patients and clinicians remain central, although the relationships of clinicians with themselves, with each other and with community are also emphasized' (Beach & Inui 2006).

Relationships between health care workers

Effective, empathic care requires health care workers commit to working together. Relationships among practitioners include those within or across disciplines, and those between practitioners and practitioners-in-training. As general practice becomes multidisciplinary, undertakes research in primary care, educates nursing and medical students and new roles for health care workers are introduced, the importance of working together is paramount. These relationships require teamwork, shared values, learning from and making use of the expertise of others, helping others learn and develop, integrating services at individual and systems levels, and setting aside issues of specialisation, hierarchy and privilege.

The best and most cost-effective outcomes for patients and clients are achieved when professionals work together, learn together, engage in clinical audit of outcomes together, and generate innovation to ensure progress in practice and service.

(Borrill et al. 1999)

Teamwork

Teamwork is described by the World Health Organisation as a

> co-ordinated action carried out by two or more individuals jointly, concurrently or sequentially. It implies common agreed goals, clear awareness of, and respect for, others' roles and functions. On the part of each member of the team, adequate human and material resources, supportive co-operative relationships and mutual trust, effective leadership, open, honest and sensitive communications, and provision for evaluations.
>
> *(Kekki 1990)*

Barriers to teamwork

Being multidisciplinary implies that several professional groups are working together as a unit such as the medical, nursing professions and allied health, however teamwork does not necessarily follow from professionals working alongside one another.

Gender issues such as doctors being predominantly male, nurses predominantly female and owners of general practice usually men may influence the degree of teamwork. Additional factors include multiple lines of management, poor communication, personality factors, perceived status differentials between different professional groups and lack of organisational systems for supporting teams (Borrill et al. 1999; Hine 2000).

The primary health care team refers to a group of professionals delivering health services in the community, at 'primary' or first point of contact with the health service. The term includes administrative staff, such as secretaries, receptionists and practice managers, and clinical staff such as GPs, nurses, physiotherapists and counsellors (Hine 2000). As practice nurses are encouraged to be part of the development of GP management plans, it is important to identify the team members involved in the patient's care. Understanding the role of each health professional is important not only for the staff members on the team but for the patient as well.

Benefits of teamwork

There is some evidence that teamwork enhances health outcomes for patients, particularly those with chronic disease. An Australian study by Proudfoot and colleagues (2007) examined whether good **team climate** for innovation as assessed by the Team Climate Inventory had an effect on care and job satisfaction. They found that team climate predicted the job satisfaction of the general practitioners and staff irrespective of the number of practice staff and was also associated with greater satisfaction by patients with their care.

The mental health of those working in teams has been found to be better than those working individually, as team members are buffered from the negative effects of organisational climate and conflict. This is thought to be due to better peer support and better role clarity (Borrill et al. 1999). Effective teamwork in primary health care teams is associated with lower stress among members. Staff retention and lower turnover was also noted in secondary health care settings from this study.

Successful work relationships

Although many practices may describe themselves as teams, Grumbach and Bodenheimer (2004) identified five key characteristics that a cohesive health care team will have. They are:

- clear goals with measurable outcomes;
- clinical and administrative systems;
- division of labour;
- training of all team members; and
- effective communication.

Talia and colleagues (2006) analysed clinical and financial outcomes in primary care across 160 practices in the United States. Using quantitative and qualitative data they explored the characteristics in successful practices that functioned well and had a high quality of care that resulted in improved health outcomes. These include:

- trust—seek input from others and openly discuss successes/failures
- diversity—encourage different viewpoints
- mindfulness—open to new ideas
- interrelatedness—sensitive to task and how it affects others
- respect—considerate, honest and tactful
- varied interaction—social and task-related relationships
- effective communication—use a variety of communication methods especially for messages of unclear meanings or emotional content.

These characteristics need to be modelled, developed and nurtured to support staff working in an environment, such as general practice, where successful teamwork has been identified as improving health outcomes for patients.

Reflections

How many of the above characteristics does you practice demonstrate?

All health care professionals recognise that communication is necessary for teams to work; however, in practice, communication is often inadequate. For example, in large general practices, separate subcultures may exist between administrative and clinical staff, which has implications for designing effective team interventions (Proudfoot et al. 2007). Providers often operate independently with poor continuity across or even within services. Overall, content and timeliness of communication between providers is poor and lack of feedback after referral inhibits collaboration (Bambling et al. 2007).

The following recommendations have been made by a forum on teamwork, which included representatives from the Royal College of Nursing, on how a team should function in general practice. Teams should:

1. Recognise and include the patient, carer, or their representative, as an essential member of the primary health care team.

2. Establish a common agreed purpose, setting out what team members understand by team working, and what they aim to achieve as a team.

3. Agree to set objectives and monitor progress towards them. Build into its practice opportunities to reflect as a team on the care provided and how it could be improved.

4. Agree on team working conditions, including a process for resolving conflict. Identify predictable problems which the team might encounter and plan ways of managing them.

5. Ensure that each team member understands and acknowledges the skills and knowledge of team colleagues and regularly reaffirm what each member contributes.

6. Pay particular attention to the importance of communication between its members, including the patient, and use, to the full, technological developments to assist this.

7. Take active steps to ensure that the practice population understands and accepts the way in which the team works within the community.

8. Select the leader of the team for their leadership skills rather than on the basis of status, hierarchy or availability, and include in the team all the relevant professions.

9. Promote teamwork across health and social care for patients who can benefit from it, using team members' joint efforts to help to reduce ill-health and social exclusion.

10. Evaluate all its team working initiatives and as a result, develop its practice on the basis of sound evidence.

11. Ensure that the sharing of patient information within the team is in accordance with current legal and professional requirements.

(Hine 2000)

Research that suggests communication as an essential component of highly functioning practices is plentiful (Proudfoot et al. 2007; Grumbach & Bodenheimer 2004; Hine 2000) but nurses may encounter difficulties in participating effectively in discussions with management and GPs who are also their employers, as they may lack negotiation and assertiveness skills.

Reflections

What strategies does your practice use to ensure that your team can achieve the Royal College of Nursing's recommendations?

Assertiveness skills

Assertiveness is the ability to express oneself and one's rights without violating the rights of others and is useful when working in a team. Assertive people tend to be open, expressive and relaxed and are able to build honest, fulfilling relationships (Dwyer 2002). They have the ability to disagree, stand up for their rights, and present alternative points of view without being intimidated and putting others down (Dwyer 2002). Acting assertively will allow nurses to feel self-confident, communicate openly, be heard and acknowledged, and will generally gain them the respect of their peers. It can increase the chances for honest relationships, and help nurses feel better about themselves and their self-control in everyday situations. It will also enhance their negotiation skills. Assertiveness basically means the ability to express thoughts and feelings in a way that clearly states their needs and keeps the lines of communication open with the other party. However, before anybody can comfortably express their needs, they must believe they have a legitimate right to have those needs (Bolton 1987). Assertive behaviour is based on high self-esteem while submissive behaviour is based on low self-esteem (Dwyer 2002).

In the workplace each person has the right to:

- their own values, beliefs, opinions and emotions—and the right to respect themself for them, no matter the opinion of others;

- not justify or explain their actions or feelings to others;

- tell others how they wish to be treated;

- express themself and to say 'No', 'I don't know', 'I don't understand', or even 'I don't care'. They have the right to take the time needed to formulate ideas before expressing them.

- ask for information or help—without having negative feelings about their needs;

- change their mind, make mistakes and sometimes act illogically—with full understanding and acceptance of the consequences; and

- have positive, satisfying relationships within which they feel comfortable and free to express themself honestly—and the right to change or end relationships if they don't meet their needs.

When nurses don't believe they have these rights, they may react very passively to circumstances and events in their lives. When they allow the needs, opinions and judgments of others to become more important than their own, they are likely to feel hurt, anxious and even angry. This kind of passive or non-assertive behaviour is often indirect, emotionally dishonest and self-denying. Further, lack of assertiveness is most certainly one of the reasons why conflicts occur in any relationships. Table 4.1 below shows a comparison between assertive and submissive behaviour.

Table 4.1 Differences between assertiveness and submissiveness

Assertive behaviour	Submissive behaviour
Satisfies own needs and those of others	Is self-denying
May achieve desired goal of others	Does not achieve desired goals
Has a positive self-concept	Feels hurt or anxious often
Makes decisions for self	Allow others to make the decisions
Is expressive	Is inhibited
Feels comfortable with and equal to others	Feels uncomfortable and of less worth than others
Is able to present a point of view and accept a different point of view	Is unable to present a point of view

Source: adapted from Dwyer 2002

Reflections

What qualities of assertiveness do you possess?

Techniques for assertiveness

The following techniques will assist practice nurses in demonstrating more assertive behaviour.

1. Be as specific and clear as possible about what you want think and feel. 'I' messages can be used to express both positive and negative feelings and demonstrate how other people's behaviour affects you. It also shows a willingness to share your thoughts and feelings with others.

    The following statements project this:

    *   'I want to…'

    *   'I don't want you to…'

    *   'Would you…?'

    *   'I liked it when you did that.'

    *   'I have a different opinion, I think that…'

    *   'I have mixed reactions. I agree with these aspects for these reasons, but I am disturbed about these aspects for these reasons.'

2. Be direct. Deliver your message to the person for whom it is intended. If you want to tell Jane something, tell Jane; do not tell everyone except Jane; do not tell a group, of which Jane happens to be a member.

3. 'Own' your message. Acknowledge that your message comes from your frame of reference, your concept of good versus bad or right versus wrong, and your perceptions. You can acknowledge ownership with personalised 'I' statements such as 'I don't agree with you' (as compared to 'You're wrong'). Suggesting that someone is wrong or bad and should change for his or her own benefit when, in fact, it would please you, will only foster resentment and resistance rather than understanding and cooperation.

4. Ask for feedback. Asking for feedback can encourage others to correct any misconceptions you may have as well as help others realise that you are expressing an opinion, feeling or desire rather than a demand. Encourage others to be clear, direct and specific in their feedback to you, for example, 'Am I being clear?', 'How do you see this situation?', 'What do you want to do?'

Self-reflection and observation

One of the major skills required to help practice nurses to improve their communication skills is the ability to reflect on their own behaviour and attitudes towards patients and other members of the team (Atkins & Murphy 1993). Attending to how one is feeling during or after an interaction with a patient or a colleague is an aspect of reflection. Noticing or becoming aware of what is happening in and around you allows you to intervene and change what is happening (Taylor 2000). For example, discussing bowel cancer screening with an elderly patient might evoke no feelings in one practitioner and yet another whose father died of bowel cancer recently may find they become quite angry if the patient chooses not to be involved in a screening program. Understanding and then adapting how you interact with the patient and other practitioners is vital for effective communication. The skills required to be reflective include:

- self-awareness;
- description of the event;
- critical analysis;
- synthesis; and
- evaluation.

Not only do practice nurses need to reflect on patient consultations, but they would benefit from reflecting on systems of communication and teamwork in their practices. Mechanisms that incorporate reflection on how a practice is functioning are vital for a team to achieve a high level of satisfaction by staff, patients and, ultimately, to improve the health care of the patient population.

Conclusion

This chapter has explored the communication skills necessary to hear and bear witness to patients' stories in primary care. With effective communication skills and a patient-centred approach nurses will improve opportunities for patients to engage in and be part of the decision-making process in their health care. With education and experience practice nurses are well placed to support psychological techniques for patients attending general practice. Practice nurses have the opportunity to demonstrate leadership and build the capacity of practices by improving their own communication skills. In turn this will help build the teams so necessary in Australian general practice.

Key messages

Effective communication and patient-centred care are important for improving patient health outcomes.

Effective communication reduces medico-legal risks.

Teamwork skills need to be developed within primary care.

All health care workers need to reflect on their communication with patients and colleagues.

Useful resources

Mood gym

> http://moodgym.anu.edu.au/

Sarah Edelman, Australian Broadcasting Corporation, *Change your thinking: positive and practical ways to overcome stress, negative emotions and self-defeating behaviour using CBT* (see reference 14 overleaf)

References

1. Atkins, S & Murphy, K 1993, 'Reflection: a review of the literature', *Journal of Advanced Nursing*, vol. 18, no. 8, pp. 1188–92.

2. Australian Nursing and Midwifery Council 2008, 'Code of Ethics for Nurses in Australia', viewed 12 January 2010, http://www.anmc.org.au/.

3. Avant Mutual Group Limited 2007, 'The absolute fundamentals of good risk management', viewed 12 January 2010, http://www.avant.org.au/retrievemedia.asp?Media_ID=1477.

4. Bambling, M, Kavanagh, D, Lewis, G, King, R, King, D, Sturyk, H, Turpin, M, Gallois, C & Bartlett, H 2007, 'Challenges faced by general practitioners and allied mental health services in providing mental health services in rural Queensland', *Australian Journal of Rural Health*, vol. 15, no. 2, pp. 126–30.

5. Barry, J 2009, 'Nurse practitioner/patient communication styles in clinical practice', *The Journal for Nurse Practitioners*, vol. 5, no. 7, pp. 508–15.

6. Beach, M & Inui, T 2006, 'Relationship-centered care: a constructive reframing', *Journal of General Internal Medicine*, vol. 21, no. S1, pp. S3–S8.

7. Bolton, R 1987, *People skills: how to assert yourself, listen to others and resolve conflicts*, Simon and Schuster, Sydney.

8. Borril, C, Carletta, J, Carter, A, Dawson, J, Garrod, S, Rees, A, Richards, A, Shapiro, D & West, M 1999, 'The effectiveness of health care teams in the National Health Service', Aston Centre for Health Service Organization

Research, viewed 12 January 2010, http://homepages.inf.ed.ac.uk/jeanc/DOH-final-report.pdf.

9. Burns, D 1980, *Feeling good: the new mood therapy*, Quill, Harper Collins, New York, pp. 9–27.

10. Chant, S, Jenkinson, T, Randle, J & Russell, LG 2002, 'Communication skills: some problems in nursing education and practice', *Journal of Clinical Nursing*, vol. 11, no. 1, pp. 12–21.

11. Charlton, C, Dearing, K, Berry, J & Johnson, M 2008, 'Nurse practitioners' communication styles and their impact on patient outcomes: an integrated literature review', *Journal of the American Academy of Nurse Practitioners*, vol. 20, no. 7, pp. 382–8.

12. Dowrick, C 2008, *Beyond depression*, 2nd edn, Oxford University Press, Oxford.

13. Dwyer, J 2002, *Communication in Business Strategies and Skills*, 2nd edn, Prentice Hall, NSW.

14. Edelman, S & Australian Broadcasting Corporation 2002, *Change your thinking: positive and practical ways to overcome stress, negative emotions and self-defeating behaviour using CBT*, Sarah Edelman & ABC Books for the Australian Broadcasting Corporation, Sydney.

15. Gath, DH & Mynors-Wallis, LM 1997, 'Problem-solving treatment in primary care', in DM Clark, CG Fairburn (eds.), *Science and practice of cognitive behaviour therapy*, Oxford University Press, Oxford.

16. Grumbach, K & Bodenheimer, T 2004, 'Can health care teams improve primary care practice?', *Journal of the American Medical Association*, vol. 291, no. 10, pp. 1246–51.

17. Greenhalgh, T 2007, *Primary health care: theory and practice*, BMJ Books, Blackwell, Oxford.

18. Gunn, J, Hegarty, K, Nagle, C, Forster, D, Brown, S & Lumley, J 2006, 'Putting woman-centred care into practice: a new (ANEW) approach to psychosocial risk assessment during pregnancy', *Birth*, vol. 33, no. 1, pp. 46–55.

19. Hickie, IB 2000, 'An approach to managing depression in general practice', *Medical Journal of Australia*, vol. 173, no. 2 pp. 106–10.

20. Hine, D 2000, *Teamworking in primary healthcare: final report 2000*, Royal Pharmaceutical Society of Great Britain, British Medical Association, Royal College of Nursing, National Pharmaceutical Association, viewed 12 January 2010, http://www.rpsgb.org.uk/pdfs/teamworking.pdf.

21. Kekki, P 1990, *Teamwork in primary health care*, World Health Organisation, in D Hine, *Teamworking in primary healthcare: final report 2000*.

22. Ketunnen, T, Poskiparta, M & Gerlander, M 2002, 'Nurse–patients power relationship: preliminary evidence of patients power messages', *Patient Education and Counseling* vol. 47, no. 2, pp. 103–13.

23. Kurtz, S, Silverman, J & Draper, J 1998, *Teaching and Learning Communication Skills in Medicine*, Radcliffe Medical Press.

24. Little, P, Everitt, H, Williamson, I, Warner, G, Moore, M, Gould, C, Ferrier, K & Payne, S 2001a, 'Preferences of patients for patient centred approach to

consultation in primary care: observational study', *British Medical Journal*, vol. 322, no. 7284, pp. 468–72.

25. Little, P, Everitt, H, Williamson, I, Warner, G, Moore, M, Gould, C, Ferrier, K & Payne, S 2001b, 'Observational study of effects of patient centredness and positive approach on outcomes of general practice consultations', *British Medical Journal*, vol. 323, no. 7318, pp. 908–11.

26. McCabe, C 2000, 'Nurse-patient communication: an exploration of patients' experiences', *Journal of Clinical Nursing*, vol. 13, no. 1, pp. 41–9.

27. Miller, W & Rollnick, S 2002, *Motivational interviewing—preparing people for change*, 2nd edn, The Guilford Press, New York, pp. 33–42.

28. Myerscough, P 1996, *Talking with patients: keys to good communication*, 3rd edn, Oxford University Press, Oxford.

29. Mynors-Wallis, LM, Gath, DH & Baker, F 2000, 'Randomised controlled trial of problem solving treatment, antidepressant medication and combined treatment for major depression in primary care', *British Medical Journal*, vol. 320, no. 7226, pp. 26–30.

30. Proudfoot, J, Jayasinghe, U, Holton, C, Grimm, J, Bubner, T & Amoroso, C 2007, 'Team climate for innovation: what difference does it make in general practice?', *International Journal of Quality in Health Care*, vol. 19, no. 3, pp. 164–9, viewed 12 January 2010, doi: 10.1093/intqhc/mzm005.

31. Robbins, S, Millett, B, Cacioppe, R & Waters-Marsh, T 2001, *Organisational behaviour*, 3rd edn, Prentice Hall, Australia.

32. Robertson, K 2006, *Advanced communication skills*, post-graduate course, University of Melbourne.

33. Stewart, M, Brown, J, Weston, WW, McWhinney, IR, McWilliam, CL & Freeman, TR 1995, *Patient-centered medicine transforming the clinical method*, Sage Press, California.

34. Sully, P & Dallas, J 2005, *Essential communication skills for nursing practice*, Elsevier Mosby, Edinburgh.

35. Talia, A, Lanham, H, McDaniel, R & Crabtree, B 2006, 'Seven characteristics of successful working relationships', *Family Practice Management*, vol. 13, no. 1, pp. 47–50.

36. Taylor, BJ 2000, 'The value of reflection', in *Reflective practice: a guide for nurses and midwives*, Allen and Unwin, St. Leonards.

Chapter five

Legal issues

by Kim Forrester

Overview

This chapter will focus on some of the legal issues pertaining to nursing in general practice, such as the law in relation to medical negligence litigation, the requirements for obtaining a legally valid consent to a health care treatment or procedure and the importance of documentation and medical record keeping.

Objectives

At the completion of this chapter you should be able to:

- understand the standard of practice required of a registered nurse in general practice;

- understand the effect of the doctrine of vicarious liability;

- identify the elements of a legally valid consent;

- understand the legal issues relevant to obtaining consent from an adult with diminished capacity or a child; and

- understand the legal significance of the medical record.

Introduction

The legal issues relevant to the provision of nursing services within the context of general practice are wide and varied. This is due to the fact that the activities in which a practice nurse may become involved are conducted in a community-based facility, and span from minimal intervention and information giving through to participation in surgical procedures. In these circumstances it is important that practice nurses are familiar with the legal principles that underpin and direct their practice. The laws that apply to the provision of nursing care within the context of general practice are derived from case law and the state, territory and Commonwealth legislation that apply in the particular jurisdiction in which the nurse is working.

Negligence

Negligence is a civil action in which a patient, client or family member sues a health professional and/or the employing health care facility and seeks money to compensate them for injuries suffered while in their care. The patient or client who initiates the negligence action is seeking to have the health professional, or health facility, responsible for the care made liable for injuries the patient has allegedly sustained. For the purpose of this chapter, a negligence action would involve a patient, client or family member commencing an action in negligence against the practice nurse and/or the general practice (as the employer or an independent entity) and seeking compensation for damages. Negligence has been defined in legislation as the 'failure to exercise reasonable care and skill' (*Civil Liability Act 2002* (NSW); *Civil Liability Act 2002* (ACT); *Civil Liability Act 1936* (SA); *Wrongs Act 1958* (Vic)). The basis of the claim is that the conduct of the nurse or health care facility fell below the standard of care appropriate in the particular circumstances and that their conduct resulted in damage, which the patient now seeks to have compensated in money. Unlike criminal proceedings, a negligence action seeks to place the injured patient (the plaintiff) in the position they would have been in had they not sustained the damage. The consequence of a finding of liability against a nurse and/or the general practice facility (the defendant) is, therefore, not considered as a punishment but rather as compensation to the injured party or their relatives. The principle underpinning this form of legal redress is to shift the loss, as far as money is able to do so, from the individual who has sustained the injury or damage to the individual or institution that is held to have caused the loss.

The patient bringing the action in negligence (referred to as the plaintiff) must be able to prove, based on the evidence, every element of the negligence action to the standard required by the courts. In a civil action this standard is 'on the balance of probabilities'. ('On the balance of probabilities' has been described as meaning more probably than not.) That is, in a civil trial (such as a negligence action), the patient (plaintiff) must prove 'on the balance of probabilities' every element of the action to succeed in their claim for compensation. To do this, the plaintiff must have evidence to place before the court in the form of documents, oral testimony and other relevant materials that is sufficient to satisfy the court to the requisite standard. If the plaintiff fails to prove any one of the elements to the required standard, the negligence action will fail. It is now appropriate to consider the elements of proof that are necessary for a negligence action to succeed.

Elements of negligence

Negligence has been defined by the courts as:

> *The omission to do something which a reasonable man, guided upon those considerations which ordinarily regulate the conduct of human affairs, would do, or doing something which a prudent and reasonable man would not do.*

> (*Blyth v Birmingham Water Works Co* (1856) 11 Exch 781 at 784)

It is important to recognise, however, that every injury which a patient suffers while under the care of the nurse will not provide the basis for an action in negligence, and not all actions, or decisions not to act, which result in an injury to the patient will be held to be negligence. The patient (plaintiff) must therefore establish, 'on the balance of probabilities', the following elements to succeed in a negligence action against the nurse (defendant):

- the nurse (defendant) owed the patient (the plaintiff) a duty of care;
- the standard of care conducted by the nurse fell below that required and the nurse thereby breached their duty of care;
- the breach of the duty of care by the nurse caused the injuries suffered by the patient (referred to as the damage); and
- the loss suffered by the patient was reasonably foreseeable.

We will now consider each of these elements.

Duty of care

As a general proposition where there is a practice nurse–patient relationship, there will also be the legally recognised relationship upon which the courts impose a duty of care (Kennedy & Grubb 1994). This is so, based on the 'neighbour principle' stated by Lord Atkin, in what is now considered the landmark case of *Donoghue v Stevenson* [1932] AC 562. In this case, the plaintiff sought compensation for the consequences flowing from drinking the contents of a bottle of ginger beer that contained a decomposing snail. Lord Atkin stated:

> *You must take reasonable care to avoid acts or omissions which you could reasonably foresee would be likely to injure your neighbour. Who, then, in law,*

is my neighbour? The answer seems to be—persons who are so closely and directly affected by my acts that I ought reasonably to have them in contemplation as being so affected when I am directing my mind to the acts or omissions which are called in question.

(*Donoghue v Stevenson* [1932] AC 580)

Though this case was specifically concerned with consumer law, it can be seen that the general practice nurse–patient relationship is one which gives rise to a duty of care. The patient is clearly a person whom the nurse can reasonably foresee as likely to be injured if reasonable care is not exercised. In an Australian case involving a medical practitioner, the majority judgement of the High Court of Australia in *Rogers v Whitaker*[1] held:

The law imposes on a medical practitioner a duty to exercise reasonable care and skill in the provision of professional advice and treatment. That duty is a single comprehensive duty covering all the ways in which a doctor is called upon to exercise his skill and judgement; it extends to the examination, diagnosis and treatment of the patient and the provision of information in an appropriate case.

The determination of the existence of a duty of care is based on an assessment of who is 'reasonably foreseeable'. This is an objective test and based on the evidence before the court; was the patient foreseeable to the nurse as an individual, or a member of a class, to whom the duty was owed by the nurse? The persons to whom a practice nurse may owe a duty of care can be quite extensive and, in the general practice context, the persons who potentially owe a duty of care to the patients and clients are not confined to the medical practitioners, nurses and allied health professionals. In the New South Wales Court of Appeal case of *Alexander v Heise* [2001] NSWCA 422 (27 November 2001), the court held that a medical practitioner's receptionist had a duty of care to make an assessment of a patient's condition, determine the urgency of the condition based on that assessment and schedule an appointment with the medical practitioner accordingly.

Duty to render assistance

As the majority of general practices are located within a community setting, the legal position in relation to the 'duty to rescue' or render assistance in an emergency is of particular relevance to general practice nurses. What are the legal obligations of the nurse in general practice when asked to assist in an emergency that is occurring outside the practice. The term 'good Samaritan' is often used to refer to a person who, in good faith and without the expectation of a fee, provides assistance or rescues another who has been injured, is at risk of being injured or requires emergency assistance. Though nurses may feel ethically compelled to render aid in such circumstances, as a general proposition, there is no common law obligation on any individual to render emergency aid, regardless of whether they are a nurse or any other health professional.[2] As stated by Windeyer J in *Hargrave v Goldman* [1963] 110 CLR 40:

> *The dictates of charity and of compassion do not constitute a duty of care. The law casts no duty upon a man to go to the aid of another who is in peril or distress, not caused by him. The call of common humanity may lead him to rescue. This the law recognises, for it gives the rescuer its protection when he answers the call. But it does not require that he do so. There is no general duty to help a neighbour whose house is on fire.*

The decision in the New South Wales Court of Appeal case of *Lowns v Woods* [1996] Aust Torts Reports 81–376 (CA NSW) was a significant departure from the traditionally held assumption that in Australia there was, at common law, no duty to rescue or assist in an emergency. In this case the Court of Appeal held that the refusal by the general practitioner, Dr Lowns, to attend to a 10-year-old boy who was suffering an epileptic seizure when requested was negligent. Further exceptions to the general principle that there is no duty to rescue would include the following:

- where there is legislation specifically directed to the imposition of a legal duty to render assistance. See Example 5.1 overleaf.

- where the person has assumed responsibility for the supervision or care of another.

- where the person requiring assistance is in an existing and special relationship with the rescuer.

- where the employer has, as part of the policy of the institution, a stated expectation that employees, in particular circumstances, will stop and render assistance. For example, the general practice may require employees who drive the practice's motor vehicle to stop and provide assistance should they come upon an accident while on work-related business.

Example 5.1

Under section 155 of the Northern Territory Criminal Code, 'any person who, being able to provide rescue, resuscitation, medical treatment, first aid or succour of any kind to a person urgently in need of it and whose life may be endangered if it is not provided, callously fails to do so is guilty of a crime and is liable to imprisonment for 7 years'. Though the Northern Territory is the only Australian jurisdiction to impose such a general duty on 'any person', where the person is the driver of a motor vehicle involved in an accident, the relevant legislation in each of the states or territories may impose an obligation to stop and provide reasonable assistance. It is noteworthy that the legislative obligation imposes the duty to stop and render assistance only on the driver of the vehicle involved in the accident and not on the drivers of other vehicles who come upon the accident.

If the nurse decides to render assistance to a person in an emergency, a duty of care arises. The standard of care, however, will be reflective of the circumstances in which the emergency care is provided. As an example, the standard of care would be that of 'any reasonable rescuer' in the environment in which the accident or injury has occurred. There is no expectation that the practice nurse, at the scene of the emergency, could deliver the same standard of care that would be anticipated in the general practice or hospital setting. Where the rescuer is confronted with an unfamiliar emergency situation that requires life and death decisions to be made urgently, the courts have been reluctant to find the rescuer liable in negligence (*Leishman v Thomas* [1985] 75 WN (NSW) 173 at 175). Provided that a rescuer acts in good faith and not in a manner that could be considered reckless, negligent or demonstrating a lack of reasonable care and skill, the courts have taken a lenient attitude.

Both Queensland and New South Wales have legislation protecting specified health professionals from legal action in the rescuer role. In Queensland, s. 16 of the *Law Reform Act 1995* protects medical practitioners, nurses or other people prescribed under a regulation who render medical care, aid or other assistance to an injured person in an emergency in circumstances in which the aid given is reasonable, given in good faith and without gross negligence or the expectation of a fee. In New South Wales the *Health Services Act 1997* s. 67I protects only members of staff of the New South Wales Ambulance Service and honorary ambulance officers. In all Australian states and territories other than Tasmania there is legislation which addresses potential claims against rescuers, good Samaritans and not-for-profit organisations.[3]

Breach of the duty of care

Once it is established that the general practice nurse (the defendant) owed a duty of care to the patient (the plaintiff) it must be proven, to the civil standard, that the action or omission of the nurse amounted to a breach of the standard of care considered appropriate. The requirements for a finding by the courts of a breach of the general duty have been legislated in all jurisdictions other than the Northern Territory. The Queensland *Civil Liability Act 2003* provides at s. 9:

1. *A person does not breach a duty to take precautions against a risk of harm unless—*

    a. *the risk was foreseeable (that is, it is a risk of which the person knew or ought reasonably have known); and*

    b. *the risk was not insignificant; and*

    c. *in the circumstances, a person in the position of the person would have taken the precautions.*

2. *In deciding whether a reasonable person would have taken precautions against a risk of harm, the court is to consider the following (among other relevant things)—*

    a. *the probability the harm would occur if the care were not taken;*

    b. *the likely seriousness of the harm;*

    c. *the burden of taking precautions to avoid the risk of harm;*

    d. *the social utility of the activity that creates the risk of harm.*

When the issue involves the standard of care required of a skilled professional, such as a practice nurse, the civil liability legislation and case law provide the benchmark standard against which the alleged conduct will be considered. Allegations made about general practice nurses involving a breach of their duty of care would most likely arise in the context of a technical blunder (for example, administering the incorrect medication to a patient or carrying out an incorrect procedure) or the failure to provide a warning to the patient about a risk inherent in, or associated with, a nursing procedure (for example, failing to warn a patient of the risks associated with syringing an ear).

The introduction of civil liability legislation in each Australian state and the ACT (the Northern Territory has no specific legislation for professionals) now prescribes the standard of care for professionals.

Example 5.2

The following sets out the legislation in New South Wales.[4] The New South Wales *Civil Liability Act 2002* s. 50 states:

50 Standard of care for professionals

1. *A person practising a profession (a professional) does not incur a liability in negligence arising from the provision of a professional service if it is established that the professional acted in a manner that (at the time the service was provided) was widely accepted in Australia by peer professional opinion as competent professional practice.*

2. *However, peer professional opinion cannot be relied on for the purposes of this section if the court considers that the opinion is irrational.*

3. *The fact that there are differing peer professional opinions widely accepted in Australia concerning a matter does not prevent any one or more (or all) of those opinions being relied on for the purposes of this section.*

4. *Peer professional opinion does not have to be universally accepted to be considered widely accepted.*

From the foregoing it is evident that, as a general principle, professionals will not be found liable in negligence if their practice is consistent with that which is widely accepted in Australia by peer professional opinion as competent professional practice.

The standard as set out in the legislation provides that professionals benchmark their own standard of practice. It is therefore against this standard, as determined by their peers, that the conduct of the particular defendant will be considered. Documents, such as unit/ward, institutional and Department of Health policies, procedures, protocols and guidelines, are therefore significant pieces of evidence which demonstrate the appropriate standard of care. In addition to these documents, there are the professional and regulatory policies, guidelines and codes which evidence what conduct 'is widely accepted ... by peer professional opinion as competent professional practice'.

The court will decide whether the conduct of the practice nurse amounts to a breach of the duty of care based on the standard of practice at the time the injury to the patient occurred. (*Roe v Minister of Health* [1954] 2 QB66; *Anna Koziol v Louise Anassson* [1997] 803 FCA; *H v Royal Alexandra Hospital for Children* (1990) Aust Torts Reports 81–100; *Black v Lipovac*, unreported 4 June 1998 FLC.) While there is no expectation that the nurse could have known something which only becomes evident after the incident, there is a clear expectation that the nurse will be practising in a manner which is consistent with the state of clinical knowledge at the time. Practice nurses must therefore ensure that they are constantly updating their knowledge and skill base in their area of clinical expertise. The civil liability legislation in New South Wales, Queensland, South Australia, Tasmania, Victoria and Western Australia provide that the liability of a professional, in providing a professional service, will be determined by the peer professional opinion 'at the time' the service was provided or at the time the act or omission occurred.

Prior to undertaking any procedure or treatment there is an obligation on all health professionals to provide the patient with the information they would require to make an informed choice. In addition, there is also an obligation to inform the patient of any information which the health professional knows, or ought to know, is particularly relevant to this patient in reaching a decision about their health care. That is, does this patient have a particular condition, pathology or injury which would potentially impact on the outcome, and therefore must be specifically addressed, prior to reaching their decision? A failure to provide such information may result in a successful claim in negligence based on a breach of the duty to warn the patient of risks associated with a certain procedure or treatment. In relation to this duty there is a lack of uniformity across the Australian states and territories. In jurisdictions that have specific legislative provisions, the obligation is imposed on medical practitioners. However, it is suggested that all nurses familiarise themselves with the legislation or case law in their own state or territory.

Damages

The injury to the patient (referred to as the damage) is the 'gist' of an action in negligence. No matter how reckless the conduct of the practice nurse, if the conduct does not result in an injury capable of being recognised and quantified by the courts there can be no claim. For example, the nurse may administer the incorrect drug to a patient. While the nurse owes a duty of care to the patient and has breached the standard of care, if the patient sustains no injury they cannot obtain compensation through a claim in negligence.

The courts recognise the following types of damage for the purpose of compensation:

- physical injury
- pure economic loss
- psychological/mental harm.

Causation

The patient must establish a causal relationship between the negligent conduct of the practice nurse and the damage the patient has sustained. That is, the breach of the duty of care by the nurse must be causally linked to the injury now claimed by the patient or no compensation will be payable. Can it be argued that 'but for' the negligence of the practice nurse the patient would not have sustained the injury?

Example 5.3

In the case of *Barnett v Chelsea and Kensington Hospital* [1969] 1QB 428, the patient presented to the emergency department complaining of being unwell after drinking tea with his work colleagues in the early hours of the morning. The nurse in the emergency department attempted to contact the doctor, however, the doctor was also ill and instructed the man to go home and contact his local doctor in the morning if he continued to feel unwell. Some five hours later the man died and it was discovered that there had been arsenic in the tea he had drunk. The widow of the man (the plaintiff in this case) sued the doctor and the hospital in negligence alleging a breach of the duty of care. Although the doctor and the hospital had a duty of care to the man and, by sending him away without examining him the doctor had breached the duty of care, the court held that the doctor was not liable. The basis of this decision was the inability of the plaintiff to prove that the man would not have died 'but for' the breach of the duty of care by the doctor. The evidence indicated that the man would have died from the arsenic poisoning even if the doctor had examined and treated him promptly.

There is now legislation in Queensland, Western Australia, Tasmania, the Australian Capital Territory, South Australia and Victoria setting out the requirement for a finding that a breach of the standard of care caused the damage now claimed.

Apologies and expressions of regret

All states and territories have introduced legislation that recognises the appropriateness of a health professional apologising or expressing regret when a patient is injured while under their care.[5] As the legislative provisions are not uniform across the jurisdictions it is recommended that practice nurses identify the legislation relevant to the state or territory in which the work. Expressions of regret and apologies form part of the National Open Disclosure process and must therefore be delivered as part of that process following consultation with the treating medical practitioner.

Vicarious liability

The doctrine of vicarious liability serves to shift the financial responsibility from the individual who has been found liable for the damage to another individual or entity that has a greater financial capacity to bear the loss. Therefore, in the context of a general practice, the doctrine of vicarious liability transfers the responsibility for compensating the patient's damages from the general practice nurse to the employer of the nurse, who may be an individual, a company or a corporation.

The doctrine of vicarious liability operates when an employee, in the course and scope of their employment, negligently injures a patient. Once the negligence is proven and an amount of damages awarded the employer becomes liable for the loss caused by their employee that occurred in the course and scope of their employment. It is therefore a necessary precondition to the operation of the doctrine that:

- the practice nurse is an employee and not an independent contractor; and
- the negligent conduct occurred within the course and scope of the employment.

Any nurse who is not an employee should have indemnity insurance. This may be obtained through professional organisations, such as the Australian Practice Nurses Association and the Royal College of Nursing Australia, or industrial organisations, such as the Australian Nursing Federation or unions in the respective states and territories. In addition, indemnity insurance may also be obtained privately through an insurance broker.

Consent

As a general principle, obtaining consent from patients or clients prior to commencing any assessment, treatment or procedures is polite and respectful behaviour and should be undertaken as a matter of course by all health professionals. When a patient gives a legally valid consent it converts what would otherwise amount to civil assault and battery into lawful touching. The action initiated by a patient when a legally valid consent is not obtained is called 'trespass to the person' (also referred to as civil assault and battery) and is a recognition by the law of the proprietary right in one's own body; the right of all adults of sound mind to determine what is, and what is not, done to their body. This legal right to self-determination is evident in the case of *Schloendorff v Society of New York Hospitals* 105 NE 92 (at 93) (1914) where Justice Cardozao stated:

> *Every human being of adult years and sound mind has a right to determine what will be done with his own body; and a surgeon who performs an operation without his patient's consent commits an assault, for which he is liable in damages.*

The legal principle is also reinforced through the Australian Nursing and Midwifery Council's codes of ethics and conduct for both nurses and midwives.

An action in trespass to the person within a health care context is rare and will most frequently be initiated as an alternative action to a claim in negligence. Assault involves the creation in the mind of another the fear of imminent and unwanted physical contact. This may take the form of using abusive and threatening language as a means of getting a patient to comply with the demands of the practice nurse. There is no requirement for any physical contact and it is sufficient to successfully prove the claim if the patient can establish that they had both a reasonable belief that the nurse intended to carry the threat and that the nurse had the means to do so. Battery is the actual physical contact. Unlike an action in negligence, it is not necessary to prove the contact was harmful, offensive or caused any physical injury. It is the actual touching of the person without their consent that constitutes an action in battery. It is not a defence for the nurse to claim that they touched the patient to bestow some benefit or carried out a procedure that was in the patient's best interests. The patient does not need to be aware at the time that the touching occurred. For example, the patient may be asleep, in a coma or under an anaesthetic. There is case law and legislation which deems consent in cases where the patient is unconscious or requires treatment as an emergency measure. However, this will only operate as a defence in circumstances where the patient has not given a legally valid refusal of treatment beforehand.

Types of consent

The law recognises that within a health care context, consent by a patient to any form of assessment or procedure may take a number of different forms depending on the circumstances in which the decision is made and the nature of the consent sought. The consent from a patient may take one or more of the following forms:

- implied consent
- verbal consent
- written consent.

A consent may be **implied** from the conduct or behaviour of a patient. For example, where the patient rolls up their sleeve prior to an injection or lifts their shirt to facilitate listening to their chest through a stethoscope consent to the procedure or examination is implied.

Practice nurses should be wary of relying on implied consent unless the patient is familiar with the procedures and treatment carried out by the practice. Where a patient is new to the general practice, or the patient is not familiar with the procedure or treatments, it is possible to misinterpret behaviours that are benign and unrelated as consent. The mere fact that the patient attends the practice does not in itself provide a valid consent for a nurse to initiate any form of assessment or treatment (*Hart v Herron* [1984] Aust Torts Rep 80–201).

A more frequent form of consent occurs when a **verbal** agreement to treatment is obtained from the patient. In the general practice context, a nurse may obtain the consent by explaining to the patient what is about to occur and allowing the patient to consider the information before verbally agreeing or refusing. Where the procedure is invasive, this type of exchange is commonly followed by the completion of a written consent form.

Consent to invasive procedures may be required to be obtained in **writing** and witnessed. In this case it is the legal obligation of the health professional carrying out the procedure (usually the medical practitioner) to ensure that a valid consent is obtained. That is, the medical practitioner may obtain the consent or may delegate the activity to another health professional, such as the nurse. The written consent form that has been signed by the patient and witnessed is a significant piece of evidence. The written consent is most important when non-routine treatments or procedures that have risks and complications attached to them are to be carried out. The benefit of having the consent in writing lies in the fact that it provides documentary evidence of the consent. Thus, a written consent makes proof of consent easier to establish. However, the existence of a written consent is not to be equated with a process of obtaining consent. If the process is defective, the consent will be held to be invalid or non-existent. Therefore, even when a patient has signed the consent form, they are not precluded from initiating an action in assault, battery or negligence if they were insufficiently informed, did not understand the content or did not have the risks explained. The need for a written consent and its superiority over implied or oral consent is questionable.

Elements of a valid consent

Where a patient initiates an action in trespass to the person, the defence of the practice nurse is that the nurse obtained a legally valid consent prior to initiating the assessment, treatment or procedure on the patient. It is therefore important to have an understanding of the following elements of a legally valid consent.

The consent is voluntarily given

The patient must give their consent to undergo an assessment, procedure or treatment freely and voluntarily. That is, there must be no coercion, duress, fraud or misrepresentation by the nurse. In a general practice setting, nurses must be mindful not to give an impression to the patients that if they do not undergo a particular treatment or procedure there will be negative or unpleasant consequences flowing directly from their refusal of treatment.

The consent must cover the procedure

The consent by a patient to a procedure is specific and does not extend to the carrying out of a different procedure. Should the nurse consider that it is necessary to undertake a different procedure, the consent requirement will only be waived where the circumstances indicate that the action was necessary to save the patient's life. That it was convenient to carry out the procedure at the time will not suffice (*Candutti v ACT Health an Community Care* [2003] ACTSC; *Murry v McMurchy* [1949] 2 DLR 442).

Example 5.4

In the case of *Candutti*, the plaintiff was admitted to the hospital for a laparoscopic tubal ligation. She had consented to a laparotomy only if an emergency arose during her surgery. Due to some difficulty inflating the plaintiff's abdomen the surgeon proceeded to undertake the tubal ligation by way of a laparotomy. The plaintiff sued the medical practitioner in trespass to the person on the grounds that she had not consented to this more invasive procedure. The court, in upholding the plaintiff's claim, determined that the particular circumstances did not amount to an emergency and, therefore, the procedure was performed without the patient's consent.

The consent must be informed

A nurse will be in breach of duty of care in failing to warn a patient or client of the 'material and significant' risks associate with a treatment or procedure, or in failing to comply with any legislative provisions which address a failure to warn of risks. There is a distinction, however, between a lack of consent prior to undertaking a procedure or treatment, which lays the basis for an action in trespass to the person, and obtaining a consent where the patient has not been adequately warned of risks which may give rise to a negligence action.

For the purpose of defending an action in trespass to the person it will be sufficient if the nurse has informed the patient in 'broad terms' of the nature of the procedure prior to obtaining the patient's consent.

The person giving the consent has legal capacity

The starting presumption should be that all adults of sound mind have the capacity to give a legally valid consent or to refuse to consent to treatment. A patient with legal capacity may make their own decisions about their health care and any attempt by a health professional to override those decisions, or impose their own decisions, may be liable in an action of trespass to the person.

Reflections

What is the policy in your practice on consent for procedures?

Legal capacity

The legal capacity to consent is defined in various ways by legislation which cover specific situations (for example, mental health Acts, various guardianship and administration Acts protecting the rights of intellectually disabled citizens, blood alcohol legislation and statutory protection for children at risk where the state may act on their behalf) and common law decisions. The law makes provision for substitute decision makers where the patient, by reason of age, mental or intellectual incapacity, may not be considered competent to provide a valid consent.

It is beyond the scope of this chapter to address all aspects of legal capacity in the context of health care decision making. The following will therefore only briefly address particular issues which are of relevance to nurses working within a general practice environment. Practice nurses must familiarise themselves with the relevant legislation and case law in their respective jurisdiction.

Children

As a general principle, a parent or legal guardian is capable of consenting to the medical and dental treatment of his or her child. Where a parent or guardian is not able to be located and a child requires emergency treatment, it may be given without a consent being obtained or, if it is only minor first aid which is required, the child may be legally capable of giving a valid consent (for example, the application of a Band-Aid on a foot). The authority of the parent is not absolute and may be overridden by the courts or through legislative provisions where it is considered that the parent is not making decisions which are in the 'best interests' of the child.

Once persons have reached the age of 18 years, they are considered at law to have full legal capacity. Prior to this age, particular legislation specifies the age at which the consent will be taken as valid at law.

In New South Wales, the *Children and Young Persons (Care and Protection) Act 1998* defines a child (for purposes other than employment) as a person under the age of 16 years and a young person as being 16 to 18 years. Similarly in the ACT, the *Children and Young People Act 1999* defines a child as being under the age of 12 years and a young person as being aged 12 to 18 years. In Tasmania the *Children, Young Persons and their Families Act 1997* defines a young person as either 16 or 17 years of age. It is clear from the decision in *K v Minister for Youth and Community Services* [1982] 1 NSWLR 311, litigated against the background of the *Minors (Property and Contract) Act 1970* (NSW), that such legislation which stipulates the age for consenting to medical treatment operates to protect medical and dental practitioners treating persons who might, but for the Act, be considered minors.

The case law is silent as to the specific age at which a minor becomes legally competent to give a valid consent to medical treatment. The case of *Gillick v West Norfolk and Wisbech Area Health Authority* [1986] AC 112; [1985] 3 All ER 402, however, gave rise to the term 'Gillick competency' to indicate that a person, under the age of majority was legally capable of giving a valid consent. In this case Lord Scarman stated:[6]

> *I would hold that as a matter of law the parental right to determine whether or not their minor child below the age of 16 will have medical treatment terminates if and when the child achieves a sufficient understanding and intelligence to enable him or her to understand fully what is proposed. It will be a question of fact whether a child seeking advice has sufficient understanding of what is involved to give a consent valid in law. Until the child achieves the capacity to consent, the parental right to make the decision continues save only in exceptional circumstances.*

The competence of a minor to consent was thereby determined on the basis of the child's capacity to understand the nature of the treatment. The High Court of Australia approved the Gillick test as to the capacity of a minor to consent to treatment in the case of *Secretary, Department of Health and Community Services v JWB and SMB (Marion's case)* [1992] 175 CLR 218 at 238.

It is therefore important for a nurse, practising in a jurisdiction in which there is no legislation which expressly identifies an age at which a person may consent to medical treatment, to undertake a clear assessment of the capacity of the minor to understand the nature of the treatment or procedure that is being proposed. That is, the nurse decides whether the child is 'Gillick competent' for the purpose of making this health care decision and documents that process and decision. It is of particular note that the capacity of a child to refuse to consent to treatment may be overridden by the courts depending on the nature of the medical intervention. Where a minor refuses a procedure or treatment, the nature of the particular treatment, the age of the minor, and their level of understanding and intelligence, will all be factors which determine what the nurse is to do. This must be determined on a case-by-case basis. Where a minor who is assessed as Gillick competent refuses to undergo a treatment, the nurse must exercise great care before making a decision whether or not to proceed. This is so, even if the parent of the minor has given consent.

Example 5.5

In a situation where a minor who is assessed as Gillick competent is refusing to be immunised even though a parent has consented to the immunisation, the nurse should not proceed. Instead, the nurse should encourage both the parent and minor to resolve the issue and not proceed until this has occurred.

Unconscious patients

Where a patient is in an unconscious state or, due to his or her condition is incapable of consenting, the common law will deem a consent for the treatment given provided that it was necessary, reasonable and given in good faith.

Impaired intellectual capacity

The issue of capacity to consent is of great concern when a patient with an intellectual impairment (including an intellectual disability, acquired brain injury or dementia) presents to a health care facility or institution for assessment, care or treatment. As a general principle nurses should work from the basis of assessing whether this particular patient has capacity to make this particular decision at this particular time. It is not correct to assume that because a person has an intellectual deficit or disability that they have no capacity to make decisions in relation to their own health care. It is incumbent on the nurse to assess (and document[7]): the following prior to the patient making a decision:

- the patient's level of understanding of the nature and effect of their decision;
- whether the patient is making their decision voluntarily and of their own free will;
- the patient's ability to communicate their decision to others; and
- whether the patient can consent on their own behalf or requires a substitute decision maker.

All Australian jurisdictions have legislation which addresses the issue of consent to medical and dental treatment, or health and lifestyle decisions, for persons with an intellectual disability. This legislation, however, only applies when the person is not capable of understanding what it is that they are being asked to consider in terms of treatment or care. It may well be that for some decisions, for example, having a wound dressed or undergoing an ultrasound procedure, the person with the intellectual disability or reduced intellectual capacity will be able to give a valid consent. However, in relation to more medically technical and complicated procedures, a substitute decision maker may be required.

Refusal to consent

All adults of sound mind have the legal capacity not only to consent to the treatment recommended by the health professional but also to withhold their consent. The patient has the legal right, even after giving a valid consent, to withdraw it and refuse to continue to undergo the procedure. Provided the patient is competent, the patient has the right to refuse all treatment regardless of whether the refusal will result in permanent physical injury or death.

Documentation

The documentation of patient and client information is fundamental to the provision of health care services and facilitates optimal patient outcomes through accurate, objective and contemporaneous observations and notations of the ongoing care and treatment of the patient or client. The medical records also enable the transfer of patient information, not only between health professionals within the same discipline, but also across disciplines. That is, the practice nurse should use the patient's medical records as a means of communicating patient information with other nurses involved in the patients care and, in addition, as a vehicle for communication with the treating doctor and allied health professionals involved in the patient's care. Patient records may also be used for research purposes, as educational tools and as documentary evidence in legal proceedings. For these reasons, it is important that nurses in general practice understand the significance of the content of any patient's medical records and the potential for the use of such documents.

Recording patient information

Though there is no Commonwealth or state legislation specifically mandating the reporting of patient care by nurses, there are clear professional obligations to maintain a record of the nursing care and treatment the patient receives. Although the Medicare Benefits Schedule is aimed at general practitioners when it states that medical records should be adequate and contemporaneous, it could be assumed that the same reasoning would apply to practice nurses.

The following are elements to consider in relation to the documentation of patient care and treatment.

- In a paper-based system of record keeping, the patient must be identified on every page by full name and identification number.

- Information should be clear, concise and accurate.

- Documentation of patient information should be contemporaneous with the event, and recorded in chronological order. The nurse in general practice should aim to document patient and client information as soon as practicable after the consultation or procedure. This not only ensures accuracy of the information but is also more likely to be interpreted by the courts as the true and correct version of an event.

- Where the nurse fails to make an entry in a patient's records in circumstances in which it would be considered accepted practice to do so, the court may infer no nursing care was given.

- All entries must be prefaced with the precise date and time of the entry.

- All entries in the records must be readily identifiable and referable to the writer of the report. For nurses working in a general practices which have a paper-based system, this requirement is satisfied by a signature at the end of the entry.

In computer-based medical records, the writer should be identified by via a PIN, access code or password. All health professionals and health workers who make entries into a patient's or client's medical records must be allocated an individual access PIN or password. It is through this mechanism that the writer of the entry is identified.

- The medical records must be legible and, if paper based, must be written in ink.

- The nurse should only write what the nurse has witnessed or accessed. Nurses should not write for any other health professionals unless the information is attributed to that individual. For example, the entry would read, 'Dr Smith informed me that the patient vomited blood'. This entry clearly conveys that the nurse did not personally witness the patient vomit blood.

- Words such as 'appears' and 'apparently' should be avoided. The nurse should provide objective and factual information as to the condition and presentation of the patient. For example, the nurse should avoid writing the patient 'appeared sad' and instead write the 'patient was sitting in the chair crying and said, 'I will never get over this".

- Never write or chart information for a patient in advance or remove and rewrite an entry at a later date.

- If the nurse makes an error while writing up the nursing entry into the patient's records, a line should be put through the error, the nurse must write 'written in error', and then sign and date the entry.

Always read the patient's medical records in their entirety if the patient is not familiar to you. Do not rely on a verbal handover or the last entry in the medical records.

Reflections

What is your practice policy on computer passwords for all staff and does it comply with the above advice?

Conclusion

The foregoing provides a brief overview of the legal principles applicable to medical negligence litigation, consent and documentation as relevant to nurses working within a general practice environment. Clearly, the scope of the chapter is such to permit only a general discussion of what are complex areas of health law. It is hoped that you will use this information as a basis upon which to pursue this area of your professional practice in greater depth.

Key messages

Practice nurses will not be found liable in negligence if their practice is consistent with that which is widely accepted in Australia by peer professional opinion as competent professional practice.

Documentation of their nursing care is essential part of nursing practice.

Any nurse who is a contractor should have indemnity insurance.

The process of obtaining consent has several elements to be fulfilled.

Notes

1. *Sidaway v Board of Governors of the Bethlem Royal Hospital* [1985] AC 871 at 893; *Gover v South Australia and Perriam* (1985) 39 SASR 543 per Cox J, adopted per Mason CJ, Brennan, Dawson, Toohey and McHugh JJ in *Rogers v Whitaker* (1992) 109 ALR 625 at 628.

2. Refer generally to Eburn, M, *Emergency Law*, Federation Press, Melbourne, 1999; Mendelson, D 2001, 'Quo lure? Defendants' liability to rescuers in the tort of negligence', *Tort Law Review*, vol. 9, no. 2, p. 130.

3. *Civil Law (Wrongs) Act 2002* (ACT) s. 5; *Civil Liability Act 2002* (NSW) ss. 56 and 57; *Personal Injuries (Liabilities and Damages) Act 2005* (NT) s. 8; *Law Reform Act 1995* (Qld) s. 16; *Civil Liability Act 2003* (Qld) s. 26; *Civil Liability Act 1936* (SA) s. 74; *Wrongs Act 1958* (Vic.) s. 31B; *Civil Liability Act 2002* (WA) Pt 1D.

4. *Civil Law (Wrongs) Act 2002* (ACT); *Wrongs Act 1958* (Vic.); *Civil Liability Act 2002* (WA); *Civil Liability Act 1936* (SA). Legislation applicable in these jurisdictions may be found on http://www.austlii.edu.au/.

5. *Civil Liability Act 2002* (Qld) s. 72; *Civil Liability Act 2002* (NSW) s. 69; *Civil Liability Act 2002* (Tas) s. 7(1); *Civil Liability Act 2002* (WA) s. 5AH; *Wrongs Act 1958* (Vic.) s. 14J (1); *Person Injuries (Liability and Damages) Act 2003* (NT) s. 13; *Civil Liability Act 1939* (SA) s. 75; *Civil Law (Wrongs) Act 2002* (ACT).

6. Ibid at 188–9 per Lord Scarman.

7. *Guardianship Act 1987* (NSW) s. 33(2); *Guardianship and Administration Act 2000* (Qld) Schedule 3; *Powers of Attorney Act 1998* (Qld) Schedule 3; *Guardianship and Administration Act 1995* (Tas) s. 36(2); *Guardianship and Administration Act 1986* (Vic) s. 36(2).

Useful resources

Australian Nursing and Midwifery Council
http://www.anmc.org.au

Royal Australian College of General Practitioners
Medico-legal Handbook for General Practice
http://www.racgp.org.au

Australian Commission on Quality and Safety in Healthcare
Open Disclosure
http://www.safetyandquality.gov.au

Australian Practice Nurses Association
http://www.apna.asn.au/

Royal College of Nursing Australia
http://www.rcna.org.au

References

1. Kennedy, I & Grubb, A 1994, *Medical Law: Text with Materials*, Butterworths, London.

2. Mendelson, D 2001, 'Quo lure? Defendants' liability to rescuers in the tort of negligence' *Tort Law Review*, vol. 9, no. 2, p. 130.

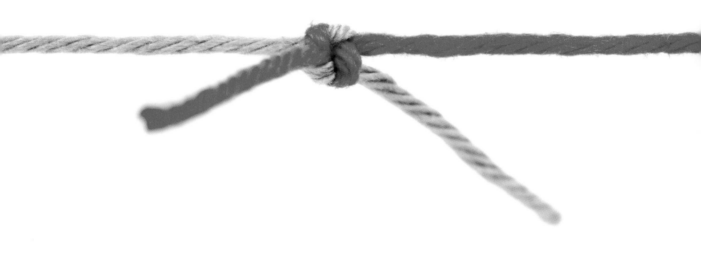

Part two

Fundamentals of practice nursing

Edited by **William Wong**

Chapter six

Triage in general practice

by Marie Gerdtz and Judy Evans

Overview

In general practice, people will make appointments to see the general practitioner or practice nurse for a wide range of conditions; some of these cases will be urgent, while many are not. Some will be unexpected emergencies while other visits will be planned. Being able to accommodate the needs of the entire practice population with limited resources is a constant challenge for all providers of health care.

The purpose of this chapter is to define the aims and discuss the process of triage and a conceptual framework for making triage decisions in general practice will be provided.

Objectives

At the completion of this chapter you should be able to:

- define the aims of triage systems;

- differentiate the concept of clinical urgency from severity of illness, clinical risk and case complexity;

- discuss the assessment approaches used for making safe triage decisions; and

- identify signs and symptoms of critical illness that may be evident at triage.

Introduction

Clinical justice (or urgency) ensures that all people who seek medical treatment receive a level of care that is both timely and commensurate with their current health status. A consistent approach to triage assessment and categorisation must therefore be based on objective clinical criteria (FitzGerald et al. 2010). Triage is the rapid systematic process that is used in health care services to determine a person's level of urgency at point-of-entry to the service (FitzGerald 2010). The aim of any triage system is to provide efficient delivery of health care and achieve equity of access to limited resources based on level of urgency and in many instances the triage role is performed by nurses.

Triage assessment involves: making observations of the patient's general appearance, collecting a brief history of the presenting complaint, identifying any chronic health problems or comorbid factors, and collecting physiological data related to airway patency, work of breathing, circulation and neurological status.

Clinical justice

Clinical justice is the central construct that is used to guide triage decision making. Urgency is defined as 'the speed of intervention that is required to achieve an optimal outcome' (FitzGerald 2000). It is dynamic and will change both over time and among patients with the same diagnosis (Whitby et al. 1997). For example a patient with asthma may present to general practice with moderate asthma and progress to severe asthma within minutes, thus level of urgency will change. Similarly, in a group of patients with asthma all may have different levels of urgency, based on their work of breathing at the time the triage assessment is conducted.

Factors that complicate the diagnosis of urgency include the severity of illness, the complexity of the case and the clinical risk of an adverse outcome (Department of Health and Ageing 2007). However, severity, complexity and clinical risk are discrete constructs that may or may not be relevant to urgency categorisation.

The context of general practice

In a general practice the first point of contact for patients is usually with reception staff who may have limited skills in assessing the level of urgency of the patient's health status. Without appropriate training, triage guidelines and ongoing support from the clinical team, decisions made at reception in the allocation of appointments and therefore access to care, may present a real risk of harm to patients.

Triage in the general practice setting can occur when the patient is in attendance or presents at the clinic, or, more commonly, triage occurs through a telephone consultation when the patient rings the practice for an appointment (refer to Table 6.1 opposite for differentiating factors). Telephone triage has emerged as a core component in the management of patient appointment needs and access to care. The telephone is an effective communication tool, but does not offer to the triage process visual clues and the observation of non-verbal communications.

After initial screening by reception staff, nurses are seen as a crucial step in further assessment which may culminate in the allocation of an appointment or the giving of advice.

Telephone triage requires an assessment of the patient's current health status using interview techniques—asking questions and interpreting the responses—without the advantage of visual cues. It involves a process of critical thinking, applying clinical knowledge and utilising skills of assessment. After this process the patient is allocated a level of priority for access to care. Depending on the established priority, the patient could

Table 6.1 Differences between face-to-face triage and telephone triage

Face-to-face triage	Telephone triage
Assessment can be rapid	Without the aid of sight and touch, gathering information can take a little longer and relies on other senses to create a mental image of the patient and the problem
Conventional triage criteria using appearance and physical assessment can be used to determine urgency	Assessment relies almost entirely on responses to questions
The patient has arrived in the place where care can be provided so that caregiver–patient relationship is established	Rapport, trust and roles need to be established with verbal communication
The triage decision usually only relates to the time frame in which the patient needs to be seen. After this the patient just waits	The triage decisions involve not only a time frame in which care must be administered but where the most appropriate care should be sought and what to do in the interim
The patient in a medical facility is in a safe location and is reassured that they are being dealt with	The patient has made contact because of anxiety about a medical problem, may feel isolated or vulnerable. Hence triage decision may be driven more by anxiety level of patient or carer
The patient can be monitored easily and reclassified	Opportunity for reassessment is more difficult and may not yield additional information
Relies on good observation skills	Relies on good listening skills

Source: Collaborative Health Education and Research Centre 2001

be offered an appointment at the general practice, advised to attend to an emergency department or to call an ambulance.

All triage requires a structure and process and this also applies to telephone triage. The main steps in undertaking telephone triage are:

1. Introduce yourself and open communication channels
2. Perform the assessment via interview
3. Make the triage decision
4. Offer advice according to protocol or established guidelines for care
5. Incorporate follow-up plans when concluding the call
6. Document the call.

Nurses performing telephone triage has been demonstrated to be safe. St George, Cullen and Branney (2003) identified that while symptomatic patients cannot often judge the urgency of their symptoms, they can be 'safely and happily triaged to the right place at the right time' by telephone contact with a nurse supported by algorithm-based decision tools.

High levels of clinical risk for disease may or may not be pertinent to a person's level of urgency on presentation to general practice. This will depend on their reason for seeking care and the signs and symptoms they exhibit at the initial point of contact with the service.

It is sometimes possible for a person to present to triage with severe disease and a high level of case complexity, but have a low level of clinical urgency. Thus, a patient with severe lung pathology presenting to a general practice may be able to wait for assessment and treatment providing vital signs are stable and pain and discomfort are minimal.

Reflections

What is the triage policy of your practice, and how does it delineate roles and responsibilities of practice staff in relation to clinical urgency?

Triage scales

A triage scale stratifies clinical urgency across a number of categories and defines each in terms of the patient's level of urgency at the time of the triage assessment (Beveridge 1998; FitzGerald 2000; Gerdtz & Bucknall 2001a;

Zimmerman 2001). Most triage scales also define time-to-treatment objectives for each category.

International research shows that the use of a five-tier triage scale is an efficient and valid method for categorising people seeking medical care in hospital emergency departments (FitzGerald et al. 2010; Beveridge 1998; Mackway-Jones 1997; Wuerz et al. 2001). While five-tier triage scales are utilised worldwide, there is substantial variability in the recommended response times across the five categories (for example, see Australasian College for Emergency Medicine 2006; Mackway-Jones 1997; Beveridge 1998).

The Australasian Triage Scale

The **Australasian Triage Scale** (ATS) is a five-tier urgency scale that is used for categorising clinical urgency in Australian emergency department populations (Australasian College for Emergency Medicine 2006). The ATS could provide a useful framework for nurses to communicate with GPs or clinicians in general practice for classifying urgency and communicating the outcomes of the triage assessment to medical staff, ambulance personnel and hospital emergency department. It should be noted, however, that the response categories for the ATS are both arbitrary, and have been devised for the emergency department context. For this reason the discussion that follows will describe the response times for the ATS in general terms, rather than provide absolute time frames. The adaptation to the scale response times is informed by FitzGerald et al. (2010).

Table 6.2 overleaf shows the five categories of the ATS, the required response and a brief description of each category.

ATS category 1

Category 1 is the most urgent level of the ATS. In this category the patient's clinical condition will be such that there is an immediate threat to life, or there is an imminent risk of physiological deterioration. These patients will require immediate resuscitation due a breach of airway patency, respiratory function or circulation.

ATS 1 is characterised by one or more of the following criteria:

- The patient is experiencing full or partial airway obstruction (for example, laryngeal oedema or limited capacity to guard the airway due to impaired level of consciousness).

Table 6.2 The Australasian Triage Scale with adaptations from specific to general response times for general practice use

ATS category	Description of category	Response
1	Immediately life threatening	Immediate simultaneous assessment and treatment
2	Imminently life threatening or Important time critical treatment or Very severe pain	Assessment and treatment within minutes
3	Potentially life threatening or Situational urgency or Humane practice mandates relief of severe discomfort or distress within 30 minutes	Assessment and treatment within an hour
4	Potentially serious or Situational urgency or Significant complexity or severity	Assessment and treatment within hours
5	Less urgent	Assessment and treatment within days

Source: Australasian College for Emergency Medicine 2006, with adaptations to response times (FitzGerald et al. 2009)

- The patient has impaired ventilation and/or oxygenation (for example, signs of impending respiratory arrest or failure).
- The patient is experiencing circulatory collapse (for example, low or no cardiac output as evidenced by bradycardia and hypotension).

Clinical descriptors for ATS 1 include, but are not limited to:

- cardiac arrest
- respiratory arrest
- hypoventilation (respiratory rate <10 breaths per minute)
- extreme respiratory distress
- hypotension systolic (BP <80 mmHg in an adult)

- severely shocked infant/child
- Glasgow Coma Score <9
- severe behavioural disorder with immediate threat of dangerous violence.

Accordingly, immediate simultaneous medical assessment and intervention (resuscitation) is required. ATS 1 patients must be transferred to a hospital emergency department by ambulance while resuscitation is in progress.

> ### Reflections
>
> *What resources and training does your practice have to manage patients in ATS category 1?*

ATS category 2

Category 2 is the next most urgent level of the ATS. In this category the patient's clinical condition will fulfil one of three criteria:

- There is an imminent threat to life because the condition is critical or is deteriorating so quickly that organ failure and death will ensue if treatment is not initiated within minutes.
- Important time critical treatment is required to significantly affect the clinical outcome.
- The patient is experiencing very severe pain.

Clinical descriptors for ATS 2 include, but are not limited to:

- severe risk to airway (as evidenced by severe stridor or drooling with respiratory distress)
- impaired circulation (as evidenced by poor peripheral perfusion, mottled skin, heart rate less than 50 beats per minute or greater than 150 beats per minute in an adult)
- hypotension
- severe blood loss
- cardiac chest pain
- hypoglycaemia (BSL <2 mmol/L)
- Glasgow Coma Score <13
- fever with lethargy
- acute acid or alkali splash to eye that requires irrigation
- major fracture or amputation

- psychiatric or behavioural problem with immediate threat of harm to self or others.

ATS 2 patients require medical assessment within minutes of arrival to a general practice and will be transferred to a hospital emergency department by ambulance while treatment is in progress.

ATS category 3

Patients in category 3 of the ATS will fulfil one of three clinical criteria:

- The condition is likely to pose a potential threat to life if medical assessment and treatment are not initiated within an hour of triage.
- There is a potential for an adverse outcome if treatment is not commenced within an hour (for example, the commencement of thrombolytic therapy).
- There is a severe discomfort or pain.

Clinical descriptors for ATS 3 include, but are not limited to:

- severe hypertension
- chest pain likely to be non-cardiac
- moderate blood loss from any cause
- moderate shortness of breath (O_2 saturation 90–95% on room air)
- hyperglycaemia (blood sugar level >16mmol/L)
- seizure (now alert)
- fever in impaired immune states (for example, patients taking steroids or receiving chemotherapy)
- head injury with brief loss of consciousness
- persistent vomiting/dehydration
- limb injury with deformity
- crush injury
- severe laceration
- psychiatric or behavioural problem with risk for self-harm
- acute thought disorder.

Patients arriving at a health service who meet ATS criteria for category 3 require medical assessment within an hour of arrival. In general practice, some of these patients will be transferred to a hospital emergency department by ambulance while others will not. For example, a person who presents to general practice in pain due to an acute ankle injury may, after receiving analgesia be safely managed at home. On the other hand, a person with acute right iliac fossa pain, fever and vomiting may be assessed by a general practitioner within an hour and then sent to a hospital emergency department with a provisional diagnosis of acute appendicitis.

ATS category 4

Patients in category 4 of the ATS will fulfil one of four clinical criteria:

- The condition is potentially serious and is likely to deteriorate if assessment and treatment do not occur within hours.
- The condition may lead to an adverse outcome if assessment and treatment are not commenced within hours.
- The presenting complaint involves significant complexity and is likely to require specialist consultation.
- Distress or discomfort requires relief within hours.

Clinical descriptors for ATS 4 include, but are not limited to:

- mild haemorrhage
- foreign body aspiration with no respiratory distress
- minor head injury with no loss of consciousness
- vomiting or diarrhoea without dehydration
- eye inflammation
- minor limb trauma (for example, ankle sprain, uncomplicated laceration)
- non-specific abdominal pain
- moderate pain with no high risk features.

ATS 4 patients will require medical assessment within hours of arrival at a general practice. Some of these patients may require hospitalisation and specialist inpatient management, while others will continue to be managed in general practice. The practice nurse, with additional education, may be able to manage those patients requiring treatment such as the application of plaster casts, assessment and suturing of simple lacerations and strapping of sprains.

Reflections

What skills do practice nurses in your practice have to enable them to manage patients in category 4?

ATS category 5

Category 5 of the ATS describes less urgent cases which include minor symptoms of an existing stable illness, minor symptoms in low-risk conditions and minor injuries. Patients presenting for scheduled reviews or requesting medical certificates are also classified under this category. ATS 5 patients may safely wait days for assessment and treatment in general practice. The majority of these patients will continue to be managed in general practice and will not require hospitalisation.

Clinical descriptors for ATS 5 include, but are not limited to:

- minimal pain/discomfort
- minor symptoms of an existing stable illness
- abrasions and lacerations that do not require suturing
- immunisation appointments
- scheduled visits to review wounds or complex dressings.

> **Reflections**
>
> *How does the triage policy of your practice allocate appointments for patients in this category?*

Triage decision making

Triage decision making is a rapid and systematic process that should take no more than five minutes (Australasian College for Emergency Medicine 2006; Gerdtz & Bucknall 2001a; Monash Institute of Health Services 2001).

Step 1 of the triage process requires the clinician to establish the reason the patient is seeking medical treatment and determine the level of urgency for that presentation. This is achieved by:

1. Observing general appearance
2. Taking a brief focused history of the illness/injury
3. Collecting a limited amount of clinical data relevant to the presentation (for example, measuring heart rate, respiratory rate, temperature).

Step 2 of the triage process involves summarising the outcomes of the assessment performed in step 1 as the 'presenting/chief complaint' and allocating a triage code.

Step 3 of the triage process involves documenting the triage decision in the medical record including the date and time, the name of the person performing the assessment, the presenting complaint and the level of urgency.

A secondary triage function involves initiating interventions to expedite care (Gerdtz & Bucknall 2001b), for example, the administering oxygen, taking bloods for pathology or performing an ECG. Such decisions should always occur after the determination of the chief complaint and the assignment of a triage category. Any interventions initiated at triage must also be documented in the patient's medical record.

Because urgency is a dynamic state, reassessment of patients who continue to wait for medical assessment requires ongoing observation in the waiting area (Australasian College for Emergency Medicine 2006). Patients should be instructed to report to reception if their condition changes and requires a reassessment by the practice nurse. Reception staff have a role in surveillance of patients in the waiting room, but will require specific instructions of when to seek assistance from the practice nurse or general practitioner.

The triage assessment

Environmental considerations

Environmental safety is critical to effective triage. This means that prior to the commencement of the triage process the care provider must ensure that all safety hazards have been considered and it is reasonable to perform the triage role. Threats to maintaining a safe environment at triage include, among others, exposure to physical violence, exposure to blood and body fluids, electrical hazards, potential injuries to staff from lifts, trips or falls (Monash Institute of Health Services 2001; Australian Commonwealth Department of Health and Ageing 2002).

Consideration should be given before placing individuals in a waiting area as patients whose condition has the potential to deteriorate must be in an area where can be easily observed.

The area in which triage occurs should have basic resuscitation equipment including a bad-valve-mask device, artificial airways equipment, and access to oxygen and suction equipment if possible. Standard precautions must be adhered to when undertaking triage: gloves and protective eyewear must be used if there is any risk of exposure to blood or body fluids.

Protocols for accessing emergency services and police should also be available in the area where triage is performed. Staff must be familiar with practice protocols so that they may effectively activate an emergency response as required.

Finally, the triage environment must afford the patient and/or accompanying person a sufficient level of privacy. Maintenance of patient confidentiality and privacy at triage are sometimes challenged due to structural aspects of the waiting area. In such environments the practice nurse should have access to an assessment room where privacy can be assured.

Reflections

Consider the physical environment of the waiting area in your practice. What structures are in place to ensure all patients in the waiting areas are safe?

Assessment of general appearance

The rapid assessment of general appearance provides much information about the patient's physiological and psychological state.

- An important initial question to consider at triage is *'Does this person look sick?'*
- At triage *'looking sick'* is a term that is used to describe the general appearance of an individual with impending critical illness.

Some of the signs of critical illness that may be observed at triage include pallor, cyanosis, diaphoresis and lethargy. This may also be reflected in abnormal vital signs, especially the respiratory rate (tachypnea and dyspnoea) and heart rate (tachycardia or bradycardia). Because infants, children and older people (65 years or older) have different physiological responses to illness, *'looking sick'* may be the first sign that critical illness is imminent.

Other aspects of the patient's general appearance that should be observed at triage include:

- **level of mobility**   Examples of questions when observing mobility include:
  - Does the patient's mobility appear acutely restricted in some way?
  - Is there evidence that pain or discomfort is acutely affecting the patient's mobility?
- **speech**   Examples of observations related to the patient's speech include:
  - Is speech clear or slurred?
  - Is there any evidence of acute dysphasia or aphasia?

- **skin colour**   Examples of observations related to the patient's skin include:
  - Is the skin normal, pale, cyanosed or ashen?
  - Is there any evidence of cyanosis around the ears, nose or lips?
- **behaviour**   Examples of observations related to the patient's behaviour include:
  - Does the patient make eye contact with you when speaking?
  - Are there signs of acute agitation?
  - Is the patient distressed, anxious or withdrawn?

Physiological measures and observations

The measurement of physiological parameters at triage follows a brief and focused process. Assessment is structured in such a way to ensure that life threatening conditions are identified and treated in order of priority—the primary survey.

The primary survey

A useful approach to the initial triage assessment is the primary survey. The primary survey is used in pre-hospital settings and in hospital emergency departments to assess and treat breaches for:

A.   Airway

B.   Breathing

C.   Circulation

D.   Disability.

Airway

Assessment of airway involves determining its patency and intervening to open and maintain the airway if it is obstructed. Where a neck injury is suspected (for example, the patient has fallen from a height of more than two metres, has sustained a hyperflexion or hyperextension injury to the head or neck, or has had an injury to the head with a subsequent loss of consciousness) care must be taken when opening the airway to avoid hyperextension of the neck.

Breathing

Assessment of breathing involves determining the work of breathing. This includes assessment of the respiratory rate, depth and use of accessory muscles for ventilation. Where there is a breach in respiratory function, interventions to support breathing include restoration of ventilation and oxygenation. This may include the commencement of assisted positive pressure ventilation and the delivery of oxygen.

Circulation

Assessment of circulation involves determining haemodynamic function and detecting haemorrhage. This is achieved by measuring heart rate, rhythm, depth and blood pressure. Where there are breaches to circulatory function, interventions must be initiated to support circulation. Interventions to support circulation include commencement of cardiopulmonary resuscitation, and advanced life support and initiation of intravenous fluids to support or restore circulation.

Disability

Assessment of disability involves determining neurological functioning. This includes determining the Glasgow Coma Score (GCS). A GCS of less than 9 represents an actual threat to airway patency and requires immediate medical intervention to open and secure the airway. A GCS of 9–12 represents an imminent threat to airway patency and requires a rapid medical response. A GCS of 12–14 will require ongoing monitoring and intervention if the level of consciousness deteriorates.

Another useful way of assessing neurological function at triage is the use of the AVPU pneumonic:

- **A**lert: the patient is alert (but may not be orientated)
- **V**erbalises/Voice: the patient responds to voice (in any way, for example, attempts to talk, opens eyes)
- **P**ain: the patient responds to a pain stimulus (nail bed pressure)
- **U**nresponsive: the patient is unconscious and unable to give a motor, verbal or eye opening response.

Assessment of disability also includes measurement of blood glucose where consciousness is impaired (as evidence by a GCS of greater than 13) or in situation where the person is a known diabetic. Another important aspect of the disability component of the primary survey is the assessment of pain. Because pain assessment is measured according to self-report this will be discussed in the following section.

Obtaining a focused history

In order to determine the chief complaint, a brief history of the acute illness or injury is required.

The first question to ask the person presenting is '*What has made you come in to see the doctor today?*' The answer to this question forms the basis of the triage interview, which should seek to establish history of pre-existing illnesses, allergies, level and intensity of pain, blood loss, mechanism and nature of injury, seizure activity and ingestion of drugs and/or alcohol.

Assessment of pre-existing conditions, illness or recent injuries

Any coexisting chronic or acute illnesses or recent injuries should be determined. Noting the patient's current prescribed medications provides a useful starting point for interviewing a patient about their current health condition.

In the context of abdominal pain and/or trauma, information about menstruation (date of last normal menstrual period, and gravida and parity if pregnant) should be determined as pregnancy may alter normal haemodynamic parameters. Acute physiological deterioration in ectopic pregnancy is not uncommon. Thus women who present to general practice with abdominal pain and/or bleeding in early pregnancy should be carefully observed and monitored. Assessment of these women by a general practitioner is recommended within one hour of arrival.

Allergy status

The existence of any allergies to medicines, foods or other allergens should be established as well as the nature of any previous allergic reactions (for example, anaphylaxis).

Pain

Pain assessment at triage should be appropriately assessed and documented. The PQRST pneumonic is a rapid approach to pain assessment that describes the:

- **P**osition of the pain
- **Q**uality of the pain
- **R**adiation of the pain to other body regions
- **S**everity of the pain
- **T**iming or duration of the pain.

The severity of the pain should be measured using a valid pain tool. Pain scales that are suitable for use at triage include the Numerical Rating Scale (NRS) and the Visual Analog Scale (VAS) (Mackway-Jones 1997).

- According to the ATS descriptors, very severe pain is consistent with an ATS of 2; moderately severe pain an ATS of 3; moderate pain an ATS of 4; and minimal pain an ATS of 5.

- For children, the Wong-Baker FACES rating scale can be utilised (Wong et al. 2001).
- For individuals with cognitive impairment, the Abbey pain scale is a useful pain assessment tool (Abbey et al. 2004).

The development of a valid and reliable approach to the assessment of pain in general practice requires individual practices to adopt pain measurement tools that are appropriate to the populations they serve. Because pain is culturally mediated, practices need to carefully consider the validity and the utility of available pain assessment tools for their practice.

Mechanism of injury

Understanding the mechanism of injury, if that is the chief complaint, provides a useful foundation for identifying actual and potential patient problems. A brief explanation of what has occurred and how long ago it happened must be sought at triage. This information may be obtained directly from the patient and/or accompanying person.

While it is uncommon for those involved in major trauma to seek care in general practice, it is worth noting the trauma criteria in your jurisdiction in order to identify those individuals who need to be triaged to a hospital emergency department. The Victorian Department of Human Services Trauma Criteria (1999) serve as an example of this and can be utilised to guide decision making. These criteria are listed below:

- Ejection from a vehicle
- Motorcyclist impact more than 30 kph
- Falls from a height >5 m
- High-speed motor vehicle accident
- Vehicle rollover
- Fatality in same vehicle
- Explosion
- Pedestrian impact greater than 30 kph
- Prolonged extrication from a vehicle of duration greater than 30 minutes.

Loss of consciousness

Although less likely when presenting to general practice, loss of consciousness can happen while attending the practice. If a patient has sustained a head strike or experienced a sudden loss of consciousness (LOC) then the time of the injury, the duration of the LOC as well as the mechanism of injuries and behaviour immediately prior to the event need to be determined.

Seizure activity

Information needs to be sought about any past history of seizure or epilepsy. In the event of an acute LOC, information from witnesses regarding any seizure-like activity should be noted. In children with a history of fever, parents should be directly asked if there has been any alteration in level of alertness or jerking or seizure-like body movements.

Ingestion of drugs and/or alcohol

At triage it is useful to obtain information in respect to prescribed drug use. As previously mentioned this information can help to inform the establishment of a chief complaint. Where acute alterations in level of consciousness are noted, information about alcohol intake and illicit drug use may be sought.

Figure 6.1 overleaf shows a schematic representation of triage decision making, which links the primary (establishing chief complaint and determining urgency) and secondary functions (expediting care).

Example 6.1

Jason, aged 17, presents to general practice requesting an appointment. He is looking pale and miserable so the receptionist requests he be triaged by the practice nurse. At triage he complains of a dull pain in the umbilical region and the right iliac fossa and states he has had diarrhoea and vomiting for a few hours.

He is in obvious pain which he rates as 6/10. He says that he hasn't felt much like eating or drinking in the last 24 hours. His skin is warm and moist. His respiratory rate is 24 breaths per minute, heart rate is 110 beats per minute and temperature 38.9°C.

1 Based on the information available in this case, the practice nurse requests that a medical assessment must occur within one hour. Do you think the practice nurse has made the correct decision?

2 Discuss how the clinical characteristics of this case can be linked to the triage decision.

3 What interventions might be initiated to expedite the management of Jason?

Answers

1 The practice nurse has made the correct decision.

2 > The patient is talking, so the airway is intact.

Continued >

Triage process   ***Example questions for triage***

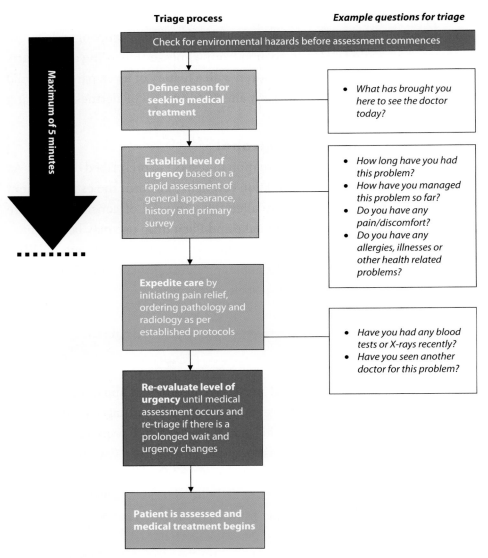

Figure 6.1 The triage process

> There is no sign of respiratory distress.

> Circulation is intact, though the heart rate is mildly elevated. This is possibly due to an elevated temperature and the pain he is experiencing.

> The patient has a moderate level of pain and requires analgesia to relieve his distress.

> The patient is febrile. This is likely to be due to an intra-abdominal cause (possibly an acute appendicitis).

3 >   The practice nurse should obtain a mid-stream urinalysis and perform a full ward test of urine.

>   The practice nurse should instruct Jason not to eat or drink anything until he is seen by the general practitioner.

Example 6.2

Bradley, aged 14 months, is brought to general practice by his mother for a second time in a week. He received a diagnosis of bronchiolitis at his last appointment two days ago. Today Bradley's mum made an appointment as she was concerned that he was not eating and has started refusing fluids in the last two hours. The receptionist calls you to triage and assess Bradley.

On examination you note that:

>   He is an alert and clinging to his mother.

>   He is quiet but makes eye contact when you speak to him.

>   There is no sign of accessory muscle use and no retraction with respiration.

>   His respiratory rate is 28 breaths per minute.

>   He has had four wet nappies today.

1   Based on the information available in this case the practice nurse should request that a medical assessment occur within what time frame?

A   Immediately

B   Within minutes

C   Within one hour

D   Within hours

E   Within days

2   Provide a rationale for your decision.

Answers

1   **D** Within hours

2 >   The airway is clear.

Continued >

> There is no sign of respiratory distress.

> His urine output is normal, though he is starting to refuse fluids now.

> The child is alert and makes eye contact when spoken to.

> Given his mother's concerns and that this is his second presentation in two days, an appointment to see the GP within hours is appropriate. Bradley's mother should be instructed to continue to offer small regular amounts of fluids.

Example 6.3

Marcus, aged 24, has a sore throat and fever. He tried to make an appointment with his regular general practitioner. He was not able to do that, however, so his mother, who regularly attends your practice, has brought him in as she is worried that he looks very sick. Marcus has previously had tonsillitis, and his mum suggests that is what the problem is today. Prior to attending the practice Marcus took some cold and flu tablets.

> When he arrives at reception he is unable to talk and is drooling and distressed.

> His mother says he has had difficulty in swallowing.

> His respiratory rate is 26 breaths per minute.

> His skin is hot and moist.

> His temperature is 39.4°C.

> He looks tired, but is alert and cooperative.

> The practice nurse assesses Marcus and asks that he make an appointment to be seen by the GP within hours.

1 Do you agree with this decision?

2 If not, why?

Answers

1 This decision is not appropriate for Marcus.

2 Marcus is at risk of airway obstruction as evidenced by his inability to speak clearly and drooling. He is also showing signs of respiratory distress. Accordingly Marcus should be assessed by a GP within minutes.

The preceding case histories (Examples 6.1–6.3, pp. 143–6) highlight that effective triage requires involvement from both the clinical and the non-clinical team. The development of policy and protocols to support a triage process need to consider that the first point of contact for care is often with reception staff. The triage process will falter if reception staff do not recognise that the patient requires further evaluation and assessment by the practice nurse or general practitioner. Reception staff need to be adequately trained to recognise potential medical emergencies and the signs and symptoms of a patient's deteriorating health.

Practice nurses can be instrumental in ensuring that the triage process is systematic and recognises the role of non-clinical (reception) staff. The development of triage policies that are inclusive of the whole practice team will contribute to mitigate the risk of harm, error or omission and are therefore an essential component of high quality care in general practice.

Conclusion

Triage is a critical component in ensuring that patients have access to care that is commensurate with their level of medical urgency. Effective triage requires good clinical decision making within a framework of applying the clinical skills of observation and assessment.

Key messages

Triage is a clinical process for determining the level of urgency at the point of entry to general practice.

Urgency is the estimated time to medical intervention in order to achieve an optimal outcome.

Triage assessment is a rapid process that should take no more than five minutes and is informed by an assessment of general appearance, history of presenting complaint, comorbid factors and basic physiological measures (vital signs).

The process for triage decision making should be structured around the primary survey.

Continued >

While no standard triage tools are mandatory across the general practice sector, the Australasian Triage Scale and the clinical guidelines for its implementation (Australasian College for Emergency Medicine 2006) may be adapted for use in general practice.

Triage requires teamwork.

Useful resources

Australian Commonwealth Department of Health and Ageing 2007, *Emergency Triage Education Kit*, Australian Commonwealth Department of Health and Ageing, Canberra, viewed 6 January 2010, <http://www.health.gov.au/>.

Australian and New Zealand College of Anaesthetists and Faculty of Pain Management 2005, section 9.9 'Acute pain in emergency departments' in *Acute pain management: scientific evidence*, 2nd edn, Australian and New Zealand College of Anaesthetists, Melbourne, pp. 178–82.

Grossman, V 2002, Telephone Triage Course, viewed 28 December 2009, <http://www.RnCeus.com/>.

Mackway-Jones, K 1997, in *Emergency Triage*, ed. K Mackway-Jones, BMJ Publishing Group, London.

Monash Institute of Health Services 2001, *Consistency of Triage in Victoria's Emergency Departments: Guidelines for Triage Education and Practice*, Victorian Department of Human Services, ISBN 0 732630061.

References

1. Abbey, J, Piller, J, De Bellis, A, Esterman, A, Parker, D, Giles, L & Lowcay, B 2004, 'The Abbey pain scale: a 1-minute numerical indicator for people with end-stage dementia', *International Journal of Palliative Nursing*, vol. 10, no. 1, pp. 6–13.

2. Australasian College for Emergency Medicine 2000, *Guidelines on the Implementation of the Australasian Triage Scale: G24* (cited 20 August 2009), viewed 23 December 2009, <http://www.acem.org.au/media/policies_and_guidelines/G24_Implementation__ATS.pdf>.

3. Australasian College for Emergency Medicine 2006, *Policy on the Australasian Triage Scale: P06* (cited 22 August 2009), viewed 6 January 2010, <http://www.acem.org.au/media/policies_and_guidelines/P06_Aust_Triage_Scale_-_Nov_2000.pdf>.

4. Australian Commonwealth Department of Health and Ageing 2002, *Triage Education Resource Book*, ISBN 0 642 82120.

5. Australian Commonwealth Department of Health and Ageing 2007, *Emergency Triage Education Kit*, Australian Commonwealth Department of Health and Ageing, Canberra (cited 20 August 2009), viewed 5 January 2010, <http://www.health.gov.au/>.

6. Beveridge, R 1998, 'CAEP issues. The Canadian Triage and Acuity Scale: a new and critical element in health care reform', Canadian Association of Emergency Physicians, *Canadian Journal of Emergency Medicine*, vol. 16, no. 3, pp. 507–11.

7. Collaborative Health Education and Research Centre 2001, 'Telephone Nurses Triage After Hours Service Delivery', Western Victoria Division of General Practice, Horsham.

8. FitzGerald, G 2000, 'Triage', in P Cameron, G Jelinek, AM Kelly, L Murray, J Heyworth (eds), *Textbook of Adult Emergency Medicine*, Churchill-Livingstone, Sydney, pp. 584–8.

9. FitzGerald, G, Jelinek, G, Scott, D & Gerdtz, MF 2010, 'Emergency Department Triage Revisited', *Emergency Medicine Journal*, In press, Accepted for publication 28 July 2009.

10. Gerdtz, MF & Bucknall, TK 2001a, 'Triage nurses' clinical decision making: an observational study of urgency assessment', *Journal of Advanced Nursing*, vol. 35, no. 4, pp. 550–61.

11. Gerdtz, MF & Bucknall, TK 2001b, 'Australian triage nurses' decision making and scope of practice', *Australian Journal of Advanced Nursing*, vol. 18, no. 1, pp. 24–33.

12. Mackway-Jones, K 1997, in *Emergency Triage*, ed. K Mackway-Jones, BMJ Publishing Group, London.

13. Monash Institute of Health Services 2001, *Consistency of Triage in Victoria's Emergency Departments Guidelines for Triage Education and Practice*, Victorian Department of Human Services, ISBN 0 732630061.

14. St George, I, Cullen, M & Branney, M 2003, 'Primary care "demand management" pilot in New Zealand: telephone triage using system-based algorithms', *Asia Pacific Family Medicine*, vol. 2, no. 3, pp. 153–6.

15. Victorian Department of Human Services 1999, *Review of Trauma and Emergency Services: Final Report*, Department of Human Services, Melbourne.

16. Whitby, S, Ieraci, S, Johnson, D & Mohsin, M 1997, *Analysis of the Process of Triage: The Use and Outcome of the National Triage Scale*, report to Commonwealth Department of Health and Family Services, Liverpool Health Service, Liverpool, NSW.

17. Wong, D, Hockenberry-Eaton, M, Wilson, D, Winkelstein, M & Schwartz, P 2001, *Wong's Essentials of Paediatric Nursing*, 6th edn, p. 1301, Mosby, St Louis.

18. Wuerz, R, Travers, D, Gilboy, N, Eitel, DR, Rosenau, A & Yazhari, R 2001, 'Implementation and refinement of the Emergency Severity Index', *Academic Emergency Medicine*, vol. 8, no. 2, pp. 170–6.

19. Zimmermann, P 2001, 'The case for a universal, valid, reliable 5-tier triage acuity scale for US emergency departments', *Journal of Emergency Nursing*, vol. 27, no. 3, pp. 246–54.

Chapter seven

Medication management

by Elizabeth Manias

Overview

The general practice setting is an environment where the medications of patients are managed through a complex set of interactions involving several health professionals. In collaboration with the general practitioner, practice nurses play an important role in medication management, including patient assessment and monitoring for safe and appropriate medication taking, communication with other health professionals and patient education.

Objectives

At the completion of this chapter you should be able to:

- understand medication management in the general practice context from the perspective of practice nurses;

- understand the concept of *medication adherence* and measures used to assess improve medication-taking behaviours;

- define the term *medication reconciliation* and describe practical strategies that can be used to facilitate medication reconciliation;

- describe the management of immediate hypersensitivity reactions; and

- outline the mechanisms of action of the most commonly used groups of medications.

Introduction

The use of medications by patients is widespread and practice nurses are working in an environment where opportunities exist for assessment and adherence to medication as well as patient education regarding the use of medication. Identification of those patients at risk of medication mishaps within the practice population and implementing strategies to enable safer use of medicines by patients, especially those patients taking multiple medicines, will be discussed in this chapter. As nurses play an increasing role in administration of vaccine medicines symptoms, the management of immediate hypersensitivity reactions is also examined. Furthermore, medication groups that are commonly used and prescribed in general practice are considered. These medication groups comprise: insulin, oral hypoglycaemic agents, analgesics, angiotensin converting enzyme inhibitors, angiotensin II antagonists, beta blockers, thiazide diuretics, anticholinergics, beta-2 agonists and inhaled corticosteroids.

National Medicines Policy

Australia launched a National Medicines Policy in 1999, which comprises the most comprehensive medicinal policy worldwide (Department of Health and Ageing 2009). The main purpose of the policy is to ensure the availability of essential affordable medications of acceptable quality, safety and efficacy. It should be noted that the policy is extremely relevant for medication management at the primary care level where the majority of health care delivery and prescribing occurs (National Prescribing Service 2006). The policy has four central objectives:

1. timely access to the medicines that Australians need, at a cost individuals and the community can afford
2. medicines meeting appropriate standards of quality, safety and efficacy
3. quality use of medicines
4. maintenance of a responsible and viable medicines (pharmaceutical) industry.

Quality use of medicines

The third objective of the policy, the quality use of medicines (QUM), has been expanded to support the development of innovative educational and professional strategies. The QUM initiative has a participatory focus, involving all stakeholders who influence medication use, including general practitioners, practice nurses, medical specialists, hospital-based nurses, pharmacists, allied health professionals, patients and family members.

There are three major principles associated with QUM (Department of Health and Ageing 2009):

1. selecting management options wisely: drug versus non-drug treatment. This principle involves the health professional deciding whether a medicine should be prescribed, recommended or self-administered, or if a non-medicinal alternative should be considered.

2. choosing suitable medicines if a medicine is considered necessary. This principle involves selecting the most appropriate medicine to be taken, after examining factors, such as the clinical condition being treated, past history of the patient, the potential risks and benefits of treatment, dosage, length of treatment and cost.

3. using medicines safely and effectively. This principle acknowledges the importance of increasing safe use and minimising misuse, overuse and underuse. Effective use means that the medicines must achieve the goals of therapy by delivering beneficial changes through positive health outcomes.

Home medicines review

Accredited pharmacists have an important role in assuring QUM by undertaking home medicines reviews (Medicare Australia 2009; Holland et al. 2008; Sorensen et al. 2004). After receiving details of patients who are targeted to have a home medicines review, accredited pharmacists visit patients at home, assess their medication regimen, and provide general practitioners with a comprehensive report. Practice nurses can liaise with general practitioners in determining which patients would benefit from having a home medicines review. For instance, warfarin requires close monitoring and practice nurses could alert accredited pharmacists to the benefit of such patients receiving a home medicines review. In collaboration with an accredited pharmacist, doctors and practice nurses can remind patients of the importance of taking warfarin exactly as prescribed, and be involved in point-of-care testing of the international normalised ratio. Examples of situations where a home medicines review would help include the following:

* patients currently taking five or more medications regularly
* patients taking more than 12 doses of medication per day
* patients with significant, recent changes to their medication regimen, including recent discharge from hospital
* patients taking medications that require therapeutic monitoring, such as warfarin or amiodarone
* patients having symptoms that imply an adverse drug reaction has occurred
* patients having difficulty in managing their own medicines because of literacy or language difficulties
* patients visiting several doctors, including general practitioners and medical specialists.

Reflections

How does your practice identify those patients who meet the above criteria for a home medicines review?

Medication adherence

Medication adherence relates to the extent to which patients conform to agreed behaviours in regard to timing, dosage and frequency of medication taking. It assumes that patients make informed decisions regarding the taking of their medications. Unfortunately, approximately 50% of patients with chronic diseases do not take their medications in the therapeutic doses recommended by their prescribers, which can result in health problems (World Health Organisation 2003).

Extensive work has been carried out on determining barriers to medication adherence. These barriers can be classified in four major areas:

1. patient factors (for example, age, gender, number of chronic diseases)
2. health professional factors (for example, prescribing by a specialist rather than a general practitioner)
3. medication regimen (for example, duration of treatment, type of medication)
4. system or environmental factors (for example, number of doctor visits, distance from doctors' practice or pharmacy, difficulty in accessing medications).

Research conducted on barriers to medication adherence has often thrown up conflicting results, depending on the methods used to analyse information and the context in which studies were undertaken (Lakey, Gray & Borson 2009; Vik, Maxwell & Hogan 2004). Nevertheless, important barriers identified in past work include the following:

*   physical vulnerability of the patient (elderly, suffering from a psychiatric illness)
*   social vulnerability of the patient (language barriers, lack of social supports)
*   complex medication regimen (use of frequent dosing when a once-daily regimen is available, increasing the number of medications used)
*   poor communication between the health professional and patient.

Practice nurses can play a valuable role in determining potential barriers to medication adherence relating to individual patients and identifying strategies through which modifiable barriers can be addressed.

Reflections

How you think some of these barriers can be overcome in your patient population?

Assessment of medication adherence

Medication adherence is very difficult to assess and assessment measures range from complex, expensive methods, such as electronic medication monitoring devices and biological markers, to more simple methods, such as self-reporting (Osterberg & Blaschke 2005). Despite problems relating to possibly overstating adherence, self-reporting measures are probably the most applicable to a general practice environment.

When asked about their medication taking, patients may not tell the truth because of their desire to please the doctor or practice nurse. They may also feel more compelled to speak to practice nurses because they are perceived to be less busy than doctors (Horrocks, Anderson & Salisbury 2002). Practice nurses can assist in assessing adherence to medications in collaboration with the general practitioner. To assist in encouraging honest and reliable answers, it is important that questions are asked in a non-judgmental way. One effective means by which patients can be encouraged to interact openly about their medication-taking behaviour is for practice nurses to begin the conversation with a statement such as, '*People forget to take their medications for many reasons*'. Figure 7.1 overleaf provides suggestions that practice nurses can use to assess medication adherence.

Practical strategies for improving medication adherence

Practice nurses have a key role in improving medication adherence. They can provide assistance and advice about administering medications. As part of the health care team approach and support from the Medicare Benefits Schedule (MBS), practice nurses are able to provide up to five sessions for complex chronic disease management where they can conduct ongoing monitoring of treatment and patient education. Often the practice nurse can identify problems with medication taking and, in conjunction with the general practitioner, identify and discuss with the patient ways which encourage medication adherence. Past work has demonstrated that an individualised education program combined

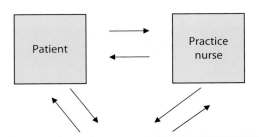

Practice nurses can assess medication adherence of patients by seeking information on the following issues. Patients should be given the opportunity to clarify issues without feeling judged.

- Ask the patient in a non-judgmental way how often they miss a dose. For instance, *'It must be hard to remember to take all your medicines regularly. How often do you miss taking them?'*
- Ask the patient if they know the reasons why they are not taking their medication regularly.
- Ask the patient if they experience side effects as a result of their medication.
- Ask the patient if they know the reasons why they have been prescribed their medication.
- Ask the patient if they know the benefits of taking their medication. Check the patient's medical history when they come in for their appointment to determine if they are taking their medication regularly.

Figure 7.1 Assessing patient adherence to medication

with a home medication review is associated with improvements in outcomes in medication adherence (Delamater 2006; Haynes et al. 2008; Holland et al. 2008; Lin & Ciechanowski 2008). Practice nurses should:

- identify the complex barriers associated with medication adherence confronting patients;
- assess patient adherence in a non-judgmental way; and
- work collaboratively with the general practitioner in implementing strategies to improve adherence.

Table 7.1 opposite contains details about the types of interventions that can be implemented by practice nurses to improve medication adherence.

Medication safety through reconciliation

In Australian health care institutions, breakdowns in communication are known to contribute to almost one-fifth of all adverse events that result in serious harm (Australian Institute of Health and Welfare & Australian Commission on Safety and Quality in Health Care 2007). Medication errors account for over one-quarter of all adverse events in health care institutions

Table 7.1 Interventions that practice nurses can use to improve medication adherence

Type of intervention	Intervention
Examinations	Review the patient's medical history to assess reasons for possible non-adherence.
	Assess patient's ability to take their medications correctly.
	Examine patient for ongoing monitoring of medication therapy, and conduct assessment for medication benefits and unwanted effects.
Activities	Encourage and facilitate the use of self-monitoring equipment for assessing various parameters, such as blood pressure and blood glucose.
	Encourage patients to use medication calendars or diaries to remind them to take their medications.
	Encourage the use of other aids, such as dosette boxes.
	Encourage the use of dose administration aids.
Collaborations	Suggest the use of once-daily regimens wherever possible to the general practitioner.
	Help patients to understand their health-related goals in collaboration with the general practitioner.
	Assist care givers in providing a supportive role to patients in their management of medications.
	Educate patients and clarify any misconceptions relating to their medications and medical conditions.
	Suggest a home medicines review to the general practitioner.
	Discuss monitoring using pathology results with the general practitioner, such as lipids, blood counts and HbA1c.

Reflections

Do you use the 'older persons' health assessment, care plans or team care arrangements as an opportunity to identify issues of medication adherence?

(Runciman et al. 2003) and over half of patients who move across transition points have medication errors associated with their treatment regimens (Rozich & Resar 2001). Transition points refer to the movement of patients through admission, transfer and discharge from hospital or other health care environments (Australian Pharmaceutical Advisory Council 2005).

Practical strategies in addressing medication reconciliation

Discharge summaries need to be written for general practitioners as patients move across environments, for example, from hospital to home. Practice nurses can play a facilitating role in comparing the list of home medications listed in medical histories with medications ordered upon discharge from hospital, and reconcile any differences. Reconciliation is the process of comparing the patient's current medications with those ordered for the patient while under the care of the organisation.

Each time a patient moves from one environment to another, the general practitioner would need to be notified as the patient's primary care provider. New medication orders sent to general practitioners and plans of care need to be examined against the most recent list of medications taken at home. This activity of reconciling medications highlights the value of ensuring accurate and current information is available on the medications taken by patients at home. It is particularly important when transferring a patient's care to another provider, from one practice to another, to ensure that any information provided is accurate, including a list of current medications and any known allergies. A variety of tools is available to support nurses in determining to what extent the patient's medications are reconciled between hospital and home. Queensland Health's Safe Medication Practice Unit (SMPU), established in January 2005, has developed a form for medication reconciliation on admission, which can easily be adopted for use in general practice environments.

Reflections

What is your practice policy regarding nurses updating medication records for both existing and new patients?

Management of allergies involving anaphylactic reactions

True allergic reactions of an anaphylactic or immediate hypersensitivity nature involve the release of immunoglobulin E. These types of reactions occur within

15 minutes from the time of exposure to the antigen, which could be penicillin, antibiotics or vaccinations. Practice nurses who are involved in administering a vaccination or another medication with a high allergic potential should ask the patient to wait in the practice setting for approximately 10–15 minutes in case of a severe allergic reaction.

Symptoms experienced by patients where a hypersensitivity reaction has occurred include the following:

- urticaria
- angioedema
- vomiting
- diarrhoea
- bronchospasm
- anaphylaxis (as demonstrated by hypotension and respiratory distress).

Practice nurses need to make sure that emergency equipment is readily available in the practice setting in case a hypersensitivity reaction occurs; the quicker the reaction develops, the more severe the symptoms are likely to be.

The management of hypersensitivity reactions involves the following measures:

- administering intramuscular adrenaline through the anterior lateral thigh
- removing the cause (if possible)
- administering oxygen by face mask at 10–15 litres/minute
- establishing intravenous access to the patient
- maintaining an adequate airway—if an obstructed airway is present, prompt intubation of the airway will be required
- administering intravenous sodium chloride 0.9% if the patient is hypotensive.

As well as managing the immediate symptoms, it is important that regular monitoring occurs during the hypersensitivity reaction. Monitoring should include the following:

- taking pulse rate
- checking blood pressure
- an electrocardiogram
- pulse oximetry.

After the hypersensitivity reaction, practice nurses should ensure that parents and informal carers of affected children are adequately informed about the nature of the reaction, the causative agent and the best course of treatment. They should also make sure that careful documentation is made in the patient's history about the symptoms encountered, the causative agent and the treatment received. Practice nurses should also check to see whether their health care setting has an up-to-date and accurate anaphylaxis protocol (Rossi 2009). Throughout Australia, Departments of Health have set up facilities to enable the reporting of adverse events following vaccinations. For instance, the Department of Health in Victoria established the Surveillance of Adverse Events Following Vaccination In the Community (SAEFVIC) in 2009. Practice nurses can be involved in the reporting of significant adverse events following immunisation through these facilities.

Reflections

Does your practice have a policy for the management of anaphylaxis? Are all staff trained in CPR?

Common groups of medications

Practice nurses cannot possibly be expected to keep up with changes that occur to individual medications. New medications regularly appear while older agents lose favour among general practitioners. However, if practice nurses know that a medication belongs to a particular group, the major characteristics of the medication can be derived (Bullock et al. 2007). Various groups of medications are commonly used and prescribed in general practice, and it is important that practice nurses have a good understanding of how these groups work and their implications for patient health care.

Insulins

Insulins are comprised of:

- ultra-short acting analogues;
- short acting agents;
- long acting agents; and
- long acting analogues.

These insulin agents are used to replenish the body's ability to metabolise glucose by:

- facilitating cellular glucose uptake;
- inhibiting glycogen breakdown; and
- promoting fat storage.

Insulins are administered in type 1 diabetes cases but they are also used to treat type 2 diabetes where diet, exercise and oral hypoglycaemics are not adequately controlling blood glucose metabolism (Rossi 2009).

Effective management of diabetes is clearly related to good control of glucose blood levels, avoiding hypoglycaemia, hyperglycaemia and long-term complications by ensuring glycosylated haemoglobin (HbA1c) levels are maintained within appropriate limits. Practice nurses can play a proactive role in informing patients about the effects of excessive exercise, illness and stress on blood glucose levels. At these times, blood glucose levels may radically change and subsequently insulin dosage will need to be altered. While there is often variability in blood glucose levels between patients, fasting blood glucose levels of less than 6 mmol/L and random blood glucose levels of 4–8 mmol/L are generally considered acceptable. Patients should be reminded to have HbA1c levels taken every 3–6 months as an indication of long-term glucose control and recommended levels are 7% or less. In ensuring stabilisation of blood glucose concentration, it is important that patients are informed about medications that may change glucose blood levels. While beta-2 agonists, thiazide diuretics and glucocorticoids can increase glucose levels, alcohol, angiotensin converting enzyme (ACE) inhibitors and high dose non-steroidal anti-inflammatory agents can decrease glucose levels (Writing Group, Endocrinology 2004).

Oral hypoglycaemics

Oral hypoglycaemics are divided into three groups:

1. sulphonylureas, such as glibenclamide, gliclazide, glimepiride and glipizide
2. thiazolidinediones, such as pioglitazone and rosiglitazone
3. other agents, such as acarbose, metformin and repaglinide.

Sulphonylureas act by increasing pancreatic insulin secretion and may also decrease insulin resistance. Thiazolidinediones work by regulating genes involved in lipid and glucose metabolism. Acarbose delays intestinal absorption of carbohydrates by inhibiting enzymes in the small intestine, and metformin reduces glucose production and increases peripheral utilisation of glucose (Bullock et al. 2007; Rossi 2009).

Metformin is considered the medication of choice for people with type 2 diabetes who do not maintain effective glycaemic control despite managing their diet and exercise. A sulphonylurea agent can be used as an alternative if metformin is contraindicated or not tolerated. Metformin is contraindicated in severe renal impairment or in hepatic failure due to the increased risk of lactic acidosis. Common adverse effects of hypoglycaemic agents include gastrointestinal symptoms, such as nausea, vomiting and abdominal pain (Writing Group, Endocrinology 2004).

In regards to clinical management, patients need to be reminded that oral hypoglycaemics are not like insulin in that they enhance the effect of insulin. An insulin formulation might be needed to supplement oral agents in times of infection, stress or surgery. It is therefore important that patients regularly monitor their blood glucose levels. The risk of hypoglycaemia from these agents can be reduced if patients have regular meals containing carbohydrates, drinking plenty of fluids and reducing consumption of alcohol.

Reflections

What is your level of knowledge of the management of diabetes?

Analgesics

Analgesics include:

- paracetamol;
- non-steroidal anti-inflammatory drugs (NSAIDs);
- opioids; and
- adjuvant agents, such as antidepressants, clonidine, antiepileptics and corticosteroids.

Adjuvant agents are those traditionally used to treat conditions other than pain, such as depression and epilepsy; however, certain properties of these agents make them amenable to reducing pain, in particular neuropathic pain.

Analgesics need to be individualised according to the severity of pain, the type of pain experienced and the characteristics of the patient (Bullock et al. 2007; Rossi 2009).

Opioid analgesics activate opioid receptors in the central and peripheral nervous systems to produce pain relief. Activation of these receptors can also lead to adverse effects, such as cough suppression, respiratory depression, constipation, sedation, nausea and vomiting. Examples of potent opioids include fentanyl, hydromorphone, morphine and oxycodone, which are often used to ease moderate to severe pain. Weaker opioids include dextropropoxyphene and codeine, which are used for mild to moderate pain (Writing Group, Analgesic 2007).

Non-opioid analgesics are comprised of aspirin, paracetamol and NSAIDs. Aspirin prevents synthesis of prostaglandins by inhibiting cyclo-oxygenase (COX) COX-1 and COX-2. Aside from its analgesic properties, aspirin has anti-inflammatory, antipyretic and anti-platelet actions. Aspirin is used to treat mild to moderate pain individually and in combination with codeine. Due to its anti-platelet effect, aspirin should generally be stopped about seven days prior to elective surgery and dental procedures (Rossi 2009).

Paracetamol produces its analgesic effect by blocking prostaglandin synthesis centrally and peripherally. It has good antipyretic properties and negligible anti-inflammatory activity. Paracetamol is used to treat mild to moderate pain individually and in combination with dextropropoxyphene or codeine. Several preparations of paracetamol are available, often with different strengths. For example, infant drops can contain 50 mg/mL or 100 mg/mL and liquid formulations can contain 24 mg/mL or 48 mg/mL. Therefore, it is very important to avoid using more than one preparation at the same time and to carefully check the strength and required dose before administration. While paracetamol is available in supermarkets and over the counter in pharmacies, it can produce hepatotoxicity if excessive dosage is administered (Bullock et al. 2007).

NSAIDs have analgesic, antipyretic and anti-inflammatory actions. They produce their effects by preventing the synthesis of prostaglandins through inhibition of COX. Non-selective NSAIDs inhibit both COX-1 and COX-2 while selective NSAIDs inhibit COX-2. While inhibition of COX-1 is associated with decreased gastric protection, both non-selective and selective NSAIDs can produce gastrointestinal adverse effects, such as ulceration, bleeding, dyspepsia and nausea. There is little difference in therapeutic efficacy between various NSAIDs. Most notably, NSAIDs can worsen existing cardiovascular disease and produce gastrointestinal effects.

To reduce the possibility of adverse effects of NSAIDs, it is important to:

- use the lowest effective dose for the shortest possible time;
- administer paracetamol concurrently to facilitate lower doses of NSAIDs;
- avoid using NSAIDs in people receiving low dose aspirin for cardio-protection or who have a high risk of cardiovascular problems (as demonstrated by a cardiovascular risk calculator); and
- administer proton pump inhibitors (for example, omeprazole) or misoprostol in patients who are at high risk of adverse gastrointestinal effects (Rossi 2009).

The World Health Organisation (World Health Organisation 2007) analgesic ladder for cancer pain is flexible and simple enough to be used for acute and chronic pain of a non-cancerous nature (Writing Group, Analgesic 2007). Treatment is provided at the most appropriate point, depending on the severity of the pain, and adjusted accordingly. There are three major categories according to the WHO ladder:

1. mild pain
2. moderate pain
3. severe pain.

For mild pain, regular paracetamol or NSAIDs are recommended. For moderate pain, tramadol, codeine, low dose oxycodone or dextropropoxyphene with a non-opioid are recommended. For severe pain, potent opioids with non-opioid agents are used.

In determining appropriate routes of administration, usually the oral route is the best choice wherever possible. Orally administered medications are, in most situations, just as effective as those that are given parenterally. On the other hand, controlled release preparations are helpful for chronic pain, such as in osteoarthritis. Controlled release preparations have a slow onset of effect, which means that rapid and safe titration is impossible. Transdermal patches containing opioids are suitable for chronic, stable forms of pain but not for acute pain because of the difficulty in titrating doses. In general, regular administration of analgesics is preferable to the use of *pro re nata* (PRN or 'as required') administration to ensure adequate, therapeutic levels of analgesia are provided (Bullock et al. 2007; Writing Group, Analgesic 2007).

Antihypertensives

Commencement of antihypertensive treatment for high blood pressure involves following recommendations of the National Heart Foundation of Australia (2008). With patients who have conditions that could be adversely affected by high blood pressure (for example, chronic kidney disease or type 2 diabetes), treatment is appropriate when blood pressure ranges between 120/80 and 140/90 mmHg or higher. For other patients, antihypertensives may be considered when diastolic blood pressure is greater than 90 mmHg or systolic blood pressure is greater than 140 mmHg. Antihypertensive agents currently used in Australia include:

- angiotensin converting enzyme (ACE) inhibitors;
- sartans;
- calcium channel blockers;
- beta blockers; and
- thiazide diuretics (Rossi 2009).

ACE inhibitors, such as elanapril, fosinopril and perindopril, are considered first-line treatment for hypertension, especially in patients who have diabetic nephropathy, heart failure or left ventricular dysfunction. These medications block the conversion of angiotensin I to angiotensin II and also inhibit the breakdown of bradykinin. They subsequently reduce vasoconstriction, sodium retention and aldosterone release. Adverse effects commonly associated with ACE inhibitors include: hypotension, cough, hyperkalaemia and renal impairment. Practice nurses need to check that potassium-sparing diuretics and potassium supplements are stopped to prevent an increased risk of hyperkalaemia and that the administration of NSAIDs are ceased to prevent renal impairment and hypovolaemia. Renal function and electrolyte levels should be checked before commencing therapy and reviewed after a few weeks. To assist with medication adherence, patients should be recommended to take once daily therapy, such as enalapril or fosinopril rather than captopril, which is taken two to three times daily (Writing Group, Cardiovascular 2008).

Sartans are also known as angiotensin II antagonists and include candesartan and irbesartan. They competitively block binding of angiotensin II to type I angiotensin AT1 receptors. As a result, they produce similar effects to ACE inhibitors by decreasing vasoconstriction, sodium reabsorption and aldosterone release. Sartans may be used as an alternative first-line treatment, especially for patients who cannot tolerant ACE inhibitors. Unlike ACE inhibitors, the sartans do not inhibit breakdown of bradykinin. The sartans, therefore, are less likely to produce cough and angioedema associated with ACE inhibitors (Rossi 2009).

Together with ACE inhibitors and sartans, calcium channel blockers of the dihydropyridine group (for example, amlodipine, lercanidipine and nifedipine) are considered appropriate first-line agents for the treatment of hypertension. These agents work by acting on vascular smooth muscle to reduce inward current of calcium into cells. Common adverse effects include headache, flushing, palpitations and peripheral oedema (Bullock et al. 2007; Rossi 2009).

Beta blockers, which include atenolol, metoprolol and propranolol, are not considered first-line agents for uncomplicated hypertension. They produce their antihypertensive effects by competitively blocking beta receptors in the peripheral vasculature. Unfortunately, beta blockers also inhibit beta receptors in the bronchi, pancreas, uterus, kidney, brain and liver. Their tendency to increase blood glucose levels, and to worsen symptoms of asthma and chronic obstructive pulmonary disease, bradycardia and second- or third-degree heart block compared with other antihypertensives, means that they are not regarded favourably in many situations. Beta blockers are, however, recommended for hypertension following myocardial infarction and in the presence of angina as they can improve cardiovascular outcomes in these conditions (Rossi 2009).

Thiazide diuretics are considered first-line agents for patients older than 65 years. Due to their link with diabetes, they are no longer recommended as first-line agents for younger people. These agents inhibit the reabsorption of sodium and chloride in the proximal segment of the distal convoluted tubule and produce an increase in potassium excretion. Examples of thiazide diuretics include hydrochlorothiazide and chlorthalidone. With thiazide medications, if two doses are required, the first dose should be taken in the morning and the second dose taken before 6 pm. The practice nurse should examine potassium levels to ensure that these are greater than 3.5 mmol/L. Potassium supplements or potassium-sparing diuretics, such as amiloride, should be considered where potassium levels are below 3.5 mmol/L (Bullock et al. 2007; Rossi 2009).

Reflections

Are you aware of the common side effects of medications to reduce hypertension? Apart from these medications, are you aware of non-pharmacological recommendations for lowering blood pressure?

Dyslipidaemic agents

Dyslipidaemic agents are more commonly known as statins. Statins competitively inhibit 3-hydroxy-3-methylglutaryl coenzyme A (HMG-CoA) reductase, which is an enzyme required for cholesterol synthesis. Their actions have the effect of:

- increasing cholesterol uptake in the liver from the blood;
- reducing concentrations of total cholesterol;
- reducing low density lipoprotein and triglyceride levels; and
- increasing high density lipoprotein levels.

These agents are used to treat hypercholesterolaemia and hyperlipidaemia and are used as a preventative measure for individuals who are at high risk of developing coronary heart disease. Examples of statins include: atorvastatin, fluvastatin, pravastatin, rosuvastatin and simvastatin. Their ability to treat hyperlipidaemia varies between agents; hence, atorvastatin, rosuvastatin and simvastatin are more potent than fluvastatin and pravastatin (Rossi 2009).

Statins are one of the most commonly prescribed medications according to statistics from the Pharmaceutical Benefits Scheme (Pharmaceutical Policy and Analysis Branch 2008) yet they can produce major problems if not used appropriately, therefore practice nurses have an important educative role to play in their use.

Common adverse effects include:

- myalgia;
- nausea;
- vomiting;
- dizziness; and
- elevated transaminase levels.

Less common adverse effects include:

- myopathy;
- rhabdomyolysis;
- renal failure;
- liver failure; and
- pancreatitis.

As some adverse effects are dose related, such as myopathy and liver failure, it is important to commence statins at low doses and to gradually increase the dosage, depending on lipid levels. Dose increments should occur in four-week intervals to facilitate maximum benefit from a particular dose. With the exception of pravastatin and rosuvastatin, statins are largely metabolised by the cytochrome P-450 enzyme system. Therefore, medications that inhibit these enzymes (for example, cyclosporine or rifampicin) can increase the serum concentration of statins, leading to an enhanced risk of myopathy and rhabdomyolysis. In minimising the risks associated with enzyme inhibition, practice nurses can monitor whether statins are administered at the lowest possible dose and monitor the patient for adverse effects. They can also recommend that creatine kinase and transaminase levels are taken at baseline administration, which can then be repeated during treatment. If patients experience severe infection, trauma, metabolic illness or are required to have surgery, it is appropriate to withhold statin treatment and carefully monitor creatine kinase and transaminase levels during this time. It is possible that these stressful situations increase the risk of myopathy, rhabdomyolysis and renal failure (Bullock et al. 2007; National Heart Foundation of Australia & the Cardiac Society of Australia and New Zealand 2005; Nelson et al. 2007; Writing Group, Cardiovascular 2008).

Reflections

What information should you give patients who are taking statins?

Medications used for chronic obstructive pulmonary disease

Chronic obstructive pulmonary disease (COPD) comprises chronic bronchitis and emphysema. Management of COPD involves preventing further disease progression and treating exacerbations. A stepwise approach is used in preventing disease progression, which involves:

- using anticholinergics and short-acting beta agonists for mild conditions; and

- the addition of long-acting beta agonists and inhaled corticosteroids for severe conditions (Rossi 2009).

Anticholinergics are the bronchodilators of choice for the treatment of COPD. Currently in Australia, two anticholinergic agents are used, and they work by inhibiting cholinergic (or muscarinic) receptors, leading to a relaxation of bronchomotor tone:

1. ipratropium is a short-acting agent
2. tiotropium is a long-acting agent (this is the first-line therapy because it only requires a once daily dose and for sustained improvement in lung function).

The most common adverse effect occurring with these agents is a mild, dry mouth, which tends to manifest in the first three to five weeks of therapy. Practice nurses should advise the patient to rinse their mouth after administration to reduce the possibility of a dry mouth (Rossi 2009; Writing Group, Respiratory 2005).

Beta-2 agonists stimulate beta-2 adrenoreceptors, which exist on the bronchial smooth muscles. Short-acting agents, such as salbutamol and terbutaline, need to be taken four times a day for sustained brochodilation. For this reason they are not used for maintenance therapy in COPD but rather as a rescue therapy to relieve severe breathlessness. Long-acting agents are used twice daily as maintenance treatment for those patients who remain asymptomatic. These agents are taken twice daily and include salmeterol and eformoterol. Practice nurses can identify poorly controlled patients by monitoring the frequency of use of rescue medication. Patients who require rescue medication more than twice a week should be referred to the general practitioner for reassessment (Rossi 2009).

Inhaled corticosteroids reduce the inflammatory response in airways and suppress bronchial hyperreactivity. They have been found to be useful at high doses in the management of moderate or severe COPD, but not in mild forms of the condition. Unfortunately, high doses of inhaled corticosteroids also increase the possibility of oropharyngeal candidiasis, dysphonia and adrenal impairment. To reduce the risk of adverse effects, practice nurses should advise patients to rinse their mouth and throat with water and to spit out after rinsing. The use of a spacer device also lessens the risk of candidiasis and dysphonia. There is little place for oral corticosteroids in COPD management as studies have only shown minimal improvement in lung function following their use (Abramson, Glasgow, & McDonald 2007; Rubins, Raci & Kunisaki 2009).

Exacerbations of COPD that show clinical signs of infection, such as increased volume and change in the colour of sputum or fever, benefit from treatment with antibiotic therapy. Since the introduction of widespread influenza immunisation for patients with COPD, viruses have become a less common cause of exacerbations. Exacerbations are more likely to be associated with bacterial causes, which can be treated with antibiotics. Recommended antibiotics include the penicillin agent, amoxycillin, or the tetracycline agent, doxycycline. An effective response is usually observed in five days; however, severe forms of COPD may require 10-day courses. Practice nurses need to inform patients about completing the full course of antibiotic therapy even if they start to feel better before this time (Wedzicha & Seemungal 2007).

Short-acting beta-2 agonists, such as inhaled salbutamol or terbulaline, in addition to maintenance medication, can be used at higher doses and frequencies to those used in stable COPD to manage exacerbation. It is important that patients are reminded not to cease their maintenance medications during this time. Often a spacer device can be used to deliver the required dose if patients with acute airways obstruction have difficulties in coordinating their breathing using a metered device (Writing Group, Respiratory 2005).

Up to two weeks of therapy with oral prednisolone has been shown to be effective in reducing the duration of exacerbations of COPD. Longer courses do not usually provide further benefit and in collaboration with the general practitioner, practice nurses can encourage patients to have a follow-up appointment to ensure they have not relapsed after two weeks. Longer courses of oral treatment can lead to adverse effects, such as hyperglycaemia or bone density loss (Wedzicha & Seemungal 2007).

Reflections

Do you have a system in the practice to identify and monitor patients with COPD to ensure optimal medication management?

Conclusion

Practice nurses interact with patients extensively in the general practice environment. They are therefore ideally positioned to play an important role in supporting patients in the management of their medications. Practice nurses need to consider a number of aspects in the safe and effective management of medications, including patient assessment and monitoring for safe and appropriate medication taking, reporting of symptoms, communication with health professionals and patient education.

Key messages

Practice nurses can play an important role in optimising a patient's health by assisting the patient in the management of their medications.

In collaboration with general practitioners, practice nurses are able to develop and implement treatment plans for managing medications effectively.

Practice nurses can support general practitioners in helping patients to adhere to their medication regimen.

Practice nurses should work within a 'quality use of medicines' framework in their everyday roles and responsibilities.

Useful resources

National Medicines Policy
> http://www.health.gov.au/internet/main/publishing.nsf/Content/
> National+Medicines+Policy-2

National Prescribing Service
> http://www.nps.org.au/

Quality use of medicines
> http://www.health.gov.au/internet/main/Publishing.nsf/Content/
> nmp-quality.htm

Australian Prescriber
> http://www.australianprescriber.com

Anaphylaxis Australia
> http://www.allergyfacts.org.au

'Quality prescribing indicators in Australian general practice—a manual for
> users', National Prescribing Service
> http://www.nps.org.au

References

1. Abramson, M, Glasgow, N & McDonald, C 2007, 'Managing chronic obstructive pulmonary disease', *Australian Prescriber*, vol. 30, no. 3, pp. 64–5, viewed 1 May 2009, <http://www.australianprescriber.com/>.

2. Australian Institute of Health and Welfare & Australian Commission on Safety and Quality in Health Care 2007, *Sentinel events in Australian public hospitals 2004–05*, Safety and Quality of Health Care Series, no. 2, AIHW, Canberra, viewed 2 May 2009, <http://www.aihw.gov.au/>.

3. Australian Pharmaceutical Advisory Council 2005, *Guiding principles to achieve continuity in medication management*, Commonwealth of Australia, Canberra, viewed 1 May 2009, <http://www.health.gov.au/>.

4. Bullock, S, Manias, E & Galbraith, A 2007, *Fundamentals of pharmacology*, 5th edn, Pearson Education Australia, Frenchs Forest, viewed 3 April 2009, <http://www.pearson.com.au/>.

5. Delamater, AM 2006, 'Improving patient adherence', *Clinical Diabetes*, vol. 24, no. 2, pp. 71–7, viewed 23 April 2009, <http://clinical.diabetesjournals.org/>.

6. Department of Health, Victoria, 2009, 'SAFEVIC, Surveillance of Adverse Events Following Vaccination in the Community', Department of Health, Melbourne, viewed 14 October 2009, <http://www.health.vic.gov.au/>.

7. Department of Health and Ageing 2009, *The National Medicines Policy document*, Department of Health and Ageing, Canberra, viewed 1 June 2009, <http://www.health.gov.au/>.

8. Haynes, RB, Ackloo, E, Sahota, N, McDonald, HP & Yao, X 2008, 'Interventions for enhancing medication adherence', *Cochrane Database of Systematic Reviews*, issue 2, art. no. CD000011, viewed 2 February 2009, <http://www.cochrane.org/>.

9. Holland, R, Desborough, J, Goodyer, L, Hall, S, Wright, D & Loke, YK 2008, 'Does pharmacist-led medication review help to reduce hospital admissions and deaths in older people? A systematic review and meta-analysis', *British Journal of Clinical Pharmacology*, vol. 65, no. 3, pp. 303–16, viewed 4 April 2009, <http://www.pubmedcentral.nih.gov/>.

10. Horrocks, S, Anderson, E & Salisbury, C 2002, 'Systematic review of whether nurse practitioners working in primary care can provide equivalent care to doctors', *British Medical Journal*, vol. 324, no. 7341, pp. 819–23, viewed 16 August 2009, <http://www.bmj.com/cgi/content/full/324/7341/819>.

11. Lakey, SL, Gray, SL & Borson, S 2009, 'Assessment of older adults' knowledge of and preferences for medication management tools and support systems', *The Annals of Pharmacotherapy*, vol. 43, no. 6, pp. 1011–19, viewed 1 May 2009, <http://www.theannals.com/>.

12. Lin, EHB & Ciechanowski, P 2008, 'Working with patients to enhance medication adherence', *Clinical Diabetes*, vol. 26, no. 1, pp. 17–19, viewed 3 June 2009, <http://clinical.diabetesjournals.org/>.

13. Medicare Australia 2009, *Home medicines review*, Australian Government, Canberra, viewed 10 June 2009, <http://www.medicareaustralia.gov.au/provider/pbs/fourth-agreement/hmr.jsp>.

14. National Heart Foundation of Australia 2008, 'Guide to management of hypertension 2008', viewed 1 June 2009, <http://www.heartfoundation.org.au/>.

15. National Heart Foundation of Australia & the Cardiac Society of Australia and New Zealand 2005, 'Position statement on lipid management 2005', viewed 2 May 2009, <http://www.racgp.org.au/>.

16. National Prescribing Service 2006, 'Indicators of quality prescribing', viewed 17 August 2009, <http://www.nps.org.au/health_professionals/tools/quality_prescribing_indicators_in_australian_general_practice/download_individual_prescribing_indicators/pdf/indicators_full>.

17. Nelson, M, Best, J, Buckley, N, Donovan, J, Dowden, J, Norton, D, Parker, S & Rossi, S 2007, 'Managing hypertension as a cardiovascular risk factor', *National Prescribing Service News*, no. 52, viewed 4 May 2009, <http://www.nps.org.au/health_professionals/publications/nps_news/current/nps_news_52/managing_hypertension_as_a_cardiovascular_risk_factor>.

18. Osterberg, L & Blaschke, T 2005, 'Adherence to medication', *New England Journal of Medicine*, vol. 353, no. 5, pp. 487–97, viewed 3 March 2009, <http://content.nejm.org/>.

19. Pharmaceutical Policy and Analysis Branch 2008, *Expenditure and prescriptions 12 months to 30 June 2008*, Pharmaceutical Policy and Analysis Branch, Department of Health and Ageing, Canberra, viewed 2 June 2009, <http://www.health.gov.au/internet/main/publishing.nsf/Content/053BB36E2A4173AACA2575910012F753/$File/PBS%20Expenditure%20and%20Prescriptions%20Report.pdf>.

20. Queensland Health Safe Medication Practice Unit 2005, *Reconciliation tool*, Queensland Health, Brisbane, viewed 9 June 2009, <http://www.health.vic.gov.au/sssl/downloads/qld_tool.pdf>.

21. Rossi, S (ed.) 2009, *Australian medicines handbook*, The Royal Australian College of General Practitioners, Australasian Society of Clinical and Experimental Pharmacologists and Toxicologists, Pharmaceutical Society of Australia, Rundle Mall, viewed 23 February 2009, <http://www.amh.net.au/>.

22. Rozich, JD & Resar, KR 2001, 'Medication safety: one organization's approach to the challenge', *Journal of Clinical Outcomes Management*, vol. 8, no. 10, pp. 27–34, viewed 10 June 2009, <http://turner-white.com/jc/abstract.php?PubCode=jcom_oct01_safety>.

23. Rubins, JB, Raci, E & Kunisaki, KM 2009, 'Managing stable COPD in 2009: incorporating results from recent clinical studies into a goal-directed approach for clinicians', *Postgraduate Medicine*, vol. 121, no. 1, pp. 104–112, viewed 3 May 2009, <http://www.ncbi.nlm.nih.gov/pubmed/19179818?ordinalpos=1&itool=EntrezSystem2.PEntrez.Pubmed.Pubmed_ResultsPanel.Pubmed_DiscoveryPanel.Pubmed_Discovery_RA&linkpos=3&log$=relatedreviews&logdbfrom=pubmed>.

24. Runciman, WB, Roughead, EE, Semple, SJ & Adams, RJ 2003, 'Adverse drug events and medication errors in Australia', *International Journal of Quality in Health Care*, vol. 15, supp. 1, pp. i49–i59, viewed 1 June 2009, <http://intqhc.oxfordjournals.org/>.

25. Sorensen, L, Stokes, JA, Purdie, DM, Woodward, M, Elliott, R & Roberts, MS 2004, 'Medication reviews in the community: results of a randomized, controlled effectiveness trial', *British Journal of Clinical Pharmacology*, vol. 58, no. 6, pp. 648–64, viewed 3 May 2009, <http://www.pubmedcentral.nih.gov/>.

26. Vik, SA, Maxwell, CJ & Hogan, DB 2004, 'Measurement, correlates, and health outcomes of medication adherence among seniors', *The Annals of Pharmacotherapy*, vol. 38, no. 2, pp. 303–12, viewed 3 May 2009, <http://www.theannals.com/>.

27. Wedzicha, JA & Seemungal, TAR 2007, 'COPD exacerbations: defining their cause and prevention', *The Lancet*, vol. 370, no. 9589, pp. 786–96, viewed 23 May 2009, <http://www.ncbi.nlm.nih.gov/pubmed/17765528>.

28. World Health Organisation 2003, 'Adherence to long term therapies: evidence for action', World Health Organisation, Geneva, viewed 2 April 2009, <http://www.who.int/>.

29. World Health Organisation 2009, 'WHO's pain ladder', World Health Organisation, Geneva, viewed 14 October 2009, <http://www.who.int/>.

30. Writing Group, Analgesic 2007, *Therapeutic guidelines: analgesic*, version 5, Therapeutic Guidelines Ltd, North Melbourne, viewed 3 May 2009, <http://www.tg.org.au/index.php?sectionid=18>.

31. Writing Group, Cardiovascular 2008, *Therapeutic guidelines: cardiovascular*, version 5, Therapeutic Guidelines Ltd, North Melbourne, viewed 3 May 2009, <http://www.tg.org.au/index.php?sectionid=42>.

32. Writing Group, Endocrinology 2004, *Therapeutic guidelines: endocrinology*, version 3, Therapeutic Guidelines Ltd, North Melbourne, viewed 3 May 2009, <http://www.tg.org.au/index.php?sectionid=44>.

33. Writing Group, Respiratory 2005, *Therapeutic guidelines: respiratory*, version 3, Therapeutic Guidelines Ltd, North Melbourne, viewed 3 May 2009, <http://www.tg.org.au/index.php?sectionid=49/>.

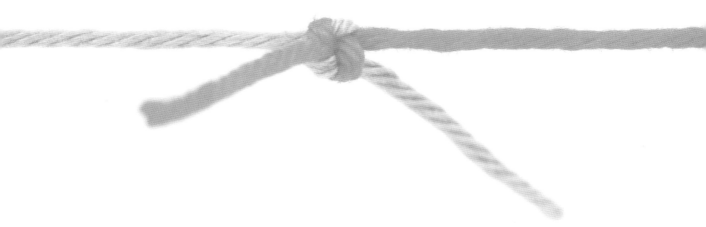

Chapter eight

Immunisation

by Michelle Wills

Overview

Immunisation forms a large part of the role of nurses working in general practice. The introduction of a Medicare Benefits Schedule item number for nurses to give vaccines has seen general practice improve and expand immunisation services. It is a role where practice nurses have demonstrated the ability to be innovative, organised, competent and show clinical leadership. This chapter will focus on the national policy aspects of immunisation and the elements that are required to deliver vaccines safely.

Objectives

At the completion of this chapter you should be able to:

- understand the role of national policy in supporting immunisation programs;

- differentiate between vaccination and immunisation;

- understand the clinical context of the immunisation encounter in general practice; and

- appreciate the various elements that are required to fulfil a safe and effective immunisation encounter.

Introduction

Immunisation and vaccination are terms that are often used interchangeably; however, they have slightly different meanings. Vaccination is the administration of antigenic material (the vaccine) to produce immunity to a disease. Immunisation is the process by which an individual's immune system becomes fortified against an agent as a result of receiving vaccine (Department of Health and Ageing 2009).

Increasing the level of immunity is essential in minimising the spread of infection within our community. Immunity to disease not only protects the individual but also protects the community. Educating the public on the importance and effectiveness of immunisation is an ongoing process as new diseases and environmental changes present ongoing challenges to our community. Immunisation is acknowledged to be among the most cost-effective and highest-impact health interventions. Nearly three million deaths worldwide are prevented each year by immunisation, and an even greater amount of illness and disability (The World Bank 2009).

As practice nurses develop an increased role in health promotion and health education, immunisation will remain a focus for both for education regarding preventable diseases, delivery of vaccines to adults and children and notification and surveillance of side effects.

Milestones of immunisation programs in Australia

There has been a long history of immunisation programs in Australia. For example, smallpox vaccination was given in New South Wales to control outbreaks of the disease as early as 1804. Routine childhood vaccination programs were established by 1953 and were the responsibility of each state or territory government. This led to differing schedules in each state and this is a phenomenon that remains with current immunisation schedules.

Significant events in immunisation in Australia have impacted and shaped the national immunisation program as it is today. Table 8.1 below shows significant milestones in Australian immunisation history.

Table 8.1 Significant milestones in Australian immunisation history

Year	Immunisation milestone
1989–90	National survey showed immunisation coverage levels of approximately 53% for children less than six years being age appropriately immunised. This rate was lower than that of some developing countries.
1993	Publication of the National Health and Medical Research Council's (NHMRC) National Immunisation Strategy which established national immunisation coverage targets.
1996	Introduction of Australian Childhood Immunisation Registry (ACIR). This national register allowed the recording of all vaccinations given to children up to their seventh birthday residing in Australia.
1997	Immunise Australia: seven-point plan

The seven-point plan arose out of the National Immunisation Strategy and was introduced to help raise the immunisation rate in Australia. It consisted of the following elements:

1. **Initiatives for parents**   A financial incentive is provided to parents as an incentive to immunise their children on time.

2. **A bigger role for general practitioners**   It was recognised that children visited their GP regularly. GPs were able to target children not immunised elsewhere and to monitor the immunisation status of all children in their care. A financial incentive is provided to GPs in the form of the GPII scheme.

3. **Monitoring and evaluation of immunisation targets**   Published data is available from the ACIR on immunisation rates.

4. **Immunisation days**   These were held at multiple sites in areas of low immunisation rates.

5. **Measles eradication**   A schools-based MMR program was held to vaccinate all school-aged children.

6. **Education and research**   Resources were developed, such as the *Australian Immunisation Handbook,* and the National Centre for Immunisation Research and Surveillance (NCIRS) was established.

7. **School entry requirements**   Some states passed legislation determining uniform school-entry requirements.

Although some of these initiatives were not ongoing, some have remained and influence immunisation services that are available currently. By June 2008, immunisation coverage rates had risen to a level which showed that the average immunisation coverage of children aged 12–15 months was 91%; 92.8% for children aged 24–27 months; and 88% for 72–75 months (Medicare Australia 2008).

The role of the nurse in general practice immunisation

A consultation for immunisation is probably the best opportunity that nurses will have to provide health promotion and disease prevention initiatives for the individual client, as well as the nation as a whole. Immunisation is an essential element of the preventive health framework that nurses in general practice work within.

The nurse's role in the provision of vaccination services is multifaceted and can support general practice in all aspects of vaccine management, including ensuring the safe storage of the vaccines. The practice nurse needs to be clinically competent to administer vaccinations, and they must be able to give up-to-date, consistent and evidence-based information about immunisation.

As well as assisting in opportunistic vaccinations within the practice, the nurse can be proactive in the development and implementation of immunisation recall and reminder systems, and the formulation of practice policies and procedures. The availability of Australian Childhood Immunisation Register (ACIR) data on overdue individual immunisations allows the nurse to be proactive in following up these children and improve coverage rates in their practice. Furthermore, practice nurses have been observed as providing significant education about immunisation to patients, nursing colleagues, general practice registrars and GPs (Phillips et al. 2008).

Nurses are able to administer vaccinations in general practice under certain circumstances:

- The practice nurse, working within their scope of practice (and subject to specific state legislation, such as medication endorsement for enrolled or Division 2 nurses), may administer the vaccines under a doctor's *written* order. The nurse may draw up and administer the vaccines without direct supervision but the doctor ordering the vaccines must remain available on the premises in case of an adverse event or anaphylaxis.

- Some states or territories have an immunisation accreditation program where the registered nurse (Division 1) may be endorsed to independently provide vaccinations in accordance with the state or territory *Drugs and Poisons Act*. At the time of publication, each state or territory had its own immunisation-provider accreditation process which is not recognised outside their jurisdiction. It is important that nurses familiarise themselves with regulations in their state or territory regarding provision of immunisations both as a registered nurse and as an independent nurse immuniser.

The ability to work as a regulated nurse immuniser expands the opportunities considerably for practice nurses. An advanced level of practice allows them to administer vaccines in various community sites, such as in workplaces, child care centres and factories, within their communities. It also allows them to establish nurse-led immunisation clinics within their practices. The establishment of such services provides better access for patients to receive immunisations, and it builds capacity for the practice and increases income. Nurse-led clinics are discussed further in Chapter 21.

Reflections

What is your role in immunisation in your practice? Are you able to expand it in any way?

National immunisation programs

Immunise Australia Program

A federal, state and territory governments initiative, the Immunise Australia Program aims to increase national immunisation rates for vaccine-preventable diseases. The Immunise Australia Program aims to increase national immunisation rates and implements the National Immunisation Program schedule. It provides free vaccination programs, administers the ACIR and educates health professionals and the public on immunisation. The Population Health Division within the Department of Health and Ageing is responsible for the development, implementation and evaluation of national immunisation policies and programs.

National Immunisation Program

The National Immunisation Program (NIP) refers to the recommended vaccines by age group which are funded by the Australian Government as they appear on the NIP schedule. The states and territories can choose whatever combination of vaccines that best suits the needs of their geographic and demographic conditions, and determine which vaccine brands they use. This has led to a variety of dosing schedules. Awareness of this becomes extremely important when vaccinating children who have had any part of their vaccination schedule administered in another state. There are also different schedules for different 'at risk' population groups. For example, the NIP schedule allows for Aboriginal and Torres Strait Islander children in areas of higher risk (Queensland, Northern Territory, Western Australia and South Australia) to have the hepatitis A vaccine as part of their funded routine childhood immunisation, but this is not available for other children. Until 2005 the NIP had been a predominantly childhood-based schedule but since then there has been an increasing number of vaccines funded for adolescent and adult programs. The adolescent immunisation programs are usually administered as school-based programs with general practice acting as a 'mop up' for those

Administering the vaccine(s)

Vaccines are classified as an S4 drug and are subject to the state or territory drugs and poisons Acts for storage and administration. As with the administration of any medication, following the 5 R rule will reduce the risk of incorrect administration (QNU 2005). The important points are:

- **R**ight person
- **R**ight time
- **R**ight vaccine
- **R**ight dose
- **R**ight route.

To administer vaccinations the nurse must work within their scope of practice. It is highly recommended that nurses who have little or no experience in administering vaccines to infants and children be mentored by an experienced immunisation provider.

It is important to ascertain that the pre-vaccination screening has taken place and consent has been obtained before administering any vaccines. The area where the immunisation is administered must also be prepared adequately. Equipment, such as adrenaline, needles, syringes and oxygen, should be available to manage an anaphylactic reaction if it occurs. If a child is the patient, age appropriate items to be used as distractions should also be available and the vaccines prepared out of the child's view. Some vaccines require mixing prior to administration and the diluent supplied with the vaccine must always be used, as this forms part of the vaccine.

The correct gauge and length of the administration needle needs to be ascertained and this will be determined depending on the child's weight. No overall rule can be given as to what size needle to use for specific age groups as there is huge variation in children's weight. It is important that the needle length will administer the correct route, either intramuscular or subcutaneous. The current schedule for the primary course of immunisations in children up to and including six months of age has a combination of both oral and injectable vaccines. The nurse must therefore be familiar with the route by which the vaccines are to be administered.

Unless the skin is visibly dirty the use of an alcohol skin wipe is not recommended, however, if a wipe is used then the area must be left to dry before administering the vaccines. In babies under 12 months of age it is recommended that the intramuscular injections are given into the anterolateral thigh at a 90° angle (Department of Health and Ageing 2009). For infants over 12 months of age, it is recommended that the intramuscular injections be given in the deltoid muscle at a 90° angle. Vaccines should never be administered into the buttocks. All vaccines that are due should be administered on the same day (Department of Health and Ageing 2009).

To allay a parent's anxiety it is essential to ensure that the parent understands the common reactions to the vaccines that have been administered, and the recommended management of those side effects is explained. The importance of remaining in the practice where medical attention is available for 15 minutes after immunisation should be explained to recipients. Paracetamol is recommended for minor reactions but not as routine prior to the immunisations (Department of Health and Ageing 2009).

Reflections

What quality and safety systems do you have in place to ensure that vaccine errors do not occur in your practice?

Documentation

Documentation of the entire immunisation encounter must be provided in the clinical notes (either hard copy or electronically). The following should be documented at every immunisation encounter:

- process of consent and who gave consent
- details of the vaccine given, including the dose, brand name, batch number and site of administration
- name of the person administering the vaccination
- date and time of the vaccination
- date the next vaccination is due.

A paper version of the child-health record is available for parents of young children. Vaccines can be documented here so that other health care providers and the parents can access the immunisation history. Children under seven years of age require timely reporting of their immunisations to the ACIR.

A paper record is also useful for adults, especially if travelling overseas.

Adverse events

An adverse event following immunisation refers to an unwanted or unexpected event occurring after the administration of the vaccine(s) (Department of Health and Ageing 2009). Such an event may be caused by the vaccine(s) or may occur by chance after vaccination, that is, it would have occurred regardless of vaccination. Most vaccines cause minor adverse events such as low-grade fever, pain or redness at the injection site and these should be anticipated (Department of Health and Ageing 2009).

Moderate to severe adverse events must be reported to the appropriate state or territory authority. Some jurisdictions will accept reports either from parents or health professionals, while others will accept a report from a health professional only. It is important that parents' concerns regarding the possibility of an adverse event are addressed, even if the concern appears trivial, as the event may negatively influence decisions about future immunisations.

Cold chain management

The aim of the national immunisation program is to increase the immunisation coverage rate; however, there is no point in high coverage rates if the vaccines being administered are not effective. Failure to follow the recommended storage guidelines can reduce vaccine potency, resulting in inadequate protection against disease. There are a number of components to vaccine management and one important aspect is vaccine storage and the 'cold chain'. The cold chain monitoring system relates to transporting and storing vaccines within a safe temperature range. It involves all practice staff, and requires equipment and procedures which ensure that vaccines are maintained at the safe temperature of 2 to 8°C (Grant et al. 2005).

It begins at the point of manufacture and continues until the actual immunisation encounter. It is important to note that the loss of vaccine potency through cold chain breaches, that is, exposure to temperatures outside the 2 to 8°C, is not reversible.

The essential elements of vaccine storage are:

* the people managing vaccine storage and distribution; and
* the equipment for storing, transporting and monitoring.

Neither of these elements can function without the other: state of the art equipment is of no value if no one is able to program it and, conversely, people cannot be expected to patch together antiquated equipment and expect it to function effectively. Vaccines are temperature-sensitive biological substances that become less effective or destroyed under certain conditions. The loss of vaccine effectiveness is cumulative and cannot be reversed so it is important to ensure that vaccines are not allowed to be frozen, exposed to high temperatures or exposed to direct sun or fluorescent light.

The Department of Health and Ageing has produced a resource, *National vaccine storage guidelines: Strive For 5* to assist in the storage of vaccines. This resource is aimed at vaccine service providers and outlines the basic principles of safe vaccine management.

Policies and procedures

It is suggested that each general practice has a nominated person (and this is usually the practice nurse) who is responsible for vaccine management within the practice, and a designated person to support this role. The nominated person is responsible for ensuring that all vaccines are managed correctly and that policies and procedures are documented. They should also have the responsibility of ensuring that all staff in the practice understand the importance of vaccine management, and that staff immediately report any concerns about potential cold chain breaches.

Vaccine management requires policies and procedures within the practice that cover the following aspects.

Vaccine ordering

The aim when ordering vaccines is to order the right amount at the right time. Monthly stocktaking will assist with this process and avoid wastage of vaccines.

Vaccine delivery

All staff must be aware of the process to ensure that the vaccines are promptly stored in the correct manner if the nominated person is unavailable.

- The nominated person should accept vaccines from the courier.
- Check dispatch date and cold chain monitors.
- Remove vaccines from larger box and polystyrene packaging, but do not remove vaccines from their individual packaging.
- Transfer vaccines to a dedicated vaccine refrigerator as soon as possible.
- Record the date, numbers of vaccines received, and vaccine type and batch numbers.

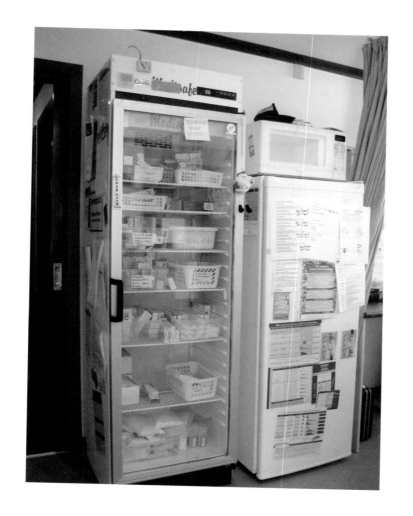

Temperature monitoring and recording

- A minimum-maximum thermometer must be in placed in each vaccine fridge to constantly monitor the temperature.

- The thermometer probe should be placed in a vaccine box (not in fluid).

- It is recommended that the thermometer is checked and recorded at least twice daily every working day. Record the current, maximum and minimum temperatures the fridge has been operating at and reset the thermometer.

- The nominated person responsible for cold chain does not have to be the person who checks the temperatures as long as the staff who are checking have been trained and understand the responsibilities of recording (and reporting) any deviations from the 2 to 8°C range).

- If cold chain breaches occur, advice should be sought from your state government authority.

- The batteries in minimum-maximum thermometers require changing at least annually. This can be aligned with a significant annual event such as when changing smoke alarm batteries or when daylight saving commences. In the case of any malfunction, check the battery first.
- If a data logger is used, instructions on use and how to download data should be easily accessible.

Power failure procedure

This procedure will be different depending on whether vaccines are stored in a domestic or purpose-built vaccine (PBV) refrigerator. *Strive for 5* has clear guidelines on what action is required in the event of power interruptions. Guidelines for power failures that occur out of hours and at weekends are recommended.

Cold chain breach

The following points should be followed in the event of cold chain breach:

- Read the instructions on who to contact as each state and territory has its own requirements.
- Isolate the vaccines but do not discard unless instructed by the relevant state/territory department.
- Record the date and time the temperature was out of the 2 to 8°C range.
- Record the maximum temperature and minimum temperature.
- Record when the minimum-maximum thermometer was last read and reset with the date and time.
- Record the numbers of vaccines and their expiry dates.
- Record any action taken to rectify cause of cold chain breach.
- Record instructions from jurisdiction.
- If shortening expiry dates on vaccines, record the new date on each vial as well as the documentation used to report breach.

Stocktaking

A monthly stocktake of vaccines will give the practice an overall indication of vaccine usage and assist in appropriate ordering of vaccines. A stocktake will involve number of vaccines, expiry dates and rotation of vaccines.

Equipment maintenance

Instruction manuals for all cold chain equipment, refrigerator, thermometer and data loggers, as well as the name and contact details of the service technician, should be easily accessible.

Maintaining the cold chain off-site

If vaccines are being transported to an off-site immunisation session the cold chain must be monitored and maintained. It is recommended that patients purchasing their vaccines from a pharmacy arrange to collect their vaccines immediately prior to their appointment. Disposable, insulated bags for transport of vaccines are usually supplied by the pharmacy and patients should inform reception staff when arriving for their appointment that they have a vaccine. This should be labelled with the patient's name and stored immediately in the vaccine fridge.

Strive for 5 recommendations

It is recommended that vaccines be stored in a PBV refrigerator; however, any refrigerator, either domestic or purpose built, must be dedicated only to the storage of vaccines. Food and drinks are not to be stored in the vaccine fridge as this can result in frequent opening of the door and potential destabilisation of the temperature.

As there are a number of different types of domestic refrigerators, such as cyclic defrost and frost free, it is possible only to offer general guidelines on vaccine storage in domestic refrigerators. If a domestic refrigerator is used, modifications need to be made to ensure temperature regulation and it is important that the nurses are aware of the properties of their specific refrigerator. Please note that it is strongly recommended that bar refrigerators are not used for vaccine storage because of their temperature instability (Grant et al. 2005).

In both PBV and domestic refrigerators it is important that there is sufficient room to store the vaccines required by the practice—noting the seasonal variations for influenza vaccine storage. Location of the refrigerator must allow a gap of approximately 10 cm between the wall and the rear of the refrigerator and the refrigerator should be away from direct sunlight. When locating the refrigerator, be aware of seasonal changes in room temperature that may affect the temperature of your refrigerator. For example, location on a west-facing wall during the summer months may affect the refrigerator's ability to maintain temperature between 2 to 8°C (Grant et al. 2005).

Travel medicine

The requirements for immunisations that constitute travel medicine are constantly changing. Vaccines and advice required will be determined not only by the destination but also by the type and length of the trip. For example, are the travellers trekking 'off the beaten track' in a developing country or are they only staying in a resort? Also of note is the duration of stay at particular destinations, for example, staying one to two weeks or travelling extensively over a number of months. It is suggested the practice determines the most appropriate immunisations for the traveller in conjunction with a travel medicine expert. As well as travel vaccines, ensure that all other NIP scheduled vaccines or recommended vaccines are current especially measles, mumps and rubella (MMR), hepatitis B and influenza. Travellers returning to Australia who are unwell are advised to telephone or visit their general practitioner (Department of Foreign Affairs and Trade 2009).

Conclusion

Immunisation is probably the optimal opportunity for nurses to provide health promotion and disease prevention initiatives for the individual client as well as the community. The nurse must possess the knowledge, skills and abilities required to promote and deliver vaccinations across a patient's life span, safely and effectively. The increasing role in health promotion and health education for practice nurses means that immunisation is a focus for education regarding preventable diseases, delivery of vaccines to adults and children and notification and surveillance of side effects.

Name of nurse
Sue Alexander

Practice
Grand Prom Medical Centre, Perth, WA

Nurses employed at the Grand Prom Medical Centre have developed an interest in immunisation and strive to provide best practice in this area. Following several national and state initiatives, several strategies were identified to improve the immunisation rate in our practice. They were:

- to design a questionnaire to measure patient satisfaction;
- to promote the uptake of the human papillomavirus vaccine (HPV); and
- to increase the vaccination rate of children having the influenza vaccine.

The strategies to improve vaccination rates varied according to the target group. For the HPV vaccine, separate invitation and reminder letters were created for that age group and once a database of regular attendees who met the criteria had been established. These were mailed incrementally so as not to overwhelm the resources that were available to meet the demand. Electronic spreadsheets were developed to maintain data which could be easily transmitted to the HPV registry at regular intervals.

A practice decision was made to promote influenza vaccine to children between the ages of six months to five years. Reception staff were educated by the nurse to be able to answer any queries from parents, ensuring that appointments were offered to appropriate children. To comply with the need for a second dose, a spreadsheet was created, reminder letters sent and follow-up phone calls to parents were made. This resulted in a 97% compliance rate of those children needing two doses.

Pre-vaccination and post-vaccination checklists have been created to increase patient's knowledge of vaccination process including side effects and their management. This has been extended to adult vaccinations as well and written information given to patients both before and after vaccination.

The results from these targeted, innovative strategies has proven valuable to the practice with an increase in the childhood immunisation rate from 86% in 2004 to current rates between 95 to 96%, a rate much higher than the local and national averages. Three hundred and seventy-five influenza immunisations have been administered to children and 750 HPV vaccinations given to young women. Travel vaccines are also stocked which attract a small profit. Diligent record keeping and written processes have ensured that adequate supplies of vaccines are always available, that there is no overstocking or wastage, and billing is appropriate to cover costs.

As well as benefits to the practice, our patient satisfaction survey showed an overall satisfaction rate of 98.5%. All practice staff were involved in the process and reception staff were responsible for recruiting responses from patients. No negative comments were received and, importantly, respondents rated 100% for the questions relating to satisfaction with the nurse-led service. This indicates that patients have a high level of confidence in the nurse immunisers at Grand Prom Medical Centre being able to provide a safe and comprehensive immunisation service.

Sue Alexander received the Australian Practice Nurses Association 'Sanofi Best Practice Award for Immunisation' in 2008.

Key messages

Immunisation is one of the most effective forms of health promotion and disease prevention at practice level.

Practice nurses should plan and implement systems as part of the general practice team to provide safe and effective immunisation for the targeted population.

People and equipment are required to manage vaccines safely and efficiently.

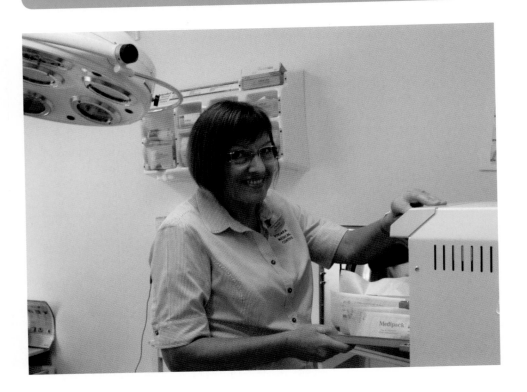

Useful resources

Australian Childhood Immunisation Register (ACIR)

http://www.medicareaustralia.gov.au/public/services/acir/index.jsp

ACIR statistics

http://www.medicareaustralia.gov.au/provider/patients/acir/statistics.jsp

The Australian Immunisation Handbook

http://www.immunise.health.gov.au/internet/immunise/publishing.nsf/Content/Handbook-home

General Practice Immunisation Incentive (GPII) scheme

http://www.medicareaustralia.gov.au/provider/incentives/gpii/index.jsp

Immunise Australia Program

http://www.immunise.health.gov.au/internet/immunise/publishing.nsf/Content/home

Strive for 5

http://www.health.gov.au/internet/immunise/publishing.nsf/content/provider-store/

National Centre for Immunisation Research and Surveillance

http://www.ncirs.usyd.edu.au/

Department of Foreign Affairs and Trade

http://www.smartraveller.gov.au/

References

1. Department of Foreign Affairs and Trade 2009, Travel Bulletin page, visited 17 January 2010, <http://www.smartraveller.gov.au/>.

2. Department of Health and Ageing 2009, *Immunise Australia Program*, visited 1 July 2009, <http://www.health.gov.au/>.

3. Grant, S, Langley, A, Peterson, K, Kempe, A, Miller, N, Bryant, V & Morton, J 2005, *National vaccine storage guidelines: Strive for 5*, Department of Health and Ageing, viewed 17 November 2009, <http://www.health.gov.au/internet/immunise/publishing.nsf/content/provider-store/>.

4. Medicare Australia 2008, *Medicare Annual Report 2007–2008*, Department of Health and Ageing, ch 2, visited 17 January 2010, <http://www.medicareaustralia.gov.au/>.

5. Medicare Australia 2009a, *Australian Childhood Immunisation Register*, Department of Health and Ageing, visited 29 November 2009, <http://www.medicareaustralia.gov.au/>.

6. Medicare Australia 2009b, *General Practice Immunisation Incentive (GPII)*, Department of Health and Ageing, visited 13 November 2009, <http://www.medicare.gov.au/provider/incentives/gpii/index.jsp>.

7.   Medicare Australia 2009c, *Table 13 – Medicare*, Medicare governance report
     2009, Department of Health and Ageing, visited 29 November 2009,
     <http://www.medicareaustralia.gov.au/about/governance/reports/07-08/files/
     mcare13.pdf>.

8.   Phillips, CB, Pearce, CM, Dwan, KM, Hall, S, Porritt, J, Yates, R, Klijakovic, M &
     Sibbald, B 2008, *Charting new roles for Australian general practice nurses:
     a multicentre qualitative study*, abridged report, Australian Primary Care
     Research Institute, visited 17 January 2010, <http://www.anu.edu.au/aphcri/
     Domain/PracticeNursing/index.php>.

9.   Queensland Nurses Union (QNU) 2005, *Reducing the risk of medication errors*,
     information sheet, visited 17 January 2010, <http://www.qnc.qld.gov.au/
     upload/pdfs/information_sheets/General/Reducing_the_risk_of_medication_
     errors.pdf>.

10. The World Bank Group 2009, *Immunization*, visited 29 November 2009,
     <http://web.worldbank.org/>.

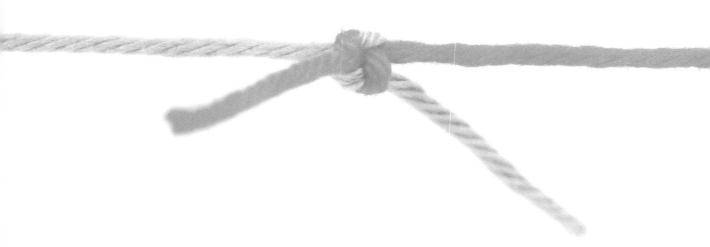

Chapter nine

Clinical organisation and infection control

by Christine Mathieson
and William Wong

Overview

Practice nurses have been identified as central to organising practice activity with tasks such as managing and ordering stock, cleaning and sterilising of instruments, maintaining a safe working environment, writing policies and procedures and clearing contaminated waste (Phillips et al. 2008). This chapter will focus on these and highlight the important role that practice nurses have in contributing to practice organisation and the delivery of safe, efficient health care.

Objectives

At the completion of this chapter you should be able to:

- understand the clinical environment in general practice and the coordination role of the nurse in this area;

- understand the principles of infection control; and

- understand how to effectively prepare for influenza season and the threat of a newly emerging pandemic.

Introduction

Leadership describes the ability to influence, motivate and enable members of an organisation to contribute to the effectiveness and success of that organisation (Griffiths et al. 2009). Nursing in general practice has a variety of roles that increasingly require leadership and the ability to motivate others to promote change. The practice nurse located in the treatment room is often central to the clinic and contributes to the nursing role as an agent of connectivity (Phillips et al. 2008). The routine thoroughfare in the treatment room, increasing need for nurse-led clinics, ordering of equipment and consumables, as well as clinical administration, are generally areas that practice nurses coordinate and manage. Historically, practice nurses have come from a background in the acute nursing sector within a large organisational structure where activities such as infection control, stock imprest and the ordering of supplies are handled by other staff. The central sterilisation departments of large hospitals manage the spectrum of sterilisation, stock rotation, and monitoring and maintaining sterilisation standards. In general practice these responsibilities often become the working domain of the practice nurse. The introduction of the Royal Australian College of General Practitioners (RACGP) Standards for General Practices in 1996 have applied a systematic approach to safety and quality which includes the maintenance of infection control and monitoring of equipment and supplies.

Standards for general practice

Improving the structure, process and outcomes of general practice has been identified as fundamental to increasing the quality of care provided by general practice (RACGP 2007). The standards recognise the aspects of general practice that support the delivery of high-quality care to patients. Included in this are the services provided, quality improvement, the rights of patients, practice management and the physical aspects of the practice. Practice nurses, because of their ability to work across all of these aspects, have been recognised as instrumental in establishing and maintaining systems to support practice capacity and improve compliance with external imperatives (Phillips et al. 2008).

Managing the clinical environment

In order to create an efficient and safe clinical environment the practice requires a systematic and well-structured approach to management. This responsibility often falls to the practice nurse. All members of the team have a role to play in establishing and maintaining resources but monitoring these has increasingly become part of the nursing role. Management of the clinical environment includes:

- developing practice policies on issues that affect patient care—for example, triage, sterilisation and cleaning;
- purchasing and maintenance of equipment;
- overseeing recall and reminder systems;
- monitoring use of medications within the practice—for example, vaccines and emergency drugs;
- maintaining and monitoring emergency equipment—for example, defibrillator and oxygen equipment;

- monitoring occupational health and safety (OH&S) practices—for example, staff immunisations and injuries; and

- supervising the ordering of consumables.

Because of their clinical knowledge and with the support of administrative staff nurses are best placed to manage policies and procedures relating to the above areas.

Policy and procedures

There are several reasons that any organisation, including general practices, may want to write policies and procedures. (Policy development is explained in more detail in Chapter 2.) Included among the reasons for having practice policies and procedures are:

- To provide staff with a framework for action that they can follow to achieve the organisational aims and thus improve teamwork

- To make decisions so that the same conversation does not need to happen repeatedly

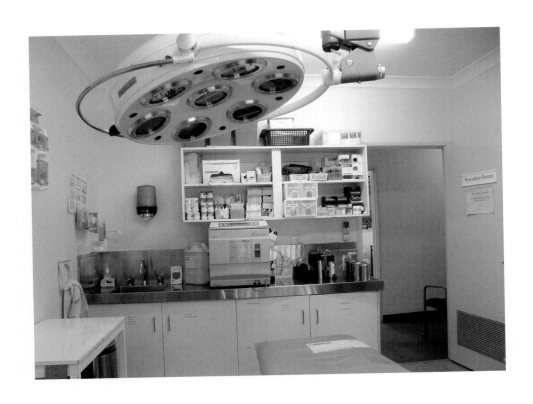

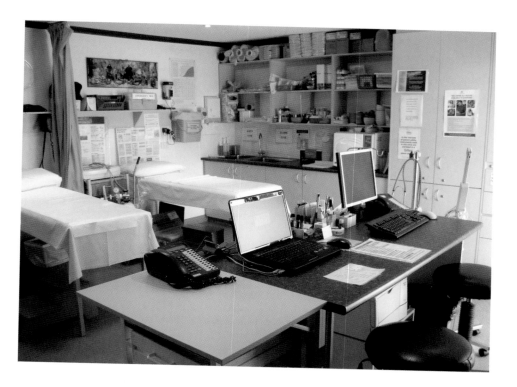

- To provide a tool for quality improvement—to improve all aspects of patient care and service delivery

- To comply with RACGP Standards of General Practices and work towards accreditation

- To comply with legislative standards—for example, Medical Benefits Schedule and OH&S requirements

- To ensure that all staff are aware of and use best practice for clinical management of patients.

Increasingly, effort is being invested in teamwork and the necessity for all staff members to understand their respective roles in contributing to patient care. A written policy will clearly outline the way in which all team members can contribute to achieving the aim of the policy, whether it be for clinical care or for smooth functioning of the organisation. The policy will outline the aim, reason and purpose of the service. It will also include what the policy is, when it applies and who it applies to.

A procedure should describe step-by-step instructions on how to successfully achieve the policy aim. It should list the responsibility for each step but avoid too much detail.

The following is an example of a framework to develop a policy and procedure. It can be adapted for either clinical management or procedure or an organisation management task such as ordering supplies or cleaning equipment. Table 9.1 below shows a template which could be used as to describe a policy.

Table 9.1 Policy template

Policy title:	
Approved by:	
Review date:	
Introduction:	
Purpose:	A concise statement of one or two sentences on why the policy/procedure exists and what it is designed to ensure.
Scope:	State all the people that this policy applies to.
Definitions:	Include an explanation of terms and abbreviations used within the policy and procedure.
Accreditation context:	For example, which criterion from the RACGP standards this policy applies to.
Policy:	The policy statement itself, what will be done.
Principles:	A general or overarching statement on the intent of the policy.
Procedure:	A description of all essential steps and explanations on how work is organised in order to achieve the stated objective, and who (position, not name) is responsible for each step, e.g. the role of the GP, the role of the practice nurse and the role of the administrative or reception staff.
Supporting documentation:	Include any references used, acknowledge other sources.
Governance:	Who is responsible for the policy? What version is it?

Source: adapted from Swinburne University of Technology 2009

Reflections

How do policies and procedures written in your practice compare to those above? Can you think of alternative suggestions?

Equipment and maintenance

The amount and type of clinical equipment varies from practice to practice and may be based on the interests of the general practitioner, the expertise of the practice nurse, the location of the practice and the practice population. Emergency equipment may be more extensive in rural practices in order to manage acutely unwell patients who cannot attend a distant accident and emergency hospital department.

Practices that perform a large number of skin checks will require dermatoscopes and skin biopsy equipment. Spirometry, ear irrigation, blood tests such as international normalised ratio (INR) testing, ankle brachial index (ABI) testing and Doppler fetal monitoring all require specialised equipment that must be maintained, and records of servicing and calibration documented. Vaccine fridges, sterilisers, oxygen cylinders, sphygmomanometers, blood glucose monitors, cast saws, defibrillators, tympanic thermometers, scales and pulse oximeters all require servicing and maintenance. A system for recording maintenance is recommended as a way of demonstrating safety of equipment and is also a requirement in meeting the Standards of General Practices and, therefore, accreditation.

Ordering of consumables

Ideally a nominated person will be responsible for ordering consumables such as dressings, syringes, needles, bandages, vaccines and all the other items of equipment necessary in the day-to-day running of the treatment room. The practice nurse is generally the person nominated to undertake this role but consideration could be given to educating administrative staff to do this under nursing supervision. With good documentation and policies in place, a non-clinical staff member could be encouraged to take responsibility for ensuring supplies are available without creating wastage from unused stock.

Relationships with surgical suppliers are important as pricing structures, delivery charges and return of unused stock is often negotiable. In order to monitor use and cost of supplies, delivery dockets and invoices need to be reconciled. With the increasing array of equipment available for use in general practice, the allocation of a budget for capital expenditure, maintenance and consumables would be ideal for controlling, updating and monitoring expenditure. Table 9.2 overleaf is an example of equipment and supplies that are needed in general practice.

Storage of vaccines is primarily the function of the practice nurse and this is discussed in more detail in Chapter 8.

Table 9.2 Maintenance of equipment and supplies in a practice

Product	Supply source	How often to order
Government-funded vaccines	State and territory public health authorities	Weekly or monthly depending on demand
Travel vaccines	Private prescription for the patient. Direct purchase from the manufacturer or a medical supplier	Demand dependent
Examination and diagnostic equipment	Order direct from medical supplier, online, by fax or phone	Demand dependent
Medications for doctor's bag	From pharmacy using appropriate doctor's bag drug order book	At the start of each month
Medications	Direct from medical supplier or pharmaceutical companies. Some purchases from local pharmacy may be cost efficient. Either order online, by fax or phone	Demand dependant
Small quantity items needed quickly	Purchase on account from local pharmacy	Demand dependent
Pathology equipment	Supplies generally supplied free by pathology companies or can be ordered through medical supplier	Demand dependent
Waste disposal equipment (sharps containers and yellow infectious waste bags)	Contract with clinical infectious waste collection services	Arrangements are made for these to be collected either weekly or fortnightly

Emergency and sample drugs

Every practice must have a basic supply of emergency drugs and equipment that is easily accessible, clearly labelled and stored safely (usually in the treatment room). General practices must have the necessary equipment for comprehensive primary health care and resuscitation. The exact types and quantities of the items should be agreed by the doctors according to practice location and clinical demand. It is often the practice nurse's responsibility to ensure that emergency supplies and equipment are checked and maintained. Generally all drugs should be checked at least monthly to ensure they have not expired and that adequate supplies are available. Practices need to develop a protocol on the appropriate disposal of expired drugs. A computer or paper-based system with a checklist of what drugs are used, when they expire, how much is in stock, when this was checked and initialled is a simple way of keeping track. This information can be arranged in a table similar to that shown in Table 9.3 below.

Table 9.3 Organisation of drugs

Drug
Strength
Amount in stock
Expiry date
Checked by
Date
Actions taken
Completion date

Emergency drugs and equipment

The list of drugs and equipment shown in Table 9.4 below is a *guide only* and should be altered according to local need. To ensure compliance with minimum standards for acceptable emergency equipment, practices need to be familiar with the current RACGP standards for general practices.

Table 9.4 Emergency drugs and equipment

Drugs	
• adrenaline	• Atrovent®
• atropine	• benzylpenicillin
• glucagen hypoglycaemia kit	• water and sodium chloride for injection
• GTN spray	• IV fluids
• aspirin	• oxygen
• Ventolin®	

Continued >

Table 9.4 *continued*

Equipment	
• Various sized needles and syringes	• IV cannulas and safesite caps
• IV giving sets	• resuscitation bag and mask for adults, children and infants
• ECG machine	
• suction and oxygen equipment (face mask and nasal prongs)	• ECG dots and paper
	• Guedel airway of various sizes
• emergency defibrillator machine	• O_2 saturation monitor

Doctor's bag list

It is recommended by the RACGP standards (RACGP 2007) that each doctor has access to a doctor's bag when consulting with patients off-site. General practitioners are able to obtain supplies of certain drugs for emergency use as listed on the Pharmaceutical Benefits Schedule. A suggested list of useful drugs and equipment in a doctor's bag is given in Table 9.5 below.

Table 9.5 The doctor's bag

Injectable preparations	Oral preparations	Consumables
adrenaline	aspirin	syringes
benzylpenicillin	Ventolin® MDI	IV cannulas
diazepam		various needles
frusemide		alcohol swabs
glycogen		Guedel oral airway kit
hydrocortisone		spacer device
Maxalon®		sharps container
morphine		urine testing strip
nalaxone		urine pathology jars
prochlorperazine		prescription pads
promethazine		S8 book for documenting the use of narcotic drugs
		practice letterhead torch

Source: Baird 2008

Pharmaceutical samples

Pharmaceutical companies often supply sample medications to be dispensed by GPs. Again, management of this is practice-specific according to consumer needs and demand. Some practices prefer not to keep these medications at all as it requires a time-consuming protocol with careful documentation and regular checks to make sure supplies are rotated, are all accounted for and have not expired. Most sample drugs are Schedule 4 drugs which require a prescription from a doctor; therefore, they should be stored safely and not freely accessible to staff who are not directly involved in patient care or patients. Often the responsibility for managing these samples falls to the practice nurse so it is recommended that all practices have a clear, written policy of the management and responsibility for such samples to ensure all perishable items are not kept beyond their recommended date and are discarded appropriately.

Infection control

The history of infection prevention and control can be traced back to 1847 when a link between the hands of health care workers and the spread of hospital-acquired disease was first established in Austria. The subsequent understanding of microorganisms and their roles in pathogenesis and recent emerging challenges, such as SARS and the H1N1 2009 influenza pandemic, has helped to refocus the importance of this topic in our health system, including general practice. However, much of the data in infection control is sourced from hospital settings. Complying with the guidelines in the RACGP Infection Control Standards for Office-based Practices will help practices meet minimum acceptable standards for infection control. Robust infection control systems are essential to ensure that patients and staff are protected from health care associated infection transmission.

Health care associated infections can occur in any health care setting. To provide safe health care, employees of general practice need to be aware of the presence of infectious agents. General practices, especially the waiting room, are places where patients who may appear well, may present with a range of different infections. This can make some patients vulnerable to exposure to disease and/or infection other than their presenting problem. An example could be a pregnant woman attending for an antenatal check who sits next to a patient with chicken pox (varicella) in the waiting room.

Successful infection control involves five elements:

1. Applying basic infection control strategies
2. Adopting quality management practices
3. Developing effective work practices that prevent the transmission of infectious agent
4. Managing specific infectious agents
5. Identifying infection control strategies in specialised health care settings.

(Department of Health and Ageing 2004)

It is recommended that any policy for the prevention of infection is structured around these elements. It is likely that the practice nurse will be the staff member most appropriate to coordinate infection control activities within the practice, including the writing of an infection control plan or policy.

Basic infection control strategies

In order for all staff to understand their role in the prevention, identification and management of infections, practices are recommended to have an overall strategy or policy in this area. All practice staff need to be educated about their role in preventing infection. The RACGP Infection Control Standards for Office-based Practices (2006 p. 3) states 'education includes the teaching of the principles of infection control, the checking of competency by observation of a person competent to check, and ongoing auditing and education to staff requirements'.

In order to manage the prevention, identification and management of infections all staff require competency in hand hygiene, standard precautions, additional precautions, managing blood or body fluid exposure, principles of environmental cleaning and reprocessing medical equipment, and where to find information on other aspects of infection control in the practice (RACGP 2006).

Standard precautions

Standard precautions are work practices required to achieve a basic level of infection control and are recommended for the treatment and care of all patients. Standard precautions include:

- hand hygiene;
- personal protective equipment;
- aseptic technique;
- safe management of sharps and other clinical waste;
- environmental controls;

- support services such as waste disposal, laundry and cleaning services; and
- effective reprocessing reusable equipment and instruments and appropriate use of cleaning products.

(RACGP 2006)

Hand hygiene

Historically, hand hygiene practices have been poor due to the workload, lack of time, not being able to see bacteria, problems with skin irritation and poorly located sinks. Hand hygiene refers to any term applying to the use of soap and water or a antimicrobial agent to the surface of the hands. It has been identified as the *single most important strategy* in preventing health care associated infections and should not be restricted to medical and nursing staff, but to all people entering and working in a health care facility, such as administration staff. Hand Hygiene Australia recommends that health care workers practice hand hygiene:

- before touching a patient;
- immediately before a procedure;
- immediately after a procedure or body fluid exposure risk;
- after touching a patient;
- after touching objects in a patient's immediate surroundings when the patient has not been touched; and
- before and after glove use.

Naturally all personal hygiene should be observed and gloves are not a substitute for hand washing. Increasingly alcohol-based rubs have been identified as an alternative to hand washing and their effectiveness against most bacteria and many viruses is better than traditional soap and water. Alcohol-based rubs take 15–20 seconds to decontaminate hands, are less irritating to the hands and do not require the use of paper towels (Hand Hygiene Australia 2009).

Aseptic technique

Aseptic technique refers to the work practices used during clinical procedures to minimise the risk of introducing and transmitting infection. Aseptic technique is used during wound dressings, minor operative procedures and venipuncture. It is achieved by:

- using standard precautions, including hand hygiene and personal protective equipment where necessary;
- using barriers (for example, gloves);

- using of water or saline to clean ulcers or lacerations;
- using skin disinfectants to prepare operative sites;
- cleaning environmental surfaces;
- using the 'no touch' technique;
- using drapes to form a 'sterile field', depending on situation and risk;
- using sterile instruments and equipment; and
- reprocessing reusable instruments and other equipment between each patient.

As practice nurses are involved regularly in wound management and minor operative procedures, an understanding of aseptic technique is fundamental to the practice nurse role.

Maintaining cleanliness in the general practice

Routine cleaning of the practice environment must meet the standards as outlined by the RACGP infection control standards (RACGP 2006) to maintain a safe, clean and healthy environment for both staff and patients. This includes the scheduling of surface and environmental cleaning as well as unscheduled cleaning required after such events as blood and/or body fluid spills. Practices should have a documented cleaning schedule that utilised by cleaning as well as practice staff. If contract cleaners are used, a cleaning schedule agreement detailing the types of cleaning products to be used, what surfaces and equipment are to be cleaned, and the regularity of cleaning, for example, daily, weekly, etc. should be included in their contract.

Effective cleaning consists of a combination of the use of mechanical action, the correct cleaning product followed by a drying action. Currently, the accepted cleaning products are mildly alkaline clinical detergents (pH 8.0–10.8). Disinfectants are not a replacement for effective cleaning. All disinfectants have been shown to fail where prior cleaning is either nonexistent or ineffective (RACGP 2006). It is recommended as part of the standards that practices have a cleaning policy that outlines:

- occupational health and safety issues;
- what needs to be cleaned;
- products to be used;
- frequency and procedures for scheduled cleaning;
- procedure for unscheduled cleaning; and
- procedure for reporting cleaning problems.

Management of linen

There is little evidence to suggest that linen, if carefully handled, is responsible for risk of cross-infection (RACGP 2007).

Staff health and immunisation

Staff need to be immunised not only to protect themselves against infection but to ensure that they do not pass on infectious agents to patients. All practice staff are at an increased risk of exposure to some vaccine preventable diseases. All health care workers directly involved in patient care should be offered vaccinations against:

- hepatitis B;
- influenza (annually); and
- pertussis.

Depending on the context of the care provided or the practice population, consideration should be given to staff receiving a hepatitis A vaccination (National Health and Medical Research Council (NHMRC) 2009).

As public health issues are raised, the health of the practice staff should be considered and vaccines offered appropriately, for example, H1N1 2009 influenza vaccine in response to the H1N1 2009 influenza pandemic. Staff who are immunocompromised or pregnant are more susceptible to infection, and hence should seek medical advice regarding their immunisation. Sometimes redeploying the worker may be necessary if the condition has occurred subsequent to employment. Health professionals displaying signs and symptoms of an infectious disease (for example, varicella or measles) or a likely exposure to an emerging infectious disease should be excluded from work until they are no longer an infection risk.

Processing reusable equipment

When thinking about using disposable and/or reusable equipment, the issues of cost and efficacy is important. Some procedures allow choice in the equipment to be used, for example, a speculum for Pap smears, or mouthpiece for spirometry. It is a balance between the quality of the instrument and ability to perform the procedure accurately and efficiently. Some disposable vaginal speculums are very flimsy and hard to manage; however, they can be disposed of immediately after use. Alternatively, some disposable speculums are very easy to use and have the luxury of an attached light source but can be very expensive. Metal vaginal speculums need to be sterilised and can be uncomfortable for women but are cheaper to use. The advantages and disadvantages, such as initial cost, cost of sterilisation, ease of use and patient preference, should be considered by individual practice preference and health care provider preference.

The reuse of equipment requires a system that is able to monitor the cleaning, sterilisation and storage of equipment. Washing and drying of instruments, loading and unloading the steriliser and storage of instruments and equipment is generally included in the role of the nurse. It is an important part of controlling the spread of infection.

The sterilisation process involves pre-cleaning through to storage when processed and ready for reuse. It is important for a practice nurse to have a good understanding of their role in all stages of this process.

Single-use equipment

Single-use equipment has several advantages, including minimising the risk of cross-infection and reducing workload associated with onsite sterilisation. Single-use equipment should not be processed for reuse (RACGP 2006).

Adopting quality management practices

Infection control is a comprehensive area and thought needs to be given to multiple areas, including education for all staff, compliance with standards, health of employees, and the auditing of infection rates and hand hygiene.

To control transmission of infection in the workplace, it is necessary to identify hazards that may impact on transmission of infectious agents in your practice. After identifying possible sources of infection, risk management protocols and strategies to ensure clear communication should be developed. For example, a triage policy which is able to identify potential patients entering the practice with infections that are easily transmissible will reduce the risk of the spread of disease from patients in the waiting room. Furthermore, there are times when precautions other than what is usual may need to be taken.

Additional precautions

Additional precautions are used when a patient is known to be or suspected to be infected or colonised with microorganisms that cannot be contained by standard precautions alone. Additional precautions are always used in conjunction with standard precautions (RACGP 2006).

Additional precautions provide additional barriers and the type of precautions used will depend on the transmission route, for example, contact, droplet or airborne.

Additional precautions can include:

- additional immunisation;
- personal protective equipment; and
- additional cleaning.

Personal protective equipment

Personal protective equipment (PPE) refers to the use of gloves, water impermeable aprons or gowns, masks and protective goggles or face shields to minimise direct unprotected contact between staff and the patient. The types and degrees of protection depend on the situation and the risk, for example, gloves where there is a risk of blood or body fluid exposure, and goggles and aprons where there is a risk of splashing or spraying of blood or bodily fluid during procedures. Masks may be used when there is a risk of droplet spread of disease, for example, from influenza. P2 and N95 masks are designed to filter out very small particles such as tuberculosis and pandemic influenza virus. These masks need to be fitted correctly to be effective.

The correct processes to put on and take off PPE are outlined below:

Put on

1. Hand washing
2. Mask
3. Goggles
4. Long-sleeved gown tied securely at the back
5. Gloves held by the edge and covering the cuffs of the gown.

Take off

1. Gloves
2. Hand hygiene
3. Gown
4. Hand hygiene
5. Goggles
6. Hand hygiene

7.   Mask

8.   Hand hygiene.

All equipment must be removed without disturbing potential contaminate further and disposed of appropriately in the waste.

Management of exposure to blood and body fluid

The practice infection policy must also detail the management of blood and body fluids exposure through spills, needle stick injury and patients presenting with infectious diseases. The role of the practice nurse can be to develop the policy and ensure that all staff are familiar with the risk, the prevention strategies and the protocol if exposure occurs. Having a spills kit will ensure that equipment is available in the event of a spill.

Practices also need to prepare for possible widespread exposure to infectious diseases. The first step in this process is a robust triage process where patients are asked questions so that if they are experiencing symptoms that may indicate an infectious disease, they are isolated quickly and staff have access to PPE. By having a kit prepared containing the necessary equipment and located close to reception will ensure that patients with potential infectious disease are managed appropriately.

Management of sharps and other waste

According to the RACGP Infection Control Standards for Office-based Practice and the NHMRC national guidelines for waste management in the health care industry (NHMRC 1999) there are three categories of waste:

1. **Clinical waste**
    * Discarded sharps (surgical blades, needles, suture needles, glass vials)
    * Human tissue (but not hair, teeth, urine or faeces)
    * Materials or solutions containing expressible blood (that is, gauze soaked in blood)

2. **Related waste**
    * Pharmaceutical waste (expired drugs, cytotoxic drugs)

3. **General waste**
    * Includes all waste materials that do not fall into the categories of clinical waste or related waste (for example, tongue depressors, disposable vaginal speculums, wound dressings) that do not have expressible blood or body substances and cannot be accessed by children.

Storage of clinical wastes

The storage area should be clean and separate from clean stores. Clinical waste containers should:

- be provided in each area of the practice where clinical waste is generated;
- be lined with plastic bags marked with a black biohazard symbol;
- have a biohazard sign affixed to the outside;
- be emptied when full and/or at the end of each day; and
- be safely located away from the reach of children.

Before collection, clinical waste must be stored appropriately:

- The waste should be double bagged.
- The bagged waste should be stored securely, preferably inside a locked, leak-proof yellow bin labelled with a biohazard symbol. There should be no public access to this area.
- The outer bag for clinical waste must be yellow to identify the contents for appropriate disposal.

Collection and disposal of waste

The disposal of clinical waste is performed by licensed contractors and requires high-temperature incineration or special burial. The practice should contact their local council or environmental pollution agencies for compliance by-laws and state or territory laws regarding disposal. If the waste is disposed of by a contractor off-site, a contract with a certificate of disposal and a certificate to state that the contractor disposes of the waste in accordance with the Environment Protection Authority guidelines is required.

Preparing for newly emerging infections

Epidemic and new pandemic viral infections pose a serious threat worldwide. Several have occurred recently, including the current H1N1 pandemic influenza (WHO 2009) and the coronavirus (SARS) outbreak that caused severe acute respiratory syndrome (Shute 2003). General practice is where the community first turns when faced with a newly emerging infection, health concern or an unspecific disease, and the general practice waiting room is a potential source of infection spread (South Eastern Sydney Public Health Unit 2001).

In responding to a pandemic, general practices need to develop practice systems that provide safety for practice staff as well as the continuation of high-quality clinical care to patients. Pandemic preparedness of a practice, clinic or health centre requires careful consideration and planning across a wide range of contingencies. This will commence with the first patient with influenza-like symptoms presenting for an appointment, through to how an acutely unwell patient is managed while in isolation in their own home (Nori & Williams 2009).

General practice planning for a pandemic falls into four functional domains (RACGP 2009):

1. clinical care for influenza and non-influenza patients
2. engaging and working with public health authorities
3. the internal environment of general practice (physical and organisational)
4. integrating general practice planning across the entire health sector.

The response to the first wave of the H1N1 pandemic in 2009 demonstrated how a practice nurse can contribute to the management of patients during a pandemic. Ideally, each practice should have a pandemic plan in place prior to the onset of a pandemic. Such a plan should identify the types of patients most at risk, how the flow of these patients will occur and what measures will be needed to contain the spread of the virus. The assessments of symptoms and signs could, in the first instance, be performed by the patient at presentation. For example, a notice could be placed on the practice door requesting that all fever patients wear a mask before reporting at the reception and wait at the designated area. At these times, appropriate triaging by the practice nurse is essential. Adequate planning will ensure that there are sufficient stocks of protective clothing and equipment to enable the practice to function effectively. Many simple and low-cost interventions, such as hand washing, masks and gloves, and advice for patients, including social distancing greater than one metre and quarantine, are found to be effective in reducing the transmission of epidemic respiratory virus (Jefferson et al. 2009).

Identifying infection control strategies in specialised health care settings

General practice is a specialised context of health care and has many unique qualities. There are, however, fundamental issues which apply to all health care settings. In order to protect patients and staff, management has the duty to ensure the following:

● Take measures to prevent the spread of infection between staff and patients.
● Constantly maintain surveillance for infections that may spread.

- Ensure comprehensive documentation to communicate risk factors of all patients attending for health care.
- Maintain adequate facilities, including cleaning of the practice.
- Monitor and maintain the effectiveness of equipment.
- Provide education in hand hygiene to all staff.
- Maintain awareness and availability of vaccines that are available to protect all staff and maintain vaccination records.
- Maintain confidentiality of patient information.

It is the responsibility of all staff to ensure that they are aware of potential infection risks and have the skills to manage those risks so that the safety and wellbeing of patients and staff are guaranteed.

Reflections

What policies and procedures does your practice have in place to monitor and manage the risk of transmission of infectious agents?

Conclusion

Practice nurses are essential to the routine organisation and management of the clinical environment. Their presence ensures a high standard of patient care, including a well-structured clinical environment that promotes both holistic and financial rewards. Nurses working in general practice have the potential to be leaders in primary care; therefore, promotion, practice support and acknowledgement of their specific roles is vital to this evolving specialty.

Infection control is a broad term and covers many areas of the general practice environment and clinical processes. All health professionals and practice staff need to have a full understanding of the risks of acquiring and transmitting infectious diseases in the health setting. There is always on ongoing risk and it is important to return to the principles of infection control to evaluate and manage the risks well. Education and communication are important elements of any infection control risk management strategy. Nurses play a key role in being the lead in the practice to ensure that the delivery of care ensures no harm to patients or staff.

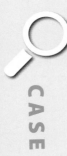

PANDEMIC PREPAREDNESS—ONE NURSE'S STORY

Name of nurse

Judy Evans, Registered Nurse Division 1

Many government agencies and health stakeholders had worked to prepare the Australian health sector for an influenza pandemic. There was no indication that a pandemic was imminent but it was expected that a pandemic was overdue and that Australia should prepare. Government planning, however, did not fully recognise the role that general practice would play in responding to such a public health outbreak. The Royal Australian College of General Practitioners (RACGP) saw this lack of engagement with general practice as a risk. Funding was granted to develop a pandemic resource kit for general practice. So, with great trepidation but enormous enthusiasm, I wrote my curriculum vitae, applied for the position and was the successful candidate. I was very excited and yet nervous with this opportunity to represent the nursing profession, work in partnership with general practitioners, and contribute to the education of general practice staff.

The expert reference group was appointed and included representation from Commonwealth and state governments, the Australian Practice Nurses Association, the Royal College of Nursing Australia, the Australian Association of Practice Managers, infection control specialists, general practitioners and key researchers in the area of pandemic planning. Little did we know that at the time of publication and dissemination of this kit we would be less than four months away from the H1N1 (2009) influenza pandemic.

My starting point was to consider my role as a practice nurse and write down the questions that I would want answered and how I could encourage clinical and non-clinical practice staff to be involved in the process of pandemic planning. The next step was a literature review to highlight what had been successful internationally, especially in relation to the recent SARS epidemic. I reviewed all the Australian Government plans and identified the gaps where general practice was not acknowledged as part of the response.

The RACGP Pandemic Flu Kit grew to become an eight-module education kit, and a workbook for practice staff to log the progress of developing their specific practice plan and the practice policies that supported it. Posters for the waiting room and treatment room were designed that demonstrated the use of surgical masks, PPE and how patients could self-identify if they had symptoms that could be infectious.

The kit was launched in December 2008, with a copy sent to every general practice in Australia. I was involved in radio and written media promoting the kit. When the news from Mexico indicated a swine influenza epidemic, and very soon after that cases were being reported in Victoria, Australia, the emergence of a pandemic was evident. By June 2009, the Australian PROTECT phase identified that this virus was mild for most but severe for many vulnerable groups. During this time the demand for up-to-date information was high and practice staff required prompt access to reliable information. Most of my days were spent dealing with the many practice enquiries.

To ensure that general practice was ready to cope with the surge of cases, and be fully aware of infection control issues in patient management and staff protection, I spent three busy weeks on a national road show armed with boxes of the pandemic kits, posters and demonstration packs of PPE to present to general practice health professionals in every state and territory in Australia. The roll out of the H1N1 vaccine and the use of multi-dose vials (MDV) required the development of guidelines and resources. These were developed through this project and would eventually be accepted and promoted by the Commonwealth as best practice when using multi-dose vials (MDVs). This process involved lengthy debate and consultation with governments and the general practice sector.

While on a personal trip to London I also was invited to speak with the Health Protection Agency for North East and North Central London, and represented the Australian response and risk management planning to a wide range of health professionals involved in the United Kingdom pandemic response.

As a practice nurse the opportunity to be involved in the early planning and then the implementation of a response to a public health alert has been invaluable. Through this process I have worked with key influencers at all levels of Commonwealth, state and territory governments, highly respected national and international researchers, and the media. However, the amazing nurses who have dealt with this pandemic at the frontline have been inspirational. To see the practical way that nurses set up fever clinics, and utilised available education and resources to manage hundreds of sick patients in any one day was inspiring. The pandemic has highlighted the vital role that nurses play in responding quickly, and with a high degree of skill, to public health alerts.

Key messages

Policies and procedures are a valuable tool in communicating roles and responsibilities of all staff.

An infection control policy will assist staff members in understanding their role in reducing the transmission of infectious agents.

Infection control is an important and essential part of safe, high quality care in general practice.

Infection control is every staff member's responsibility.

Useful resources

Feather, A, Stone, SP, Wessier, A, 2000, Boursicot, KA & Pratt, C 2000, "Now please wash your hands': the handwashing behaviour of final MBBS candidates', *Journal of Hospital Infection*, vol. 45, no. 1, pp. 62–4.

Hand Hygiene Australia
http://www.hha.org.au/

Health Emergency
http://www.healthemergency.gov.au/internet/healthemergency/publishing.nsf/Content/home-1

RACGP Pandemic Flu Kit
http://www.racgp.org.au

Royal Australian College of General Practitioners
http://www.racgp.org.au

Sondergaard, J, Vach, K, Kragstrup, J & Anderson, M 2009, 'Impact of pharmaceutical representative visits on GPs' drug preferences', *Family Practice*, vol. 26, no. 3, pp. 204–9.

World Health Organisation
http://www.who.int/en

Yeung, WKY, Tam, WWS & Wong, TW 2007, 'A review of the evidence for hand hygiene in different clinical and community settings for family physicians', *Hong Kong Practice*, vol. 29, part 4, pp. 157–63.

References

1.   Baird, A 2008, 'Emergency drugs in general practice', *Australian Family Physician*, vol. 37, no. 7, pp. 541–6, viewed 17 January 2010, <http://www.racgp.org.au/afp/200807/200807baird.pdf>.

2.   Department of Health and Ageing 2004, *Infection control guidelines for the prevention of infectious diseases in the healthcare setting*, viewed 20 January 2010, <http://www.health.gov.au/>.

3.   Griffiths, P, Renz, A, Hughes, J & Rafferty, A 2009, 'Impact of Organisation and management factors on infection control in hospitals: a scoping review', *Journal of Hospital Infection*, vol. 73, issue 1, pp. 1–14.

4.   Hand Hygiene Australia 2009, Grayson, L, Russo, P, Ryan, K, Bellis, K & Heard, K (eds.), *5 moments for hand hygiene*, viewed 20 January 2010, <http://www.hha.org.au/UserFiles/file/Manual/ManualJuly2009v2(Nov09).pdf>.

5.   Jefferson, T, Der Mar, C, Dooley, L, Ferroni, E, Lubna, A, Bawazeer, G, van Driel, M, Foxlee, R & Rivetti, A 2009, 'Physical intervention to interrupt or reduce the spread of respiratory virus: systemic review', *British Medical Journal*,

vol. 339, no. b3675, doi: 10.1136/bmj.b3675, viewed 17 January 2010, <http://www.bmj.com/>.

6. National Health and Medical Research Council (NHMRC) 1999, *National Guidelines for Waste Management in the Health Care Industry* (rescinded), viewed 19 January 2010, <http://www.nhmrc.gov.au/publications/synopses/eh11syn.htm>.

7. National Health and Medical Research Council (NHMRC) 2009, *The Australian Immunisation Handbook*, viewed 19 January 2010, <http://www.immunise.health.gov.au/internet/immunise/publishing.nsf/Content/handbook-home>.

8. Nori, A & Williams, M 2009, 'Pandemic preparedness—risk management and infection control for all respiratory infection outbreaks', *Australian Family Physician*, vol. 38, no. 11, pp. 891–5, viewed 20 January 2010, <http://www.racgp.org.au/>.

9. Phillips, CB, Pearce, CM, Dwan, KM, Hall, S, Porritt, J, Yates, R, Klijakovic, M & Sibbald, B 2008, *Charting new roles for Australian general practice nurses: a multicentre qualitative study*, abridged report, Australian Primary Care Research Institute, visited 17 January 2010, <http://www.anu.edu.au/aphcri/Domain/PracticeNursing/index.php>.

10. Royal Australian College of General Practitioners (RACGP) 2006, *Infection Control Standards for Office-based Practices*, 4th edn, RACGP, South Melbourne, viewed 20 January 2010, <http://www.racgp.org.au/>.

11. Royal Australian College of General Practitioners (RACGP) 2007, *Standards for General Practices*, 3rd edn, RACGP, South Melbourne, viewed 19 January 2010, <http://www.racgp.org.au/>.

12. The Royal Australian College of General Practitioners (RACGP) 2009, *The Pandemic flu kit 2009*, viewed 8 August 2009, <http://www.racgp.org.au/>.

13. Shute, N 2003, 'SARS hit home', *US News and World Report*, vol. 134, no. 15, pp. 38–42, 44.

14. South Eastern Sydney Public Health Unit 2001, 'Outbreak report: Measles cluster in south-eastern Sydney with transmission in a general practice waiting room', *Community Disease Intelligence*, vol. 25, no. 1, p.19, viewed 20 January 2010, <http://www.health.gov.au/internet/main/publishing.nsf/Content/cda-2001-cdi2501-pdf-cnt.htm/$FILE/cdi2501.pdf>.

15. Swinburne University of Technology 2009, *Swinburne Policies and Procedures: policy and procedure development tools*, viewed 19 January 2010, <http://www.swinburne.edu.au/corporate/registrar/ppd/tools.htm#4>.

16. World Health Organisation (WHO) 2009, *Global alert and response: pandemic (H1N1) 2009*, <http://www.who.int/csr/disease/swineflu/en/>.

Chapter ten

Promoting health in primary care

by Rhian Parker

Overview

This chapter will discuss the key concepts underpinning health promotion, describe health promoting strategies and identify areas where a nurse can contribute to these activities. It will discuss the role of prevention and examine some groups in our community that may require individual and specialised strategies to ensure access to effective health care delivery.

Objectives

At the completion of this chapter you should be able to:

- describe the key concepts and strategies that underpin health promotion in primary care setting;

- be aware of strategies for effectively communicating health promotion messages to patients;

- identify practice areas where preventive activities can be undertaken for specific conditions; and

- understand the challenges of health promotion and prevention for specific populations.

Introduction

The health reform agenda in Australia has put increased emphasis on preventing illness and promoting healthy lifestyles. It has also brought into focus the fact that, although most chronic conditions are preventable, the health system still focuses on treatment rather than prevention with only 2% of the health budget being allocated to prevention (Harris & Mortimer 2008). The burden of disease from preventable conditions is costly in health consequences for the population and in health expenditure for the health system (Australian Government Preventive Health Taskforce 2009).

General practice is in an ideal position to support the current health reform agenda and deliver prevention activities to the Australian population. Many of the activities currently undertaken in general practice are preventative activities, in particular, screening for specific conditions. However, nurses in general practice can play a wider role in supporting these preventative activities and in offering other health promotion services to their patients.

Principles of health promotion

In 1946 the World Health Organisation (WHO) defined health as 'a state of complete physical, mental and social well-being rather than a mere absence of disease or infirmity' (WHO 1946, p. 1). This definition provides an underpinning to health promotion principles and practice. Health is seen as more than an absence of specific conditions or diseases but is related to the social, behavioural, economic and environmental conditions that contribute to health and illness. Social and economic disadvantage impact on where we live, how we live and whether we have equitable access to the services we need at a cost that we can afford. On average, a girl born in Australia today can expect to live to 80 years. However, in other countries her life expectancy could be under 45 years (WHO 2008a).

The WHO defines health promotion as a process that facilitates people taking control over their health and its determinants and, as a consequence of this, improving their health. It further identifies that health promotion is guided by the following principles:

- Health as a fundamental human right and sound social investment;
- Equity and social justice in health promotion;
- Social responsibility of the public and private sectors in promoting health;
- Partnerships, networking and alliance building for health;
- Individual and community participation as a prerequisite;
- The individual has a social responsibility over their own health;
- Empowerment of the individual and communities for health promotion;
- Development of infrastructure for health promotion;
- Integration of health promotion activities across sectors;
- Professional ethics and standards.

Health and promoting good health is not just the responsibility of the health system but of an integrated community sector and government policies which support the promotion of healthy lifestyles. However, an individual's opportunity to live a healthy life is governed by their access to adequate income, healthy foods, sanitation and education. As already mentioned, an individual's health is, to some extent, socially determined. Although we are relatively affluent in Australia compared to other countries in the world, our health and wellbeing are still determined by where we were born, what our income is, what access we have to nutritious food and health services and how much education we have. The World Health Organisation states that '...there is now ample documentation—not available 30 years ago—of considerable and often growing health inequalities within countries' (World Health Organisation 2008b.) So, despite the fact that Australia is an affluent country, not everyone has equal access to care or to the resources to maintain good health.

Health professionals, including practice nurses, need to consider all these factors if they are to successfully fulfil their role in health promotion. They also need to think about what health promotion requirements their particular patient population needs given the socio-demographic profile of the area their practice serves.

Health promotion can take place at three different levels:

1. individual level
2. community level
3. state or country level.

Health promotion principles and health professionals address health issues by doing things *with* people and not on their behalf. A key feature of health promotion is that people take control over conditions that affect their health and wellbeing. Systematic health promotion practice should have empowerment, principles of social justice and equity, inclusion and respect at its heart.

There are a number of elements that contribute to effective health promotion:

- health communication
- health education
- self-help
- community engagement
- policy development.

Although practice nurses may not be familiar with all these elements in detail, it is important to recognise that each of the elements will have an impact on the role of the practice nurse, at an individual and practice level, and at a national and professional or organisational level.

Reflections

How do you think these elements of effective health promotion affect your role in promoting health to patients in your practice?

Health communication

Health messages are often communicated to us through the media, through government-sponsored campaigns and through pamphlets and posters produced by not-for-profit organisations. These messages aim to point out the benefits of certain behaviours and the risks of other behaviours. Many such pamphlets and posters are available for general practice and other primary care organisations. In particular, pamphlets and posters promoting recommended

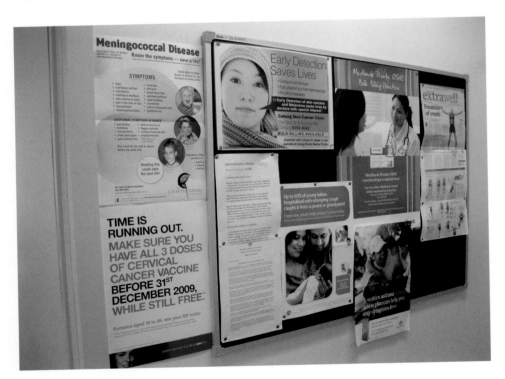

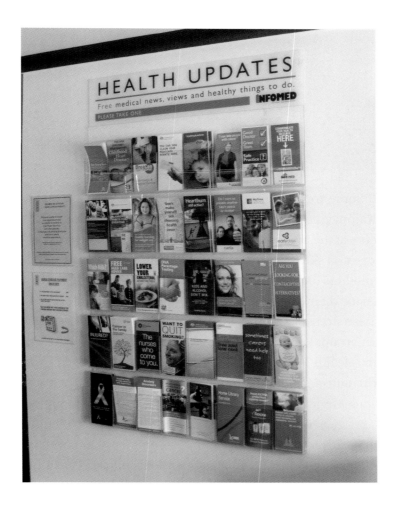

daily intakes of fruit and vegetables are often available in health centres and clinics as are pamphlets about screening programs.

The nurse working in general practice is in an ideal position to identify what significant health issues are current in their communities and practice populations. There is good evidence to show that nurses communicate well with patients at an individual level (Keleher et al. 2009) and once having identified the health issues in the practice population, the nurse can then endeavour to provide clear and reliable health information

Health education

Health education describes strategies to improve health literacy, improve knowledge about health and healthy lifestyles for the community and the

Look at some of the publications available in your workplace. Choose one that is about prevention, one that encourages screening participation and one that is about treatment. Which of these publications is aimed at the public and which is for health professionals? How effective do you think they are at informing these two groups?

individual. Some form of communication is required to do this but, unlike the larger campaigns mentioned earlier which are population based, these are targeted more at the individual or small group and focus on more specific level of knowledge and skill development. For instance, sessions provided to young expectant mothers on the care of babies or to people with type 2 diabetes about how to manage their condition.

Often these strategies require skill development and knowledge acquisition in the target group. Participants in these groups often learn from and support each other. Health education can also be learner-directed where people seek information and knowledge about specific issues that concern them. Opportunities are available for practice nurses to facilitate group education in general practice, either providing education themselves or sourcing other specialised health professionals. With the emphasis on multidisciplinary care in the report of the National Health and Hospitals Reform Commission (NHHRC 2009), nurses will more often be required to work with a range of health professionals to provide care to patients.

Self-help

Self-help groups are run by group members and focus on the concerns of the group. These groups are usually established by professionals such as a nurse. For instance, support groups for people with arthritis or who have suffered a stroke. Family and carers can also be involved in these groups. It is important that groups such as these have the support of community or health organisations so that they are sustainable; however, they do not always need the input of a professional once they are well established. An innovative example has seen a practice nurse commence a walking group as a means of encouraging patients to exercise as well as decreasing social isolation (Medical Observer 2009).

Community engagement

Working with the community to help in the process of identifying and addressing their particular health concerns is an important health promotion strategy. Significant health promotion documents and charters, such as the Ottawa Charter (WHO 1986), stress the importance of community involvement in the development of health promotion initiatives. The definition of 'community' can be as *broad* as the town or area you live in or it can be more *specific* and focus on people from the same ethnic background, the same religious beliefs, the same sexual orientation, or shared interests. The most important characteristics of a 'community' are that members feel they belong to that particular group and have something in common with the group.

Empowering communities to take control over their own health and wellbeing is a cornerstone of community development. For example, promoting healthy eating in a refugee population may encourage the pooling of resources to buy fresh fruit and vegetables in bulk which could also improve community engagement across other areas of significance to that community. It is important for the practice nurse to know the composition of their communities including marginalised groups. Knowing which community services are available to assist these groups is essential so that appropriate referrals can be made to assist patients becoming involved in and taking responsibility for their own care.

Reflections

What marginalised groups exist in your community? How does your practice meet their needs?

Policy development

Healthy public policy includes legislation, taxation and financial measures that are developed and implemented by governments to promote the health of individuals and communities to help people adopt healthy lifestyles, discourage people from adopting unhealthy practices, and create healthy physical and social environments. For policy development to be successful, the population needs to be aware of the activities that policy aims to address and the health consequences of those activities, and to be supportive of change. For example, smoking has had significant policy intervention over the past two decades with smoking advertising being banned, smoking in public places limited and taxes on cigarettes increased. Often there needs to be a range of policies developed to address one issue, therefore, policies need to be developed and implemented across different levels of government.

> ### Reflections
>
> *Think of health promotion strategies in your community that focus on the individual and, more broadly, the policies at community level. Do you think that primary care provides health promotion 'beyond its responsibility for providing clinical and curative services'?*

Health promotion in primary care

In order to work effectively in promoting health and preventing illness, primary care practitioners need to understand the underpinnings of health promotion. However, they also need to appreciate that directing people as to what they should do or what's good for them isn't likely to succeed. Health professionals need to work *with* patients to improve their health and address unhealthy behaviours thus empowering people to make sensible and well-informed choices about their health.

Fundamentally there are broadly three types of prevention:

1. **Primary prevention**—avoiding disease by reducing susceptibility or controlling risk factors which includes immunisation, encouraging a healthy diet and adequate exercise and avoiding risky behaviours

2. **Secondary prevention**—avoiding irreversible damage through early detection and therapy, which includes screening and health checks

3. **Tertiary prevention**—avoiding complications, disability or dependence in irreversible states, such as type 2 diabetes.

Clarification of these types of prevention is necessary because different strategies may be adopted to achieve appropriate disease prevention. Nurses working in general practice have many opportunities to be involved in both primary and secondary prevention but probably less so in tertiary prevention.

Primary prevention

Nurses are at the forefront of providing timely immunisation in primary care. Australia's vaccination coverage is high, particularly for children, and outbreaks of many common childhood diseases are now relatively rare, although they do exist. Australia's Indigenous community has a lower immunisation rate than the total Australia population and nurses have a role to play in helping to improve these rates. The development of new vaccines, such as the HPV vaccine which immunises against strains of the human papilloma virus and helps protect against development of cervical cancer, means that the transmission of the virus can be controlled. (More details on immunisation are provided in Chapter 8.)

Other primary prevention activities aim to help patients stop risk-taking behaviours that have the potential to cause disease and have long-term adverse consequences on their health. Here, we will deal briefly with three of these behaviours: alcohol consumption, smoking, and overweight and obesity.

Alcohol consumption

The Australian Institute of Health and Welfare (AIHW 2008a) reports that the most significant health risks for Australians are smoking, high blood pressure and being overweight. Four per cent of the worldwide global burden of disease is attributable to alcohol. This accounts for almost as much death and disability as tobacco and hypertension (Kaplan 2004). According to the National Alcohol Strategy 2006–09, more than 3000 people die every year in Australia from alcohol abuse and 72 000 are hospitalised (Ministerial Council on Drug Strategy 2006). The annual cost to the Australian community is $7.6 billion. The strategy was developed as a response to the patterns of high-risk alcohol consumption that are prevalent in Australia.

Alcohol consumption guidelines (National Health and Medical Research Council 2009) recommend Australian men should limit their consumption of a maximum of four standard drinks of alcohol per day (28 per week). They also recommend Australian women should limit their consumption to two standard drinks per day (14 per week).

Asking patients about alcohol consumption can be sensitive and patients can react defensively, so it is important to be non-judgmental. Brief interventions to reduce alcohol consumption should be offered to all patients drinking at potentially risky or high-risk levels. Education concerning the link between drinking and health problems should be made. From 14 years of age, at three-yearly intervals it is recommended that patients be asked about the quantity and frequency of alcohol intake and number of alcohol-free days they have each week. Reassessment of alcohol consumption in at risk groups, such as pregnant women, and patients with hypertension, liver disease or mental health problems, is recommended yearly.

Smoking

Smoking is the risk factor responsible for the greatest burden of preventable disease in Australia, accounting for 12% of the burden in males and 7% in females, with an increased burden among low socioeconomic status groups. It is estimated that smoking kills at least half of long-term users (Peto et al. 2006). Evidence of the carcinogenic properties of tobacco smoking was apparent in the 1950s when the link between smoking and death and disease was established (Cancer Council Australia 2007).

By 2004 there was sufficient evidence to infer a causal relationship between smoking and cancer of the:

* bladder;
* cervix;
* kidney;
* larynx;
* oesophagus;
* oral cavity and pharynx;
* pancreas;
* stomach; and
* acute myeloid leukaemia.

In Australia, tobacco smoking kills around 15 500 Australians every year (Cancer Council Australia 2007). Each year more Australians are killed by tobacco than by breast cancer, AIDS, traffic and other accidents, and murders and suicides combined. As primary care providers, practice nurses have a role to play in educating patients on the detrimental effects of smoking and assisting them to undergo strategies to adopt healthier lifestyles.

Smoking cessation

Although levels of smoking in Australia continue to decline, smoking is far more common among people in lower socioeconomic groups and among

Indigenous Australians (Australian Institute of Health and Welfare 2008a). One model that has been investigated to assess whether smokers are ready to quit smoking is the Readiness to change model (Zimmerman, Olsen & Bosworth 2000). This model categorises smokers into five groups by increasing readiness to change: pre-contemplators, contemplators, determination, action and maintenance. This model can predict when people are ready to stop smoking and when they are not. The Royal Australian College of General Practitioners (RACGP 2004) provides succinct information for practitioners about smoking cessation pharmacotherapy and outlines the readiness to change model. This model is explained in Chapter 16.

A strategy that is complementary to the readiness to change model is motivational interviewing. Motivational interviewing can be utilised as a strategy for other risk behaviours, such as hazardous alcohol use, and for supporting patients who want to lose weight. In motivational interviewing, the patient needs to recognise their current situation, and the practitioner needs to align themselves with the patient's view and work with them to create change.

There are five main motivational interviewing skills. These are:

1. Asking open-ended questions
2. Practicing reflective listening
3. Eliciting self-motivational statements
4. Affirming client effort
5. Provide summary statements.

Again, more information on key aspects of motivational interviewing can be found in Chapter 16.

There is some evidence to show that nurses can motivate smokers to quit (Rice & Stead 2008). Knowledge of the above techniques can assist practice nurses in targeting smokers for smoking cessation counselling or referral to other organisations such as QUIT.

Overweight and obesity

The AIHW reports that 7.4 million adult Australians were overweight in 2004–05, and of these, one-third were obese. There are two ways in which overweight and obesity are measured—body mass index (BMI) and waist circumference (AIHW 2008a).

BMI is a measure of body fat that is based on the height and the weight of a person. The following BMI figures indicate if a person is of healthy weight:

- underweight = <18.5
- normal weight = 18.5–24.9
- overweight = 25–29.9
- obese = BMI of 30 or greater.

There are limitations to this measure and these include overestimating body fat in people who have a muscular build, for example, athletes. Waist circumference is another measure that can indicate if a person is at higher risk of type 2 diabetes, hypertension and cardiovascular disease. A waist circumference of more than 102 cm in men and more than 88 cm in women increases the risk of these conditions. Indeed, a large waist circumference has been shown to have health-related risks among both overweight and normal weight people.

Despite the prevalence of overweight and obesity, there is limited evidence of the effectiveness of interventions. Warin et al. (2008) suggest that this may be due, in part, to the fact that existing approaches to obesity management fail to take into account the gender and class-based experiences of those who are overweight and obese and how these factors contribute to individual notions of embodiment. Thus, universal health promotion messages are ineffective in addressing the issues that are part of the everyday lives of those most likely to be overweight and obese. These issues include food insecurity, beliefs about food and eating, poverty and educational disadvantage.

Cochrane database reviews of interventions designed to improve patients' knowledge and skills to manage chronic disease, with particular reference to nursing contribution and practice (Summerbell et al. 2003; Rice & Stead 2008), found that nurses were involved in 77% of these interventions. Educational programs have definite benefits for patients suffering from asthma and are promising for interventions in areas such as diabetes mellitus, epilepsy and mental health. Unfortunately, what the active ingredients of many successful interventions are remains unclear (Coster & Norman 2009).

Current policy in Australia regarding weight is focused on children and young people, and overweight and physical activity (National Obesity Taskforce 2008). This policy aims to support healthy eating and healthy weight in the home and in a wider community context. Whilst the policy does not explicitly mention this, it is mothers who are at the core of this strategy as they are generally actively engaged in the nutrition of their children. It is, therefore, crucial to understand the understanding these women have of good nutrition if we are to develop health promotion programs that address their needs and, in turn, the needs of their children. Conducting the Healthy Kids Check is one opportunity that practice nurses can use to discuss childhood eating patterns and weight with parents and their children. This will be covered in Chapter 12.

What works in obesity prevention?

Harvey et al. (2002) state that '...there are few solid leads about improving obesity management, although reminder systems, brief training interventions, shared care, inpatient care and dietitian-led treatments may all be worth further investigation'.

Whilst the cause of obesity is fairly simple to identify, that is, we take in too many kilojoules and don't expend enough energy, the solutions are complex. For instance, given the complex range of factors that are resulting in overweight children, it is not surprising that interventions, even when they target a range of obesity promoting behaviours, have a limited effect (Summerbell et al. 2003).

Thus, the impact of a single program of prevention activity is very likely to be swamped by a multitude of other factors. For instance, if a school intervention promotes eating fruit and vegetables then this must be supported in other areas of the child's life. Using consultations, such as those for immunisations, may also provide the practice nurse with an opportunity to reinforce the messages delivered by broader widespread health promotion strategies.

Although not replicated in Australia, an example of a successful nurse-led primary care program for weight management was implemented in the United Kingdom in 2004—the Counterweight Programme (Counterweight Project Team 2005). This model takes a whole of practice approach in recruiting patients who are obese (Counterweight Project Team 2004). The intervention is nurse-led, and practice nurses are trained and educated in providing support, counselling, and nutrition and exercise information to engage the patients in weight management. A moderate amount of weight loss, 5–10% of weight, significantly reduces physical complications, such as joint pain, and results in clinical improvements, such as reductions in blood pressure and blood lipid levels (Counterweight Project Team 2008a). The Counterweight Programme outcomes include an achievement and maintenance of weight loss within a primary care setting (Counterweight Project Team 2008b).

For delivering health promotion in primary care, the practice nurse will be able to contribute to patient outcomes by:

- looking beyond the individual to aspects of environment that support the development of overweight;
- conducting intervention and commitment at every level of society; and
- providing strategies for the targeted population as a whole but emphasising those groups most at risk of being overweight.

Although it is the individual who will gain weight, a huge range of factors is brought to bear on the individual's diet and activity patterns. Some in society are far better placed to modify these influences than others and the most at risk of obesity are those who are most disadvantaged socially.

Physical activity and obesity prevention

Physical inactivity is responsible for 7% of the total burden of disease and accounts for approximately 8000 deaths in Australia per year. It is an important risk factor for overweight, obesity and many chronic diseases. Physical fitness reflects cardiovascular endurance, strength and mobility that results from a variety of factors including physical activity (RACGP 2004). The benefits of physical activity are numerous and practice nurses can incorporate this health message into numerous aspects of their work.

Reflections

How does your practice team incorporate health messages regard smoking, alcohol consumption, overweight and obesity, and physical activity into their respective roles?

Secondary prevention

Nurses in general practice are increasingly becoming involved in screening for disease and in assessment of patient health status. There are various ways screening can be undertaken:

- Opportunistically—when patients present with another medical condition
- Anticipatory—through using recall and reminder systems; for example, for Pap tests

- Proactively—that is, targeting high-risk individuals, such as those who have family history of certain conditions.

Communication and information technology systems in general practice which are able to easily identify patients suitable for screening are becoming the domain of the practice nurse. As new initiatives become available to support prevention, such as bowel screening and standard health assessments, practice nurses are learning to integrate clinical knowledge of disease and preventive health messages by using a systems approach to prevention. Practice nurses in Australia are closely involved in the maintenance of recall and reminder systems in their practices and this is an important role in supporting preventive activities in general practice.

Screening

A screening test is a procedure (history, examination and/or a test) that is performed to detect the presence of a specific disease. Any population-based screening program needs to be:

- safe, simple to administer and acceptable to patients;
- have clear guidelines and management protocols;
- effective in preventing the development of disease or detecting disease and, therefore, improving morbidity and mortality; and
- cost effective.

In the process of screening patients for disease, health professionals are offered an opportunity to deliver key health messages for disease prevention. The practice nurse is well placed to become involved in practice screening programs on a systematic level.

However, screening can also have unintended consequences including creating anxiety in patients and being costly for the community if guidelines for screening are not adhered to. In all screening activities the benefits must always outweigh the harm. All people undergoing screening tests should be made aware of any costs, limitations and risks involved.

Examples of national screening programs include:

- breast screening;
- cervical screening; and
- bowel screening.

Breast and cervical screening will be covered in Chapter 13. Bowel cancer is the most common and potentially fatal cancer in Australians and is expected to increase in incidence by more than 30% over the next five to ten years as our population ages. Population-based screening for bowel cancer, currently being introduced in Australia, is expected to reduce mortality by 30–40% in the screened population (AIHW 2008b). Its aim is to detect abnormalities at an early stage and, where cancer has developed, to detect it early in order to maximise the effectiveness of treatment.

Because bowel cancer is associated with modifiable (lifestyle) risk factors, practice nurses can contribute significantly to the identification and education of patients in need of lifestyle modification.

Reflections

How does your practice promote existing screening programs and what other screening can practice nurses initiate or contribute to?

Health promotion and specific populations

Certain population groups present specific challenges. They are difficult to reach but have specific and often predictable health promotion needs. These groups include:

- young people
- people from culturally and linguistically diverse backgrounds
- Aboriginal and Torres Strait Islanders
- refugees.

Health promotion with adolescents

Adolescence is a time of experimentation and risk taking, in particular, young people experiment with smoking, drinking and drug use and have unprotected sex. Suicide is the leading cause of death for Australian young people (Patton et al. 2009). Young men living in rural and remote areas are at particular risk as are young people from Indigenous communities. Despite this, the evidence suggests that young people are often reluctant to access general practice care because of concerns about confidentiality and cost, and because general practices are often not 'youth friendly' (Sanci, Kang & Ferguson 2005).

The World Health Organisation has developed a framework for the development of youth-friendly health services (WHO 2001). The framework states that services need to be equitable, accessible, acceptable and appropriate. For nurses in general practice to be effective in health promotion to young people, some of these key barriers need to be addressed. In particular, young people need to:

- be assured of confidentiality at all times;
- be given enough time in a consultation;
- be communicated with appropriately;
- not feel judged; and
- be involved in any decision about their health.

Many of these are more difficult to implement in the business of general practice and they have to be seen from the young person's perspective. The developmental stages of adolescents vary significantly and this must be taken into account when discussing health issues. Keep in mind that adolescents do not have the experience of adults that allows them to understand how the health system works or how to engage with a practitioner in shared decision making.

Example 10.1

Tamara (aged 16) comes into the surgery at 5.30 p.m. on a Friday evening. She doesn't have an appointment but wants to see a doctor. There is no doctor on duty. Tamara seems very upset. You walk into the reception area and agree to speak to her and you take her into a consulting room. It transpires that Tamara thinks she is pregnant but refuses to say more.

> How would you as a practice nurse deal with this situation?
> How would you explain Tamara's options to her?
> Do you think that other girls like Tamara would feel comfortable in attending your practice for advice about their health?
> How could you make your practice more youth friendly?

People from culturally and linguistically diverse backgrounds

The Australian population is one of the most culturally diverse in the world. Nearly one quarter of the Australian population was born overseas

(AIHW 2008a) and more than 60% of these were born in non-English speaking countries.

Migrants to Australia are usually as healthy as other non-Indigenous Australians, except for refugees. Refugees tend to 'have a high rate of long-term physical and psychological problems, due in large part to their exposure to conflict and oppression' (RACGP 2009, p. 3) and also to their experience as dispossessed refugees. The Royal Australian College of General Practitioners has developed guidelines on refugee health.

For some migrant populations there are particular barriers to accessing health care. These include religious, cultural and linguistic barriers, to name a few. For instance, Muslim women may be very reluctant to see a male health practitioner and may need to have a husband or other relatives present at a medical appointment. The health literacy of these populations is often poor, in particular, their understanding of how the Australian health care system works, and how the health system can help promote wellness and not just treat illness.

Female nurses can play an important role in explaining to these women how the health system works, how to access it and gain consent for screening (performing Pap tests if trained) and other preventive health checks, such as breast health and blood pressure monitoring.

Conclusion

Nurses have a significant role to play in health promotion and preventative activities in general practice. The national health agenda is moving towards more prevention (NHHRC 2009) and encouraging Australians to be more concerned with their health and wellbeing. Good communication skills, reflective listening and an understanding of motivational interviewing principles are a prerequisite of supporting patients in behaviour change. Developing relationship-centred care will enable you as a nurse to partner with your patients and support them in healthy behaviours and in maintaining good health across their lifecycle.

Name of nurse
Jenny Donaldson

Practice
Family Medical Centre, Melbourne, Vic.

Family Medical Centre is a medium-sized clinic in outer metropolitan Melbourne, Victoria. A nurse-led service was introduced to assist in reducing the burden of smoking-related conditions on our patients' health as there was no other service of this kind in the area.

AIM

The primary aim of this service was to ensure that all patients would have their current smoking status recorded on their file so that they could be recognised as benefiting from smoking cessation counselling. Smoking cessation was seen by the practice as a priority in the management of chronic illnesses present in those patients identified as smokers. It was agreed that in order to reduce numbers of smokers in the practice, all staff including general practitioners would participate in this project and referrals would be made to the practice nurse leading the clinic. GPs in particular were asked to assess the patient's smoking status at each consultation and, recognising that they may not have time to address this, they were encouraged to refer the patient to the nurse.

NURSE ROLE

As well as providing counselling, Jenny's role included marketing this service by developing invitation templates, advertising, speaking to local groups, making sure that brochures and flyers were available in the waiting room and creating a smokers' register in the practice. Jenny also advised and educated other staff, including GPs, other nurses, reception staff and allied health staff that were employed by the practice, and any medical and nursing students that undertook placement in the practice.

One of Jenny's main roles was to offer patient appointments, follow up non-attenders and generally offer face-to-face or telephone support and encouragement to those patients wishing to embark on a 'Quit' smoking attempt. It was stressed to the patients that planning their quitting and identifying trigger times were important parts of this process.

TEAM APPROACH

GPs were asked to update the patient's smoking status in their history at each visit and were encouraged to follow the 5A's framework for counselling patients. Reception staff were asked to hand out a smoking questionnaire to each new patient to the program, to be filled in while they were in the waiting room. Specific 'Quit' appointment times were allocated to this service to allow adequate time and the privacy required. All staff had access to promotional material to inform patients of the service.

BENEFITS

The patient benefits of this service included a program tailored to suit each patient's individual goals, and follow-up by a familiar staff member for 12 months to track long-term results. The practice became known within the area as a place to seek preventative health advice, including smoking cessation assistance, and attracted patients from outside our usual patient population. It also established better links with other health providers such as the local community health centre and Quit Victoria. Delivering education sessions in collaboration with Quit Victoria was beneficial as was the data that Quit collected regularly on numbers of patients enrolling in the program.

FUNDING

Several methods were tried with one of them being an out-of-pocket payment from the patient. We finally settled on a practice nurse/GP consultation with the client, and the patient was subsequently bulk billed. Having a payment attached to the service did not seem to restrict patient's access to this service.

Testimonial

The service became a source of immense job satisfaction for me, as I was able to run it autonomously, undertake continuous professional development and expand my scope of practice. Working with Quit Victoria to support other practice nurses in this role has also been a worthwhile experience. Above all though, the comments and support from the patients themselves about the positive health outcomes achieved have been a major incentive to continue and expand this service.

Key messages

Health promotion is undertaken at different levels.

Different population groups should be targeted for delivery of key health messages.

Practice nurses have many opportunities to promote key health messages to patients in their practice and communities.

Useful resources

Caring for refugee patients in general practice
  http://www.racgp.org/

Putting prevention into practice (The Green Book) 2nd edition 2006
  http://www.racgp.org.au/

Guidelines for preventive activities in general practice (The Red Book)
  7th edition 2009
  http://www.racgp.org.au/

Australian guidelines to reduce health risks from drinking alcohol
  http://www.nhmrc.gov.au/

Nutrition and physical activity guidelines
  http://www.health.gov.au/

References

1.   Australian Government Preventative Health Taskforce 2009, *Australia: the Healthiest Country by 2020. National Preventative Health Strategy—the roadmap for action*, Department of Health and Ageing, viewed 19 January 2010, <http://www.preventativehealth.org.au/>.

2.   Australian Institute of Health and Welfare (AIHW) 2008a, *Australia's Health 2008*, AIHW, Canberra, viewed 19 January 2010, <http://www.aihw.gov.au/>.

3.   Australian Institute of Health and Welfare (AIHM) 2008b, *National Bowel Cancer Screening Program monitoring report 2008*, AIHW, Canberra.

4.   Cancer Council Australia 2007, *National Cancer Prevention Policy 2007–09*, Cancer Council Australia; viewed 20 January 2010, <http://www.cancer.org.au/>.

5.   Coster, S & Norman, I 2009, 'Cochrane reviews of educational and self-management interventions to guide nursing practice: a review', *International Journal of Nursing Studies*, vol. 46, no. 4, pp. 508–28.

6.   Counterweight Project Team 2004, 'A new evidence-based model for weight management in primary care: the Counterweight programme', *Journal of Human Nutrition and Dietetics*, vol. 17, no. 3, pp. 191–208.

7.   Counterweight Project Team 2005, 'Empowering primary care to tackle the obesity epidemic: the Counterweight programme', *European Journal of Clinical Nutrition*, vol. 59 (Suppl. 1), S93–S101.

8.   Counterweight Project Team 2008a, 'Prevalence of CVD risk factors by body mass index and the impact of 10% weight change', *Obesity Research & Clinical Practice*, vol. 2, pp. 15–27.

9.   Counterweight Project Team 2008b, 'Evaluation of the Counterweight programme for obesity management in primary care: a starting point for continuous improvement', *British Journal of General Practice*, vol. 58, no. 553, pp. 548–54.

10. Harris, A, & Mortimer, D 2008, *Preventative Priorities Advisory Committee and Prevention Benefits Schedule for Australia*, options paper prepared for The National Health and Hospitals Reform Commission, Centre for Health Economics, Monash University, Melbourne.

11. Harvey, EL, Glenny, AM, Kirk, SFL & Summerbell, CD 2002, 'An updated systematic review of interventions to improve health professionals' management of obesity', *Obesity Reviews*, vol. 3, issue 1, pp. 45–55.

12. Kaplan, W 2004, *Alcohol Use Disorders: Alcoholic Liver Diseases and Alcohol Dependency. Opportunities to Address Pharmaceutical Gaps*, World Health Organisation, Geneva.

13. Keleher, H, Parker, R, Abdulwadud, O & Francis, K 2009, 'The effectiveness of primary and community care nursing in primary care settings. A systematic literature review', *International Journal of Nursing Practice*, vol. 15, issue 1, pp. 16–24.

14. Medical Observer 2009, Practice Nurse, website, viewed 20 January 2010, <http://www.medicalobserver.com.au/PracticeNurse/>.

15. Ministerial Council on Drug Strategy 2006, *National Alcohol Strategy 2006–2009*, Department of Health and Ageing, viewed 20 January 2010, <http://www.alcohol.gov.au/internet/alcohol/publishing.nsf/content/nas-06-09>.

16. National Health and Hospitals Reform Commission (NHHRC) 2009, *A Healthier Future for all Australians*: final report of the National Health and Hospitals Reform Commission, Department of Health and Ageing, viewed 20 January 2010, <http://www.nhhrc.org.au/>.

17. National Health and Medical Research Council (NHMRC) 2009, *Australian Guidelines to Reduce Health Risks from Drinking Alcohol*, DS10, viewed 20 January 2010, <http://www.nhmrc.org.au/>.

18. National Obesity Taskforce 2008, *Healthy Weight 2008: Australia's Future. The National Action Agenda for Children and Young People and their Families*, Department of Health and Ageing.

19. Patton, GC, Coffey, C, Sawyer, SM, Viner, RM, Haller, DM, Bose, K, Vos, T, Ferguson, J & Mathers, CD 2009, 'Global patterns of mortality in young people: a systematic analysis of population health data', *The Lancet*; vol. 374, no. 9693, pp. 881–92.

20. Peto, R, Lopez AD, Boreham J & Thun, M 2006, *Mortality from smoking in developed countries 1950–2000'*, 2nd edn, viewed 20 January 2010, <http://www.deathfromsmoking.net/>.

21. Rice, VH & Stead, LF 2008, *Nursing interventions for smoking cessation*, Cochrane Database of Systematic Reviews 2008, issue 1, art. no. CD001188, doi: 10.1002/14651858.CD001188.pub3.

22. Royal Australian College of General Practitioners (RACGP) 2004, *Smoking, Nutrition, Alcohol and Physical activity (SNAP): a population health guide to behavioural risk factors in general practice*, Royal Australian College of General Practitioners, Melbourne.

23. Royal Australian College of General Practitioners (RACGP) 2009, *Caring for refugee patients in general practice*, p. 3, 2nd edn, Royal Australian College of General Practitioners, Melbourne.

24. Sanci, LA, Kang, M & Ferguson, BJ 2005, 'Improving adolescents' access to primary health care', *Medical Journal of Australia*, vol. 183, no. 8, pp. 416–17.

25. Summerbell, CD, Ashton, V, Campbell, KJ, Edmunds, L & Kelly S EW 2003, *Interventions for treating obesity in children*, Cochrane Database of Systematic Reviews, issue 1, art. no. CD001872, doi: 10.1002/14651858.CD001872.pub23.

26. Warin, M, Turner, K, Moore, V & Davies, M 2008, 'Bodies, mothers and identities: rethinking obesity and the BMI', *Sociology of Health and Illness*, vol.30, no. 1, pp. 97–111.

27. World Health Organisation (WHO) 1946, *Constitution of the World Health Organisation*, p. 1, WHO, Geneva.

28. World Health Organisation (WHO) 1986, 'Ottawa charter for health promotion', *American Journal of Health Promotion*, vol. 1, pp. 1–4.

29. World Health Organisation (WHO) 2001, *Global consultation on adolescent health services a consensus statement*, Department of Child and Adolescent Health and Development, WHO, Geneva.

30. World Health Organisation (WHO) 2008a, *The World Health Report: primary health care now more than ever*, WHO, Geneva.

31. World Health Organisation (WHO) 2008b, *Closing the Gap in a Generation: health equity through action on the social determinants of health*, WHO, Geneva.

32. Zimmerman, GL, Olsen, CG & Bosworth, MF 2000, 'A 'stages of change' approach to helping patients change behavior', *American Family Physician*, vol. 61, pp. 1409–16.

Chapter eleven

Wound management

by Jan Rice

Overview

Patients presenting to general practice with a wound are a common occurrence. The principles of determining the underlying cause of the wound and whether there is an underlying pathology are paramount to successful outcomes. The general health and clear identification of bacterial load potentials are very important in the overall assessment and management of patients presenting with wounds. The introduction of Medicare Benefits Schedule (MBS) funding for wound management has seen practice nurses embrace wound management as part of their expanding role.

Objectives

At the completion of this chapter you should be able to:

- understand normal physiology of wound healing;

- understand common aetiologies of wound formation and factors influencing wound healing, including wound bed preparation concepts in general practice;

- appreciate **tissue assessment tools**, including 'TIME' and 'CDE';

- be familiar with products and devices used in managing wounds; and

- appreciate the importance of documentation and evaluation of treatment plans.

Introduction

Wound management is a marriage of science and artistic endeavours. Discoveries over the past 30 years have unravelled some of the science related to the physiology of wound healing and the approach taken to solve the problems of chronic wound development. The challenge for contemporary clinicians is to implement these findings while tailoring wound management to the individual needs of the client. This challenge, coupled with modern societal demands on general practitioners and practice nurses, mandates the need for an understanding of current wound management principals and actions. This chapter provides a foundation for ongoing development in this area.

Wound care is not just about treating a wound; it is about assessing, evaluating and treating the whole person. Regular consideration needs to be given to the patient's health conditions and comorbidities, as well as ongoing assessment of their present health status, including nutrition and mental status, as these impact on wound healing. The case history in this chapter will also demonstrate the importance of holistic care resulting from teamwork in helping a patient acquire the knowledge towards self-management and improved health outcomes, and the eventual healing of persistent leg ulcers.

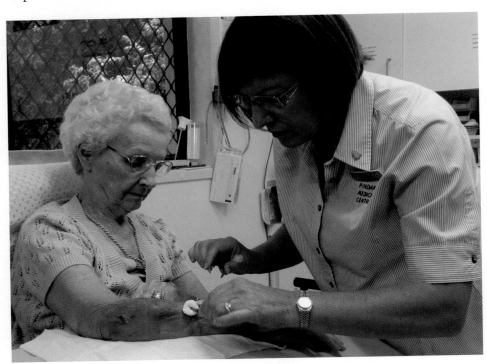

Normal wound healing physiology

Irrespective of the type of wound and the extent of the tissue loss, the healing of all wounds takes place in phases or stages which overlap and may at times be difficult to differentiate. The phases or stages of healing are described by Ovington and Schultz (2004) as involving:

- haemostasis;
- inflammation;

- matrix synthesis;
- angiogenesis;
- epithelialisation; and
- remodelling.

Haemostasis, as the name suggests, eliminates haemorrhage from the wound using the normal clotting cascade centred on the activity of platelets.

The inflammatory phase follows the same process as any other inflammatory process, specifically, dilation and increased permeability of the infiltrating blood vessels under the influence of histamine. This, in turn, leads to a fluid shift from the vascular compartment to the interstitial area, accompanied by the infiltration of phagocytes (neutrophils and latter macrophages). The intent is to provide protection from infection. It is during this phase that any necrotic tissue is removed by the phagocytic action.

Once the necrotic tissue has been removed the body begins to replace the granular tissue (matrix synthesis) infiltrated with new blood vessels (angiogenesis). Fibroblasts provide the necessary cellular activity for this process.

Once the new granular tissue has been formed, the epithelial cells begin to multiply and migrate over the granular bed (epithelialisation and remodelling) from the wound margins and hair follicles within the wound bed. Orchestration of the above process is provided by soluble proteins (known as cytokines) and growth factors that attach to cells and initiate a specific process; for example, the maturation of macrophages. Each of these phases or stages can be influenced in a negative way with an end result of failure or delayed wound healing.

Factors influencing healing

Three principle findings underpin the contemporary view of delayed healing pathology:

1. the identification of an inflammatory cycle
2. the presence of proteolytic enzymes in large volumes
3. the creation of a biofilm.

The inflammatory process is believed to be a result of two principle processes: the *trapping* of leukocytes and changes to fluid shear within the blood vessels supplying the wound (Thomas, Nash & Dormandy 1988). Studies have identified that leukocytes are adhered to, and in some instances have migrated into, the wall of affected veins (Takase, Schmid-Schönbein & Bergan 1999). Trapped leukocytes, in turn, release oxygen free-radicals and proteolytic enzymes which damage the capillary walls. This increases the wall permeability leading to further trapping of leukocytes.

Fluid shear stress refers to the sliding forces applied to the wall of the vein by blood passing over that wall. This is a normal physiological process that assists the transfer of nutrients and gases, and is believed to promote the release of factors that reduce inflammation and the formation of free radicals (Bergan et al. 2006), principally nitric oxide (Leach 2004). In patients suffering from delayed healing the force may be lower, have a turbulent flow, and in some instances, flow in the reverse direction (Weber 2003). Changes to fluid shear reduce the release of nitric oxide which, in turn, increases the release of factors that initiate inflammation.

Proteolytic enzymes break down protein chains and enable the neutrophils and macrophages to phagocytose necrotic tissue. In wounds with delayed healing it has been found that large amounts of this enzyme are present in wound fluid and for a sustained length of time. It is felt that the presence of the enzymes leads to ongoing breakdown of any newly formed granular tissue.

An examination of the bioburden carried by slow to heal wounds has revealed the presence of a biofilm. This forms when bacteria clump together and produce a polysaccharide matrix that forms an impenetrable barrier to the phagocytes. This affords the bacteria some protection enabling them to multiple to large numbers. This, in turn, places additional metabolic demands on the wound bed and delays healing.

In addition to the above findings a number of other factors have been found to influence healing (Carville 2005) and they include:

- age;
- underlying disease;
- vascularity;
- nutritional status;
- obesity;
- disorders of sensation or movement;
- psychological state;
- radiation therapy; and
- medications/drugs.

The local factors include:

- over- or under-hydration of the wound;
- wound management practices;

- wound tissue temperature;
- further trauma, e.g. pressure, shear, friction;
- foreign bodies; and
- wound infection.

This list is not exhaustive; however, it is recommended that the practice nurse concentrates on some of these factors at the initial consultation and expands on them as the assessment and reviews take place. Accurate assessment allows a comprehensive wound management plan to be established that will take into consideration these factors and aim to rectify any abnormalities.

> **Reflections**
>
> What systematic process of assessing wounds do clinical staff use in your practice?

Tissue assessment

A number of authors have addressed the process of tissue assessment by creating acronyms to ensure all the important factors are taken into consideration when assessing any wound. One such acronym is TIME, which stands for:

T = tissue

I = infection and/or inflammation

M = moisture balance, not too wet, not too dry

E = epithelialisation and wound edge.

Another commonly used acronym is CDE, which will be discussed in detail below. Both acronyms are very similar but with a slightly different emphasis.

C = colour of tissue

D = depth

E = exudate volume and type.

Although none of these systems account for wound aetiology they form a basis from which to commence tissue and wound assessment. Many companies produce product information based on these systems.

Tissue colour

Green tissue or exudate, yellow and black tissue are perhaps the worst seen within wounds as they imply necrosis, destruction of tissue and possible infection. Red tissue is considered a sign of healing, especially if the wound initially contained the aforementioned tissue colours. Not all red is good however. If the red is a pale red, the client may be anaemic; if it is very bright red, it may indicate a streptococcal infection, so the degree of redness and the strength of that tissue impact on definition of healthy or poor granulation tissue.

Healthy granulation tissue is beefy red and firm. If the tissue is very friable, very bright red and exuding moderately then bacterial load can be high or the tissue is hypergranulated due to tissue hypoxia or excessive oedema (Butcher 2006). Hypergranulation requires attention as epithelium fails to grow up and over this tissue.

Epithelium is the new skin progressing from the sides of the wound and any healthy skin appendages to complete the healing process. In the very early days of wound healing, this is transparent and may be easily disturbed, so observation techniques to identify this tissue are paramount. One such technique is the 'wrinkle test' in which, if a cotton bud is placed over the tissue and wrinkles are seen, then there is a new layer of epithelium present but possibly only one or two cells thick and so easily injured.

Wound depth

There are many tools available to assist in actually measuring wound depth; however, most that can measure this accurately are used in research and are either too expensive or too cumbersome for general practice. The best method to determine the greatest depth of a wound is to insert a pre-moistened cotton bud into the cavity and then pinch it at the level of the surrounding tissue and compare it against a linear ruler. Undermining can also be assessed using a similar technique. A pre-moistened cotton bud is inserted at the end point into undermined space (*do not force*), gently push upward until there is a bulge in the skin, mark the points with a pen and connect them, measure two diameters, as in length by width.

Wound exudate

Wound exudate will be mentioned within its role of wound bed preparation. The clinician is required to determine if the volume and type of exudate is consistent with normal wound healing. High volumes of exudate are often linked to oedema or infection or both. Wound exudate is necessary for cellular movement, however, excessive exudate, particularly chronic exudate, may be detrimental to the surrounding skin and requires management. Dressings designed to manage exudate may be listed as super-absorbers, foams or foam-like products.

A comprehensive assessment must be made of the patient, the wound and the environment in which the wound is going to be placed, for example, is the patient is going back to work in the garage or in a wet area. The treatment aim can vary and must be established in consultation with the patient, the attending clinicians and any other relevant allied health care providers. Wound management is a multidisciplinary field of health practice, and the practice nurse and the general practitioner have an opportunity to contribute to a team approach in this area. The following information may be seen as a guide to determining use of dressings but is not prescriptive:

- Black: if aiming to heal (cleansing dressing)*
- Green: antimicrobial dressing
- Wet yellow: antimicrobial dressing
- Dry yellow: rehydrating dressing
- Red: protect
- Hypergranulation: antimicrobial dressing
- Pink: protect.

*If the wound is dry, black and ischaemic or cachexia is involved, then keeping the black dry is the rule—select dry dressings and consider using a skin antiseptic to remove surface bacteria.

Reflections

How do you go about formulating a plan of management for wound care in your practice?

Once an assessment has been completed a plan of management can be developed. While a management plan will be individualised, certain key interventions are common to most types of wounds.

Wound bed preparation

The concept of 'preparing the wound bed' was first described in 2000 by Sibbald et al. and Falanga (2000). Traditionally clinicians used dressings that were later seen to be quite traumatic to tissue so that when the moist wound

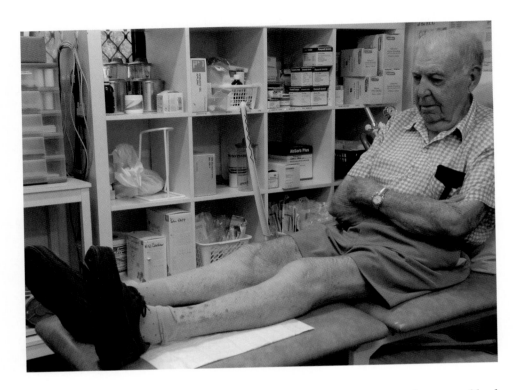

healing concepts were adopted there was a sense of do as little to the wound bed as possible for fear of damaging viable cells. Falanga encourages the clinician to take a holistic approach and if healing is the goal then active preparation of the wound bed tissue is to be encouraged.

Nursing interventions aimed at preventing an acute wound from becoming chronic include:

- preparing the wound bed to receive the next dressing;
- maintaining cellular moisture and temperature;
- reviewing known individual factors that may influence healing and where possible correcting these;
- empowering the patient to take an active role in the wound care;
- minimising pain and discomfort; and
- addressing any depression and other psychological problems associated with a chronic wound.

Schultz, Ladwig and Wysocki (2005) encourage clinicians to identify senescent tissue in the wound and remove it as quickly as possible at each dressing change. This removes the damaging components of inflammation and restoring the balance between the matrix metaloproteases (MMP) and tissue inhibitors of matrix metaloproteases (TIMP).

A structured approach to this concept is recommended to guide the clinician in focusing on five major components:

1. Restoration of bacterial balance
2. Management of necrosis
3. Management of exudate
4. Correction of cellular dysfunction
5. Restoration of biochemical balance.

(Vowden & Vowden 2002)

Restoring the bacterial balance implies that a holistic patient assessment has been conducted. The standard equation of bacterial virulence and host defence has been taught for many years, however, the emphasis has been on the bacterial virulence. Vowden and Vowden (2002) are encouraging the clinician to focus on the wound and the patient as a whole and to have a defined aim.

Restoration of bacterial balance is one such aim which may be achieved in several ways. Wound cleansing is an area of limited good evidence, however, there would be little argument from any clinician that wounds require cleansing; just what is used to perform this cleansing is a topic of much debate. Sibbald et al. (2006) have stated that there may be some benefit in using antiseptics especially in wounds that may be deemed non-healable or where the local bioburden is of greater concern than the stimulation of healing. Supporting host resistance may thus be achieved by reducing bacterial bioburden, the theory being that once bacterial bioburden has been controlled, there will be less necrosis. Other ways to manage necrosis, apart from managing the bacterial bioburden, may be:

- mechanical;
- autolytic;
- enzymatic; or
- biosurgical.

Clinical staff will select the most appropriate method to manage necrosis based on the patient, the wound and the care setting. A clear aim should be determined—is debridement necessary to rid the area of the tissue causing malodour or is it a step necessary in promoting healing? Set a clear defined time line—mechanical debridement using a share instrument, such as scalpel, is the quickest but, depending on the setting, may also consume the greatest amount of resources. The selection of method is dictated by many factors and all these must be clearly articulated in the rationale for the final method chosen. Clear rationale is particularly relevant in general practice where, due to the part-time nature of the practice nurse role, several clinicians may be involved in the patient's ongoing care.

Mechanical debridement

Mechanical debridement implies the physical removal of debris from the wound. The most complex form of this technique is surgical debridement, requiring surgeons and generally an operating theatre. The simplest method is the use of wet-to-dry gauze dressings. Each method has both positive and negative factors to be considered. The older traditional wet-to-dry method has been shown to be cost ineffective and also is very time consuming. Furthermore, it causes pain to the patient, and is non-selective, causing damage to viable tissue (Sibbald et al. 2000) and as a result this method is generally unacceptable to most clinicians.

Autolytic debridement

Autolytic debridement employs the natural processes of macrophage and endogenous proteolytic activity encouraging selective liquefaction, separation and digestion of the eschar and wound debris (Meekes 2001). The creation of a moist environment is believed to encourage this process. Some dressings, such as alginates, are believed to exert a bioactive effect by stimulating the macrophages to generate TNF-alpha and interleukin-1, 6 and 12 aiding to restore balance of the MMP and TIMP (Stewart 2002).

Enzymatic debridement

Enzymatic debridement relies upon the topical application of exogenous enzymes that work synergistically with the endogenous enzymes. A recent addition to the Australian market has been Flaminal® which is glucose oxidase and lactoperoxidase enzymes in an alginate gel. White (2006) cites a clinical trial by de la Brassinne et al. comparing Flaminal with Intrasite Gel® in the management of leg ulcers. Two groups of 10 patients were treated for 28 days. The Flaminal group achieved greater area reduction ($p < 0.01$) at day 14 and 28 than the Intrasite group.

Biosurgical debridement

The larvae from *Lucilia sericata* have been used for **biosurgical debridement** in more recent times with great success (Thomas & Jones 2001). These exquisite scavengers digest only necrotic tissue and excrete enzymes and calcium salts on the tissue to make it more digestible (Blake et al. 2007). This process would not be considered ideal in general practice, as most patients undergoing formal biosurgical debridement require hospitalisation.

The above methods of debridement address several aspects of the structured approach suggested by Vowden & Vowden (2002); however, there are several more factors the clinician should target in order to achieve maximum healing of the acute wound before it becomes chronic. Managing exudate is seen both as a priority for the nurse and the patient.

Wound exudate management

In normal wound healing the exudate appears to promote cell proliferation. The MMP are present mainly in an inactive form; however, the opposite is seen in chronic wounds with the exudate containing elevated levels of inflammatory mediators and activated MMP (World Union of Wound Healing Societies 2007). Exudate management products are available and when combined with other strategies, particularly addressing the underlying pathology of the wound, progress in healing and patient comfort are restored.

In vitro studies of some dressings show that, for example, carboxymethyl cellulose fibres and some alginates trap bacteria and exudate components, such as enzymes, in a process termed sequestration. Dressings that produce a uniform coherent gel appear to have enhancing effects on this sequestration (Newman et al. 2006).

Ideally:

- if the tissue is black and the aim is to debride then there should be granulation buds appearing within three weeks of commencement of treatment;
- green exudate should cease after two weeks of antibiotic treatment combined with antimicrobial dressings;
- wet yellow tissue should be less wet within two weeks if correct oedema control and antimicrobial therapy have been undertaken;
- dry yellow tissue should be rehydrated, and almost gone after two weeks of correct hydrating therapy;
- healthy red tissue should show signs of epithelial edges within two weeks of using products to maintain some moisture and prevent any shear and friction to the good tissue; and
- hypergranulated tissue should be less so after five days of using an antimicrobial and removing any occlusive dressings.

Dressings play a vital role in the general practice setting; therefore, nurses must be very familiar with the constituents of the various dressings available and the way in which each dressing will interact with the tissue and cells.

Wound care products and devices

Product selection may be determined by many factors external to the above assessment. These factors generally come down to product price or availability (Ovington & Eisenbud 2004). These issues must be addressed within each practice setting. Generally speaking, products are either classified by their basic components (pharmacology) or by function and the way they influence the wound. Ideally all clinical practice team members will have an understanding of both concepts.

Classification by pharmacology:

- Impregnated mesh dressings, e.g. Adaptic®, Cuticerin®
- Low-adherent pads, e.g. Melolin®, Interpose®
- Super-absorber pads, e.g. Absorb® plus, Zetuvit® plus
- Polyurethane film wipes and film sheets, e.g. No Sting Barrier® wipes, Opsite®, Tegaderm
- Polyurethane foams, e.g. Allevyn®, Mepilex®
- Hydrocolloids, e.g. DuoDerm®, Comfeel®
- Calcium alginates, e.g. Kaltostat®, Algisite M®
- Hydrogels, e.g. Solosite®, DuoDerm® gel
- Hydrofibres, e.g. Aquacel®
- Medical silver based dressings, e.g. Atrauman® Ag, Acticoat®
- Cadexomer Iodine products, e.g. Iodosorb®
- Medicated honey products, e.g. Comvita®, Manuka®
- Enzyme based agents, e.g. Flaminal®
- Tea-tree based agents, e.g. BurnAid®, Wound Aid® gel
- Hypertonic salt dressings, e.g. Mesalt®, Curasalt®.

Classification by function:

- Wound protection
- Wound rehydration
- Exudate management
- Antimicrobial
- Debriding/cleansing.

Reflections

Given the number of products available and their cost, what criteria does your practice use to determine usage of wound care products?

Achieving treatment goals within an appropriate time frame

The aim of treatment and the selection of dressing products and devices is essential for best outcomes. The decisions determining patient appointments, cost of dressings, home visits and the billing structure will be determined differently for each practice, and are based on resources and staff that are available. Having a practice policy which clearly outlines how a wound management service is structured is beneficial to all staff as it clearly defines the roles and responsibilities of each team member. All team members, including reception staff, can work more effectively with good communication and designated roles; however, the practice nurse will play an important role in the leadership of such a service and in educating other practice staff.

Understanding how wound care products work and what to expect from them comes with experience and practice. Ensure that if the patient is removing the dressing and showering prior to coming to clinic, the practice nurses should request that the removed dressing be brought in for examination to ensure it has been effective in achieving the aim.

The aim of using a dressing is to create the environment for the body to heal. Every endeavour must be made to restore many of those general factors influencing healing as suggested by Carville (2005). By setting a time frame and reviewing the assessment regularly, any reasons for delayed healing, such as an incorrect diagnosis, poor nutrition or other factors which have been overlooked on initial assessment, will be identified.

Common wound presentations

The variety of wound presentations to general practice is very broad. General practice is not only the first contact in some instances for patients receiving an injury, it is also used often as a follow-up after patients have presented to emergency departments or private specialists for wound management. Some of the typical presentations may include:

- lacerations and abrasions;
- skin tears;
- superficial partial thickness burns;
- venous leg ulcers;
- arterial leg ulcers;
- ulcers of mixed aetiology; or
- post-operation follow-up to review lesion removals by specialists.

Lacerations and abrasions

Where possible, the injured area will need to be thoroughly cleaned to remove embedded debris. The use of any local anaesthetic should be discussed with a general practitioner. Warmed cleansing solution is more comfortable for the patient and in the case of very soiled wounds; washing under running warm tap water may be indicated. If the patient's immune status is a concern it may be advisable to use an antiseptic solution, rinsing off after two to five minutes. If the patient's wound is a tetanus-prone injury, it is also important to check their vaccination status to determine if any immunisations are required.

Assessing the depth of the wound and whether nerves and tendons are functioning normally will guide management. If the wound is deep, suturing or using a device, such as Leukosan SkinLink® strips, will be required. A secondary non-adherent pad should be used to cover the wound and the dressing should be supported with a crepe bandage and tubular support bandage which will reduce oedema and guide the inflammatory phase of healing. Review will be within 72 hours to check the dressings are clean, bleeding has ceased and no signs of infection exist.

Some GPs prefer to cover suture lines with a waterproof dressing but as many acute wounds are initially 'dirty' it is important they can be easily inspected. For this reason, adhesive products should be avoided at this time. Following review of the wound (and providing healing is occurring) it may be appropriate to apply a waterproof dressing. Re-dressing of cuts and abrasions is generally conducted twice weekly or weekly and are generally expected to heal in two to three weeks.

Skin tears

Because skin tears are caused by trauma, their initial management has a big impact on the viability of the skin flap and for this reason, accurate assessment is vital. Skin tears can be categorised into three main types:

1. Category 1a and 1b (approximation of the skin edges without undue tension)
2. Category 2a and b (the skin edges cannot be approximated)
3. Category 3 (the skin flap is completely absent).

The commonly accepted STAR skin tear classification tool is used to describe skin tears and provides a structured framework from which standard protocols for all clinical staff working in the practice can be established.

For **category 1**, flexible adhesive support strips covered with a light, low-adherent product, crepe bandage and elasticated tubular bandage—distal to proximal. For **category 2 and 3** skin tears, if the skin edges cannot be approximated then using the mesh dressings similar to the dressing mentioned above for burns will protect the raw area without over-hydrating the tissue or desiccating the area.

There is another widely used treatment option becoming standard practise in acute care facilities which involves the use of silicone foam products such as Allevyn® Gentle, Biatain® Soft Hold and Mepitel Border®. These treatment options are yet to be adopted by general practice staff due to the perception of higher costs associated with these products. With the right protocols in place, the silicone foam regimes have proven very cost effective.

A review of skin tears in three to four days is recommended. It is advisable to be highly suspicious of possible infection, especially in the elderly. Skin tears will leak serum for a few days and, therefore, an absorbent pad such as those mentioned for managing burns may be required over the mesh dressings if not using the silicone foam products. The mesh dressings are then managed as for burns. If the skin flap is stable, re-dressing once or twice weekly is sufficient with an aim to have the wound healed in two to three weeks.

If a localised or systemic infection is suspected then an antimicrobial dressing, such as Iodosorb® powder or ointment, and an absorbent pad, such as Melolin, covered with a pad and bandage as previously mentioned or flexible tape, such as Mefix® or Hypafix®, should be used.

Do not use occlusive dressings on suspected locally or systemically infected wounds.

Superficial partial thickness burns

Superficial partial thickness burns are painful, with blisters and/or shedding of the upper layers of the epidermis and partial dermis. It is important to estimate the surface area involved and the region in order to determine if further assessment is required at a burns unit.

Immediate action involves cooling the burn area with cool running water if possible. If this is not possible or has been done but there is still some discomfort, tea-tree based agents, such as BURNAID®, can be placed on the area while awaiting further assessment by the GP.

Ideally, burns of greater than 10% of body surface area should be assessed in an acute care facility other than general practice. Burns of the perineum, feet, hands or face and circumferential require assessment by someone used to managing burns. Based on the scope of practice of all practice staff, it is a recommended that each practice has a written protocol outlining what injuries, such as burns, can be managed within the practice.

If the burn is to be managed in the practice and has been deemed clean then some of the newer mesh dressings (Urgotul®, Hydrotul® and Mepitel®) can be placed over the burn, covered with an absorbent pad such as Zetuvit Plus®, Mesorb® or Exudry® bandaged in place and covered if possible with an elasticated tubular bandage—distal to proximal—to control oedema.

The patient will require a review in three days. Take the dressing down to the primary mesh layer but do not remove this. It is possible to observe the state of the tissue beneath the mesh to determine how the wound is progressing. If no erythema or purulent discharge is evident then cover the wound with a fresh absorbent pad, apply the bandage and tubular bandage and review the patient again in three to four days. Repeat the procedure and if all is well, review the wound using the same techniques in one week. At this time the mesh dressing is usually dry and lifts off the wound to reveal the healing beneath.

Once healed, the area is very sensitive to heat so the practice nurse should advise the patient to take care, apply moisturiser daily and use sun protection if required. A clean superficial partial-thickness burn should be healed within two to three weeks.

Reflections

What is outlined in the wound management policy for your practice?

Venous and arterial leg ulceration

Australia's national health expenditure on wounds such as leg ulcers is said to be in the vicinity of $365 million to $654 million (Baker et al. 1991; Santamaria,

Austin & Clayton 2002). For the patient, delayed wound healing has been shown to impact on personal finances, employment prospects and general quality of life. Phillips et al. 1994 found that 30% of cases surveyed spent between $101 and $1000 per annum. A further 8% of participants estimated out-of-pocket expenses to be greater than $1000 per annum. Smith and McGuiness (2006) identified that participants spent on average $114 per month on the treatment and management of their ulcer, resulting in a personal cost of $1368 per annum. In addition, clients report social isolation because of the exudate and odour associated with their wounds. Wet shoes and stockings, and the accompanying odour, often interfered with normal social or family interactions (Persoon et al. 2004). Equally, the prevalence of pain has been found to be high among this client cohort (Yamada & de Gouveia Santos 2005).

Wound management, for the patients, the family and the general practice is often not straightforward, and it is essential that a correct diagnosis be made of the underlying issues related to healing. A simple skin tear on the lower leg may become a venous ulcer if there is underlying venous hypertension.

Differentiating between a true venous ulcer and an arterial ulcer requires the clinician to know the risk factors and identifying characteristics of each. There are several factors which increase a patient's risk of developing venous hypertension. These include:

- a past history of deep venous thrombosis (DVT)
- multiple pregnancies, surgeries or trauma
- family history of varicose veins, vein surgery or DVT
- an occupation requiring prolonged standing or sitting
- obesity.

Risk factors for arterial occlusion and stenosis are generally those associated with arterial disease more broadly and may include:

- past history of atherosclerosis
- smoking
- hypertension
- advanced age
- diabetes.

A comparison of the characteristics of venous and arterial ulcers is shown in Table 11.1 overleaf.

Table 11.1 A comparison between characteristics of venous and arterial ulcers

Venous ulcer	Arterial ulcer
The ulcer is located on the lower third of the lower leg.	The ulcer is located anywhere on the leg, although most commonly higher up or on the foot.
The ulcer edges when tracing are ill defined and irregular.	The ulcer edges when tracing are well defined and regular.
The ulcer is not excessively necrotic and more often has just a fibrin layer covering a granulating base.	The ulcer is necrotic and may often involve tendon and bone.
The ulcer is wet and weeping.	The ulcer is dry unless infected.
The leg may have pitting oedema and resemble an inverted champagne bottle shape.	There may also be changes in the toenails.
The ulcer may be uncomfortable but not excessively painful (unless infected).	The ulcer may be very painful, also the patient may complain of leg pain on activity.
Infection is not as common in this type of ulcer.	Infection is common in this type of ulcer.
If oedema is present it is easily reduced by leg elevation.	The skin is often thin and shiny, with minimal evidence of hair.
Pulses are palpable or heard with a hand-held Doppler.	Pulses are poor or not felt at all.

Managing chronic lower leg ulcers requires a degree of persistent vigilance. If underlying factors such as ischemia have been treated and local wound factors have been resolved, the wound is more likely to heal. Failure to heal is often linked to insufficient perfusion, oedema or persistent infection or bacterial colonisation. Often simple interventions, such as removing oedema or applying a topical antimicrobial dressing, produce dramatic changes in healing rates.

The management of ulcers caused by underlying arterial problems is distinctly different from those which are used to manage venous disorders. A thorough patient history is needed in order to ascertain a correct diagnosis and prior to beginning therapy, the clinician must be sure the diagnosis is correct by validating their diagnosis with the inclusion of listed factors previously mentioned.

Management of venous ulceration

Venous ulceration is treated with an appropriate primary dressing over the ulcer and then compression or support therapy to restore valvular function. The tissue seen in venous ulcers is usually a superficial yellow fibrin layer and all that is required is an absorbent non-adherent dressing. Absorbent non-stick dressings may include:

- polyurethane foams or silicone foams, for example, Allevyn, Mepilex® or Biatain
- gelling foams, for example, Versiva® XC
- hydrofibre dressings such as Aquacel.

If there is any thought that the ulcer may have bacterial bioburden or infection issues then consideration is given to systemic antibiotics alone or in conjunction with topical antimicrobials such as cadexomer iodine, silver or hypertonic salt dressings.

If there is good quality granulation tissue the aim is to protect and encourage epithelial growth. There are a number of zinc paste bandages available to achieve this aim. These products may include Steripaste™ bandages or ZipZoc™ bandages.

The compression or support therapy seen in general practice is often limited to straight elasticated tubular bandages. These products are not known to deliver the higher pressures often required to heal venous ulcers, however, compliance, costs and discomfort at higher pressures have all been reported as factors inhibiting the use of the ideal pressures. This should not deter the clinician in general practice as with some compression and support, education and a modified activity level healing can be achieved.

A trend emerging in general practice is the use of three layers of straight elasticated tubular bandages, each layer shorter than the previous:

- first layer—toes to knee crease (two fingers below knee crease to be precise)
- second layer—toes to two-thirds of the lower leg
- third layer—toes to one-third of the lower leg.

The patient may remove one or two layers prior to sleeping as long as they replace them before getting out of bed for the day. This system is said to deliver approximately 15–18 mmHg at the ankle with 12 mmHg at the calf and 6 mmHg at the knee—thereby achieving distal to proximal graduation. It is important to stress that this is well below the figures quoted to achieve increased venous flow velocity, however, the ideal therapy is painful and restrictive, and patients may refuse or remove the garments, in which case, treatment is about establishing other methods to assist with venous drainage.

Other methods to encourage include good walking techniques and elevation of the lower limb as often as is possible when sitting, with the foot above the level of the hip. Ankle exercises and blocks beneath the foot end of the bed to assist drainage when in bed are helpful.

Management of arterial ulceration

Management of arterial ulcers should ideally involve a vascular surgeon as restoring premium blood flow is the aim. While awaiting a surgical review a dry wound should be kept dry by painting it with Betadine lotion daily and covering with a light non-adherent dressing.

However, if the wound is wet and necrotic, the aim will be to aid autolytic debridement and reducing damage around the wound while awaiting a review. Topical antimicrobials or enzymes to aid this process may include cadexomer iodine, Flaminal hydrogel and silver dressings.

The patient with an arterial wound should not have high-compression bandages applied for fear of causing further ischaemia. One layer of straight elasticated tubular bandage may be used, with instructions given to the patient to remove it if uncomfortable. In end stage arterial disease, oedema may be present due to leg dependency. These patients are unlikely to elevate their limb due to severe pain and rest with the leg down 24 hours per day. In these situations the role of the clinician is to provide adequate pain relief and reduce the risk of infection. Palliative pain teams may be used for these patients to maintain a balance between adequate analgesia to allow normal functioning and reduce pain to tolerable levels.

Documentation

In order to maintain continuity of care and record an ongoing history of the progress of healing, it is important to keep comprehensive and descriptive notes from each consultation. Included in the patient file should be:

- aetiology of the wound
- date of initial assessment or injury
- location of the wound
- size, including maximum length and width
- depth—using the technique described previously in the burns assessment
- volume of exudate
- type of exudate
- tissue colour—if necessary using percentages of each type
- state of the surrounding skin.

If all staff are able to maintain comprehensive records, patients will benefit by having a regular review of the wound using the same criteria for assessment. Issues restricting healing are more likely to be identified and addressed in a timely manner.

Conclusion

Wound management is a science and discoveries are being made in this area every day. The practice nurse is in the position to offer first aid as well as ongoing management of wounds that present to general practice from a variety of causes and from patients of all ages. They must have good knowledge of the current science and be able to apply this into clinical practice, so that the holistic needs of the patient are addressed. The overarching principles of wound management are correct diagnosis and aetiology. Recognising the underlying factors that may influence healing is fundamental in ensuring wounds heal as efficiently as possible with the aid of a variety of wound care products that are now available.

C A S E   S T U D Y

Name of nurse
Susan Halsey
Practice
Pindara Medical Centre, Gold Coast, Qld

INTRODUCTION

Wound care is not just about treating a wound; it is about assessing, evaluating and treating the whole person.[1] Regular consideration needs to be given to the patient's health conditions and comorbidities, as well as ongoing assessment of their present health status, including nutrition and mental status, as these impact on wound healing. This case history demonstrates the importance of holistic care resulting from teamwork in helping a patient acquire the knowledge towards self-management and improved health outcomes, and eventual healing a venous leg ulcer.[2]

MRS B

Mrs B is a 58-year-old woman who first presented with a non-healing ulcer on her left lateral malleolus while visiting family in October 2008. The ulcer had been present since removal of sutures following internal fixation of a fractured tibia and fibular in May 2008. The wound had been treated with all manner of products but the ulcer failed to heal. When Mrs B presented, her ulcer measured 1.8 cm × 1.5 cm, was shallow, and showed some slough evident in the wound base. Inflammation extended 2–3 cms beyond the wound edge. The patient

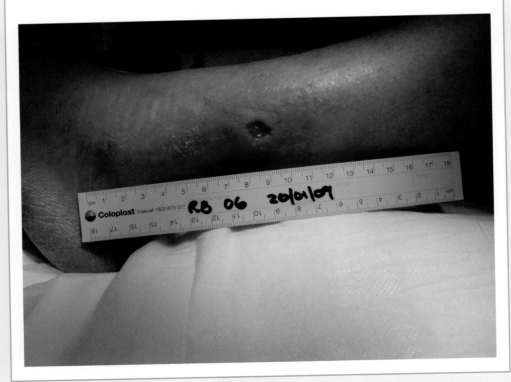

complained of increasing pain and exudate. It was evident there was localised infection together with increasing systemic infection and a course of antibiotics was prescribed. At this time the wound was debrided of slough and cleaned, zinc was applied to the surrounding skin edges for protection, and Acticoat 3-day applied to the ulcer and secured in place with an absorbent secondary dressing. Rationale for the use of Acticoat was its bactericidal effect at the wound bed. The patient was instructed to continue to dress the wound twice weekly with Acticoat 3-day for two weeks. She was given a letter for her usual GP outlining our care.

In January 2009 Mrs B again presented and the practice was asked to take over her care. Her circumstances had changed and she was relocating following a relationship break-up. A comprehensive health history and assessment, including nutritional status and wound assessment were undertaken. Mrs B is a patient with insulin-dependent type 2 diabetes mellitus: her random blood glucose was 18.6 mmol. She was depressed, hypertensive and obese with oedema present in her lower limbs, a sign of incompetent leg veins. Following the treatment in October Mrs B had been treating her ulcer twice weekly by flushing the ulcer to clean and using simple dressings of a hydrogel and tulle gras. The ulcer now measured 1.2 cm × 1.1 cm, the base contained some slough and granulating tissue was evident but presented as dark red. The skin edges were not undermined and the peri-wound area was inflamed to 1–2 cm. A small eczematous area possibly due to venous stasis existed distal to the ulcer. Exudate was moist indicating localised bacterial burden. The patient described the pain as constant and 'niggly'. Ankle brachial index ratios were performed and were within normal limits.

The TIME framework was used to optimise healing by reducing or correcting abnormalities which contribute to impaired healing. Her history determined the treatment, as the team needed

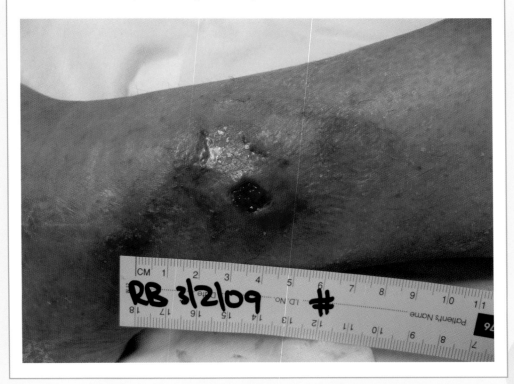

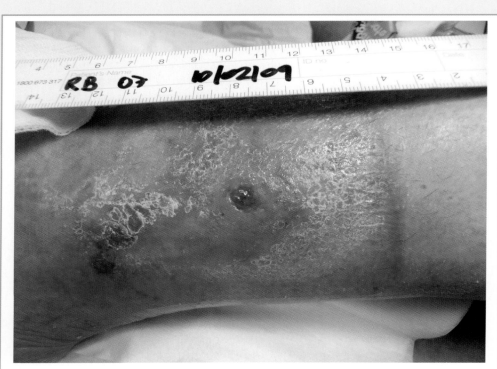

to optimise her host response by helping her to manage her condition and comorbidities.[3] In this case, gaining glycaemic control and reducing oedema were initial priorities in her immediate treatment because they impact significantly on wound healing. Therefore, urgent referrals to a diabetes educator and a dietician were arranged to gain glycaemic control and increase the patient's knowledge and understanding and so improve compliance to treatment.

The ulcer was debrided of slough and then dressed with a silver sulfadiazine impregnated hydrocellular occlusive dressing (Allevyn Ag Adhesive) and in the short term a graduated shaped-support tubular-form compression bandage of appropriate size was applied to the lower leg until class two moderate compression stockings (25–35 mmHg) were acquired. Mrs B was reviewed at the wound clinic four days later, at which time she appeared happier and the ulcer bed appeared healthier. The ulcer was re-dressed with the same product to be left in situ until review seven days later. Moderate (Class 2 25–35mmHg) below knee compression stocking therapy was commenced to her left lower leg.

Eleven days after initial presentation, during which time the diabetes educator was managing Mrs B's insulin therapy, she had several hypoglycaemic episodes: random blood glucose was 8.9 mmol. There was a marked reduction in ankle oedema following continued use of the compression stocking. The ulcer bed was clean and healthy granulation tissue was present and wound measurements were 0.8 cm × 1.1 cm. But there was evidence of a local reaction to the dressing as there was a noticeably inflamed, raised area in the shape of the hydrocellular padding surrounding the wound. A cortisone ointment was prescribed to be applied to the inflamed area twice daily. Dressings were changed to a simple hydrogel and fine tulle gras (Adaptic) secured in place with a non-occlusive island dressing. This dressing could be applied by the patient and she could also remove it to apply the cortisone ointment when necessary.

Mrs B attended the wound clinic weekly for review over the following eight weeks. Improvements were made in her glycaemic control, and she appeared happier and compliant to her treatment regime including the wearing of the compression stocking. She was delighted to see the progressive decrease in the size of the ulcer, albeit slowly. The cortisone ointment was ceased after two weeks and instead zinc applied to the area. Dressings were attended to by the patient once during the week by simple cleaning under running water, gentle drying, and dressing with hydogel and tulle gras—all secured in place with a non-occlusive island dressing.

After two months, Mrs B once again relocated to another area to care for her mother. She was much better prepared to manage her own care, particularly in relation to her diabetes and the impact the diagnosis has on healing. When she left our care her ulcer measured 0.3 cm × 0.7 cm—it was quite small.

In July, Mrs B was once again visiting family and her wound was reviewed. She appeared well, she had improved control of her diabetes and she was wearing her compression stocking. There had been little significant change in her ulcer since March. Mrs B rang us on 3 August just to let us know how she was and that her ulcer was at long last healed.

CASE CONCLUSION

This ulcer healed after 14 months, it was a long journey for Mrs B. The case history demonstrates the importance of assessing, re-evaluating and treating the whole person. It also illustrates collaborative care in helping a patient acquire the knowledge to make changes to improve health outcomes and achieve self-management of their condition.

Notes

1. Harding, K 2008, (ed), *Principles of best practice*, cited in *Wound infection: an international consensus*, MEP Ltd, London, pp. 2–3.
2. Vowden, P, Apleqvist, J & Moffat, C 2008, *Wound complexity and healing*, cited in European Wound Management Association, position document, *Hard-to-heal wounds: a holistic approach*, MEP Ltd, London, pp. 2–9.
3. Falanga, V 2004, *Wound bed preparation: science applied to practice*, cited in European Wound Management Association, position document, *Wound bed preparation in practice*, MEP Ltd, London, p. 2.

Key messages

Always apply the basic principles when assessing and managing a wound.

Always look for 'common' before 'unusual'.

Most wounds require oedema control.

Seek a further opinion in four weeks if wounds do not demonstrate any signs of healing.

Useful resources

Burns protocol
> http://www.rch.org.au/

Wounds West
> http://www.health.wa.gov.au/WoundsWest/home

Silver Chain (STAR skin tear classification tool)
> http://www.silverchain.org.au/

World Union of Wound Healing Societies
> http://www.wuwhs.org/

European Wound Management Association
> http://www.ewma.org/

References

1. Baker, SR, Stacey, MC, Jopp-Mckay, AG, Hoskin, SE & Thompson, PJ 1991, 'Epidemiology of chronic venous ulcers', *British Journal of Surgery*, vol. 78, no. 7, pp. 864–7.

2. Beitz, J 2004, 'Practice development and the role of advanced practice nurse', in M Morrison, LG, Ovington & K Wilkie (eds), *Chronic wound care: a problem based learning approach*, Mosby, Philadelphia, pp. 334–49.

3. Bergan, JJ, Schmid-Schönbein, GW, Coleridge Smith, DW, Nicolaides, AN, Boisseau, MR & Eklof, B 2006, 'Chronic venous disease', *New England Journal of Medicine*, vol. 355, no. 5, pp. 488–98.

4. Blake, FAS, Abromeit, N, Bubenheim, M, Li, L & Schmelzle, R 2007, 'The biosurgical wound debridement: Experimental investigation of efficiency and practicability', *Wound Repair and Regeneration*, vol. 12, no. 5, pp. 756–61.

5. Butcher, M 2006, 'Progression to healing', in S Bale & D Gray (eds), *A pocket guide to clinical decision making in wound management*, Wounds, UK, pp. 21–46.

6. Carville, K 2005, 'Factors that inhibit healing', in K Carville (ed.) *Wound care manual*, 5th edn, Silver Chain, Osborne Park, WA, pp. 39–48.

7. Falanga, V 2000, 'Classifications for wound bed preparation and stimulation of chronic wounds', *Wound Repair and Regeneration*, vol. 8, no. 5, pp. 347–52.

8. Leach, MJ 2004, 'Making sense of the venous leg ulcer debate: a literature review', *Journal of Wound Care*, vol. 13, no. 2, pp. 52–6.

9. Meekes, JR 2001, 'Autolytic debridement', in GW Cherry, KG Harding & TJ Ryan (eds), *Wound Bed Preparation*, Royal Society of Medicine Press Ltd, London, pp. 105–8.

10. Newman, GR, Walker, M, Hobot, JA & Bowler, PG 2006, 'Visualisation of bacterial sequestration and bactericidal activity within hydrating Hydrofiber® wound dressings', *Biomaterials*, vol. 27, pp. 1129–39.

11. Ovington, LA & Eisenbud, D 2004, 'Dressings and cleansing agents', in M Morrison, LG Ovington & K Wilkie (eds), *Chronic wound care: a problem based learning approach*, Mosby, Philadelphia, vol. 8, pp. 117–28.

12. Ovington, LA & Schultz, GS 2004, 'The physiology of wound healing', in M Morrison, LG, Ovington & K Wilkie (eds), *Chronic wound care: a problem based learning approach*, Mosby, Philadelphia. pp. 83–100.

13. Persoon, A, Heinen, MM, van der Vleuten, CJM, de Rooij, MJ, de Kerkhof, PCM & van Achterberg, T 2004, 'Leg ulcers: a review of their impact on daily life', *Journal of Clinical Nursing*, vol. 13, no. 3, pp. 341–54.

14. Phillips, T, Stanton, B, Provan, A & Lew, R 1994, 'A study of the impact of leg ulcers on quality of life: financial, social, and psychologic implications', *Journal of the American Academy of Dermatology*, vol. 31, no. 1, pp. 49–53.

15. Santamaria, N, Austin, D & Clayton, L 2002, 'A multi-site clinical evaluation trial of the Alfred/Medseed wound imaging system prototype', *Primary Intention*, vol. 10, no. 3, pp. 120–5.

16. Schultz, G, Ladwig, G & Wysocki, A 2005, *Extracellular matrix: review of its roles in acute and chronic wounds*, viewed 27 April 2009, <http://www.worldwidewounds.com/>.

17. Sibbald, RG, Orsted, HL, Coutts, PM & Keast, D 2006, 'Best practice recommendations for preparing the wound bed: Update 2006', *Wound Care Canada*, vol. 4, no. 1, pp. 6–18.

18. Sibbald, RG, Williamson, D, Orsted, HL, Campbell, K, Keast, D, Krasner, D & Sibbald, D 2000, 'Preparing the wound bed—debridement, bacterial balance and moisture balance', *Ostomy Wound Management*, vol. 46, no. 11, pp. 14–35.

19. Smith, E & McGuiness, B 2006, *Managing venous leg ulcers in the community: financial cost to sufferers*, La Trobe Alfred Clinical School, Melbourne.

20. Stewart, J 2002, *Next generation products for wound management*, viewed 10 May 2009, <http://www.worldwidewounds.com/>.

21. Takase, S, Schmid-Schönbein, GW & Bergan, JJ 1999, 'Leukocyte activation in patients with venous insufficiency', *Journal of Vascular Surgery*, vol. 30, no. 1, pp. 148–56.

22. Thomas, PR, Nash, GB & Dormandy, JA 1988, 'White cell accumulation in dependent legs of patients with venous hypertension: a possible mechanism for trophic changes in the skin', *British Medical Journal* (Clinical research edn), vol. 296, no. 6638, pp. 1693–5.

23. Thomas, S & Jones, M 2001, 'Wound debridement: evaluating the costs', *Nursing Standard*, vol. 15, no. 22, pp. 59–61.

24. Vowden, K & Vowden, P 2002, *Wound bed preparation*, viewed 27 April 2009, <http://www.worldwidewounds.com/>.

25. Weber, C 2003, 'Novel mechanistic concepts for the control of leukocyte transmigration: specialization of integrins, chemokines, and junctional molecules', *Journal of Molecular Medicine*, vol. 81, no. 1, pp. 4–19.

26. White, R 2006, 'Flaminal®: a novel approach to wound bioburden control', *Wounds UK*, vol. 2, no. 3, pp. 64–9.

27. World Union of Wound Healing Societies 2007, *Principles of best practice: Wound exudate and the role of dressings. A consensus document*, MEP Ltd., London.

28. Yamada, BFA & de Gouveia Santos, VC 2005, 'Quality of life of individuals with chronic venous ulcers', *Wounds*, vol. 7, pp. 178–89.

Part three

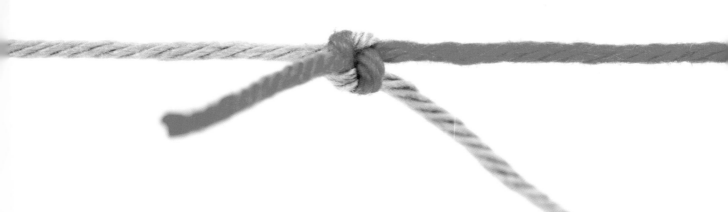

Clinical skills and management in practice nursing

Edited by Doris Young

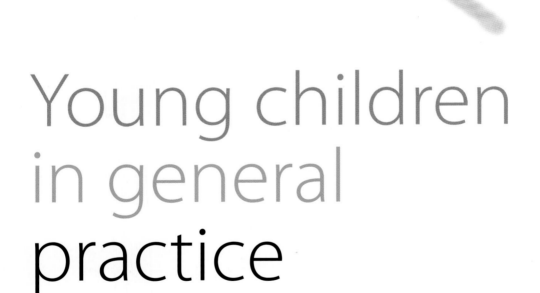

Chapter twelve

Young children in general practice

by Gerry Silk

Overview

The Australian Government has recognised the importance of children's health by introducing several national initiatives, including the 'Healthy Kids Check'. This chapter will focus on assessment and management of the 'sick' child presenting to general practice. The importance of effective communication with children is also discussed as well as highlighting a comprehensive assessment tool, the Parents' Evaluation of Developmental Status (PEDS) which practice nurses can use as part of the Healthy Kids Check.

Objectives

At the completion of this chapter you should be able to:

- have an increased understanding of communicating with children;

- be aware of some of the physical differences between children and adults;

- perform a physical assessment of a sick child;

- identify a child who may be at risk of serious illness; and

- understand the components of the Healthy Kids Check.

Introduction

It is in early childhood that the foundations are laid for good health in the long term. In the early period of their lives, children acquire a range of skills and behaviours as they learn from their family, their social environments such as preschool and child care, and are influenced by the biological factors that impact on an individual's health. Children attend general practice for a variety of reasons including acute illness, injuries, planned presentations, such as immunisations, management of long-term conditions and for screening purposes such as the Healthy Kids Check. Opportunistic consultations may arise when children present with a parent or adult receiving care. It is important to look at childhood presentations to the practice that are the most likely and to understand your practice paediatric population.

Health status of children

The definition of health as not merely the absence of disease applies to children as well as adults. Children are also affected by the many determinants of health that have been discussed in Chapter 10. As adults suffer from acute and chronic illnesses, injuries, obesity and mental illness, so do children. Forty-one per cent of Australian children were estimated to suffer from a long-term condition, including allergies and hayfever (Australian Bureau Statistics 2006). Nine per cent of children aged 4–14 years were thought to have a mental or behavioural problem, including attention deficit hyperactivity disorder (ADHD), or depressive or conduct disorders as a long-term condition (Australian Institute of Health and Welfare 2009). In 2007, 22% of children aged 2–12 years were estimated to be overweight or obese (Australian Institute of Health and Welfare 2009).

It is acknowledged that some children spend more than the recommended time in front of a video screen, are overweight or obese, and are not eating recommended amounts of vegetables. In addition to this, unfortunately, some are homeless or at risk of homelessness, or are victims of assault (Australian Institute of Health and Welfare 2009). Indigenous children are far more likely to be disadvantaged across a broad range of health and socioeconomic indicators and children living in remote areas have higher death rates; higher rates of neural tube defects; lower rates of cancer survival; worse dental decay; and are less likely to meet minimum standards for reading and numeracy, than those in major cities.

Furthermore, statistics reveal that:

- 8% of children have a disability;
- 52% of children with a disability have a profound core activity limitation;
- 7% of all hospitalisation rates in 2005–6 were for children;
- the most common reason (17%) for hospitalisation among children is for respiratory conditions;
- injury and poisoning accounted for 13% of childhood hospitalisation in this period;

- 9.8% of hospitalisations for children aged 0–4 years were for infectious and parasitic diseases; and

- Australia is in the top 10 countries for numbers of children with type 1 diabetes.

(Australian Institute of Health and Welfare 2008)

Assessing the needs of children and how best to provide care can be a challenge for nurses who are not used to caring for children. Every visit to a clinic is a learning experience for a child and how the current visit is managed will have an impact on how they approach any future visits.

> ### Reflections
>
> *How do the above statistics affect the practice nurse? What types of observations may you be prompted to make and what questions should you ask when a child presents to you?*

Communicating with children

Communicating with children is very different from communicating with adults, as they think differently and common words that may be used by nurses may have very different meanings for children. Simple phrases like 'I'm going to take your temperature' may cause concern for a three-year-old as they are egocentric and very possessive; they may not know what you want to take, but to take anything of theirs can be threatening. Rephrasing the sentence to 'I am going to see if you are warm (or hot) today' may appear less threatening to them. If using a tympanic thermometer you can make fun of it by asking if they can hear the ringing noise in their ear, just like a phone. Putting a dressing on a boy may cause concern as boys don't wear dresses; it may be more appropriate to refer to the wound covering as a big band-aid or bandage as those terms are more familiar to children and are less likely to be misunderstood.

Using closed questions to a young child, such as asking if you can 'do' something, such as 'Can I take off your shirt to listen to your chest?' or 'Can I look in your ears?' may result in a firm 'no'. This then leaves you in a dilemma for in order to make an accurate assessment you are required listen to their chest or look in their ears. State what you want to do but give them some choices: 'I want to listen to your chest—would you prefer me or mummy to take your shirt off?' or 'I need to look in your ears; which ear would you like me to look in first?' They may not answer but by phrasing the questions in a friendly way and offering them choices, they at least feel they have some control over the situation.

Young children are usually interested in what you are doing and may ask many questions about what a piece of equipment is for or why you are using it. If children have past health care experiences, they will often relate those to the present situation. They are often interested in learning about how the body works and this interest can be used to engage them in the examination or treatment they are receiving.

If you are using any equipment to examine a child, such as a stethoscope or tympanic thermometer, allowing them to become familiar with the equipment by getting them to touch and look at it first and explanations such as 'it will feel cold' may be useful.

Reflections

What strategies do you use in your practice to improve communication with children?

Children are different

Children are usually healthy individuals with a very different and unique set of anatomical, physical and developmental characteristics. Children are smaller than adults, for example, their airways are much smaller, which makes them more prone to obstruction. A 12-month-old has a trachea with a diameter of approximately 4 mm, usually the size of their little finger, so small obstructions due to swelling as seen in croup, or the inhalation of a foreign body can have a significant impact on the ability to move air in and out of the lungs. The body responds to the narrowing of the airway by using increased effort during inspiration resulting in marked tracheal tug or sternal recession. As the ribs are not fully formed in young children, the sternum is relatively flexible and the sternal recession can be half the depth of the chest.

Also, infants and children become dehydrated due to fluid loss more quickly than adults. Their body surface area to weight ratio is much larger allowing evaporative loss as well as heat loss. Daily turnover of water in an infant is more than half of the extracellular fluid volume, compared to one-fifth in adults (Rogers 1998). The small intestine of a child is six times their body length or height, compared to an adult's small intestine which is only four times their height. The implication for this physiological difference is that a child with a condition such as gastroenteritis will lose relatively more fluid than an adult will, and as their large intestine is proportionately the same length as an adult's, there is no ability to reabsorb more fluid. Hence, dehydration will occur much more rapidly in a child compared to an adult. This is made more complex by the fact that the kidneys of a young child are less developed than adults so they are unable to adequately concentrate urine. An infant passes two millilitres of urine per kilogram of body weight per hour, compared to one millilitre per kilogram in a child and half a millilitre per kilogram in an adult (Smith 1988; Silk 2006).

As infants are born with antibodies that are transferred through the placenta from the mother they have passive immunity against some diseases. These antibodies progressively decline to the lowest levels about six months after birth. The infant's own antibody production is slow to develop and immunoglobulin A (IgA), the secretory antibody in the respiratory tract and gastrointestinal tracts, does not reach adult levels until the second year of life (Mok 1999). This explains the frequent infections in their early years, but does in turn act to improve their immunity, along with immunisation. By the age of four years most children have acquired good levels of immunity as a result of the frequent infections and immunisation (Silk 2006; Mok 1999).

Reflections

Can you think of other differences between adults and children which will affect your care for them?

Assessing the sick child

Determining whether a baby or young child is unwell may be obvious, but assessing the severity of the illness may be more difficult. In their first six months, most babies will have one or more infections, usually caused by a virus and the number of infections will increase as the baby grows older. The average, healthy toddler will have 8–10 viral infections a year but that number can double if the child attends child care. The expected response to the infection is for the child to look flushed, to cry more, sleep less and generally demand more attention (Hewson & Oberklaid 1994).

Research on infants has shown that it was not the presence of fever, cough, diarrhoea or increased crying that indicated serious illness, but how the baby responded to these problems (Hewson & Oberklaid 1994; Morley et al. 1991). Although the research was carried out on babies younger than six months of age, similar features are seen in all babies and young children with serious illness.

The common signs and symptoms of serious illness in babies and young children are best summarised by the **A, B, C, Fluids in and Fluids out** system (Hewson & Oberklaid 1994; Morley et al. 1991).

A is for decreased activity and alertness and poor arousal.

B is for breathing difficulty.

C is for poor circulation.

Fluids in—feeding less than half normal amount over 24 hours.

Fluids out—fewer than four wet nappies in 24 hours.

These signs and symptoms may be commonly present but the more features that are present, the higher the risk that the infant or child will be seriously ill.

A—Activity and alertness

When babies and children are awake they are normally alert and active and respond to their environment. They may be contented, or irritable, but they can be seen to respond in a number of ways. Sick babies and children become drowsy and respond less to normal stimulation. They may be floppy, have reduced movement of the limbs and may exhibit a weak whimpering cry. They will also generally have little or no eye contact with their carers.

The tenet of 'beware the quiet child' is very true when assessing whether a baby or child may be seriously ill or injured. It takes effort and energy to be able to cry, and if they are able to cry loudly, they may be in pain but their airway is patent. This will indicate that they are breathing normally and their circulation is adequate. Seriously ill children don't have the strength to cry loudly, they don't cry at all or they just whimper. Children who have significant chest or abdominal injuries also don't cry as it is generally too painful.

B—Breathing

Healthy babies and children breathe easily and shallowly. The presence of specific noises or excessive effort may indicate serious illness. The noise may be a grunt, wheeze or stridor.

A grunt indicates that they are breathing out against a closed glottis, and effectively applying PEEP (positive end expiratory pressure) in order to inflate congested alveoli as in pneumonia. They may also be splinting their diaphragm if they have significant abdominal pathology such as peritonitis, a bowel obstruction or injured viscus.

A wheeze on expiration indicates lower airway problems, most commonly bronchiolitis in infants and asthma in children.

A stridor indicates an upper airway narrowing, most commonly seen in infants or children with croup but may be as a result of foreign body aspiration.

Tracheal tug, sternal recession, intercostal or subcostal recession are all indicators of excessive effort in breathing and are usually associated with serious illness.

Tachypnoea without recession in the awake baby or child is not indicative of serious illness (Hewson & Oberklaid 1994; Morley et al. 1990) but the presence of central cyanosis is a predictor of serious illness.

C—Circulation

The skin colour of babies and children is a good indicator of their health status. If they look pale all over, as assessed by their parents, they are more likely to be seriously ill; parents of dark-skinned children will also notice a change in the skin colour of their child. Parents are often concerned when their baby or young child has cold hands or feet, but this is a common occurrence with minor illnesses. The child may have a high temperature and still have cold hands and feet. This can be quite normal, but if the legs are cold up to the knees it may indicate that the child is seriously ill.

Fluids in

If the child is taking less than 50% of their normal fluid intake it should be considered as a sign of serious illness.

The total volume of fluid taken in over a 24-hour period needs to be calculated as a percentage of the baby or child's normal intake. If a baby is breast fed, the frequency of feeding and the duration of active sucking needs to be considered. Although this may appear difficult, mothers of breast-fed babies are generally able to assess their baby's fluid intake as accurately as those who bottle feed. The mother needs to consider how long the baby sucks for and how strongly the baby sucks and compare that to the baby's normal feeding patterns.

Fluids out

Fewer than four wet nappies in the past 24 hours indicates a higher risk of serious illness, as does more than five episodes of vomiting in a 24-hour period. However, some babies vomit regularly—the 'happy chuckers' who vomit a number of times a day but are happy, sleep well and are gaining weight normally. In these babies considerably more than five episodes of vomiting in 24 hours would be significant in assessing the presence of illness.

A further five features were also identified (Hewson & Oberklaid 1994; Morley et al. 1990). These are uncommon but if present may indicate a high risk of serious illness so they need to be assessed carefully. In these cases the practice nurse should refer the child to the general practitioner (GP) as soon as possible.

1. **Seizure(s).** There are many causes of seizures in infants and young children, from hypoglycaemia or electrolyte disturbances, to cardiac arrhythmias, trauma or epilepsy. Febrile convulsions are the most common cause of seizures in children from six months to six years of age. They occur in about 3% of children and of these, 25–30% will have further febrile convulsions. Febrile convulsions are due to a rapid rise in temperature, usually at the beginning of an illness when the parent is not even aware the child is sick. These seizures are benign, but can cause great concern for parents whenever the child has an infection (Grattan-Smith 2006).

2. **Apnoeic episode(s).** Apnoea literally means 'no breath'. The baby or child may stop breathing for 10–20 seconds resulting in transient cyanosis. The most common reason for this in babies is gastro-oesophageal reflux, but in some cases may be due to pertussis or bronchiolitis. In older children sleep apnoea may be due to adenotonsillar hypertrophy, obesity or structural airway abnormalities, including craniofacial abnormalities or Down syndrome (Rogers 1998; Great Ormond Street Hospital 2005).

3. **Green vomiting.** This is very rare but when it does occur it is more likely in the first two weeks of life. However, sometimes older children, more commonly between nine and eighteen months of age, may present with green vomiting—the colour of grass. It may be a sign of obstruction in the intestine, specifically volvulus and requires urgent surgical intervention. The green colour of the vomit is unlike any other vomit and the child needs urgent referral to hospital.

4. **Lump larger than 2 cm.**   Any lump that is larger than 2 cm in young babies, except for an umbilical hernia, should be examined by a doctor. This feature is more relevant to infants under 9 or 12 months because as children start to walk, they will fall over many times and may develop lumps greater than 2 cm that will not be serious.

5. **A petechial or purpuric rash.**   These types of rash may indicate meningococcal disease or other forms of sepsis. Petechiae are small (< 2 mm) flat round red spots under the skin surface caused by bleeding into the skin. Purpura are larger (> 2 mm) areas of bleeding into the skin that begin as red areas that become purple and later brownish-yellow (Silk 2006). The rash is flat and does not blanche when pressed. The baby or child will be unwell before the rash appears and have many of the 'A, B, C, Fluids in, Fluids out' signs present.

The febrile child

Fever is one of the most common reasons children present to their GP (Crocetti, Moghbeli & Serwint 2001). Fever is a symptom of an underlying infection, and is the body's natural way of fighting infection. As previously mentioned, young children are prone to many infections. The majority of these will be caused by viruses, but up to 1% of young children without an obvious focus of infection will have a bacterial infection, most commonly pneumococcal. The rate is higher in unimmunised children (Royal Children's Hospital 2008).

A fever does not always indicate that a baby or young child may be seriously ill. Some babies or young children will have a high fever, above 39°C, with a minor viral illness, while others may have a serious infection with a fever of only 38°C. The height of the fever does not indicate how sick a baby or young child is, nor does how the fever responds to analgesia. It is more important to look at how the child is behaving, and the presence of the features of 'A, B, C, Fluids in, Fluids out'. A child with a fever above 39°C and who is pale and lethargic is more of a concern than one who is flushed and irritable.

It is not always necessary to give medicines to lower the fever for this reason alone. However, if the child appears to be in pain, analgesics (such as paracetamol or ibuprofen) may be given in the recommended dose. Many infections cause pain, such as an ear infection (otitis media) or an upper respiratory tract infection causing a headache and aching limbs. If a child is significantly overweight the dose of paracetamol should be calculated according to the expected weight for their age, not their actual weight (Russell et al. 2003). A child who is obese has a heavier body weight but most of that

Table 12.1 Screening tool for young children presenting with acute febrile illness

Underlying chronic respiratory, cardiac, neurological or other illness? Yes ☐ No ☐			
	Low risk (green)	Intermediate risk (amber)	High risk (red)
Colour	– Normal colour of skin, lips and tongue	– Pallor reported by parent/carer	– Pale/mottled/ashen/blue
Activity	– Responds normally to social cues – Content/smiles – Stays awake or awakens quickly – Strong normal cry/not crying	– Not responding normally to social cues – Wakes only with prolonged stimulation – Decreased activity – No smile	– No response to social cues – Appears ill to a health care professional – Does not wake or if roused does not stay awake – Weak, high-pitched or continuous cry

Respiration	– None of the amber or red symptoms or signs	– Nasal flaring
		– Tachypnoea:
		  – RR > 50 breaths/minute, age 6–12 months
		  – RR > 40 breaths/minutes, age > 12 months
		– Oxygen saturation ≤ 95% in air
		– Crackles
			– Grunting
			– Tachypnoea: RR > 60 breaths/minute
			– Moderate or severe chest indrawing

Hydration	– Normal skin and eyes – Moist mucous membranes	– Dry mucous membranes – Poor feeding in infants – CRT ≥ 3 seconds – Reduced urine output	– Reduced skin turgor
Other	– None of the amber or red – symptoms or signs	– Fever for ≥ 5 days age 0–3 months, temperature ≥ 38°C – Age 3–6 months, temperature ≥ 39°C – Swelling of a limb or joint – Non-weight bearing/not using an extremity – A new lump > 2 cm	– Non-blanching rash – Bulging fontanelle – Neck stiffness – Status epilepticus – Focal neurological signs – Focal seizures – Bile-stained vomit

Source: The Royal Children's Hospital 2008

weight is in fat—their liver will be the same size as a child of normal weight. A dose of paracetamol according to their weight would be too much for their liver to metabolise and after a few doses may damage the liver (Russell et al. 2003). To calculate a child's expected weight the formula [(Age + 4) × 2] may be used. If a child is underweight medications should be given according to their actual weight (Silk 2006).

Fever is the body's natural way to fight the infection and research has shown that giving medications that lower the temperature may prolong the duration of the illness and does not prevent febrile convulsions occurring (Royal Children's Hospital 2008; National Institute for Health and Clinical Excellence 2007). If the infant or child is 'hot and happy' it is best to manage their illness with fluids and extra cuddles.

Table 12.1 opposite shows a screening tool for young children presenting with acute febrile illness and has been developed for health practitioners by the National Institute for Health and Clinical Excellence in England in 2007. This has many similarities to the 'A, B, C Fluids in and Fluids out' tool.

Reflections

Do you feel confident in recognising when a child may be seriously ill, compared to those with common viral infections? What triage processes do you have in your clinic either face to face or by telephone to assess children who present with a fever?

Healthy Kids Check

Regular childhood checks are carried out from the time of birth through to commencement of school and in some areas, for longer. The maternal and child health care (M&CHC) service in each state performs the majority of these checks but many families stop attending for regular checks for second or subsequent children. For example, in Victoria only 60% of children have a three-and-a-half-year check with their M&CHC nurse (Colahan 2009). The Healthy Kids Check can be carried out by a number of different health professionals—a M&CHC nurse (or equivalent in each state and territory), a general practitioner or a practice nurse who has had education in this area and is competent to do so.

There is substantial national and international evidence that comprehensive early intervention programs for children and their families have long-term benefits for physical and mental health, educational achievement and emotional functioning (MBS Online 2009). As a result of this, the Healthy Kids Check was introduced in Australia in July 2008 for all four-year-old children who are permanently resident in Australia. It is to be delivered in conjunction with the immunisation for four year olds. This immunisation may be provided slightly earlier or later than four years in some states and territories, so the Healthy Kids Check may be carried out if the child is over three years of age and under five years of age (Department of Health and Ageing 2009). If a parent conscientiously objects to a child being immunised, the Healthy Kids Check can still be carried out despite the immunisation not being administered. In this case the consultation does not attract a fee from Medicare. The purpose of the Healthy Kids Check is to ensure every four-year-old child in Australia has a basic health check to see if they are healthy, fit and ready to learn when they start school. It promotes early detection of lifestyle risk factors, delayed development and illness, and introduces guidance for healthy lifestyles and early intervention strategies (Department of Health and Ageing 2009).

Components of the Healthy Kids Check

Although a childhood check is not restricted to the following criteria, Medicare has determined that these are minimum requirements needed in order to fulfil Medicare requirements. The Healthy Kids Check is based on information collection, assessment, interventions and health advice. Mandatory items included in the health check include:

1. **Collection of information**, including taking or updating the child's history. Any history must include:
   - family relationships
   - environmental factors
   - care arrangements.

2. **Medical and social history**
   - care by paediatrician.

3. **Lifestyle risk factors**
   - eating habits
   - physical activity or inactivity.

4. **Examinations and investigations** as required. Investigations should be undertaken or arranged as clinically indicated in accordance with relevant

guidelines. Detailed activities according to evidence-based guidelines can be obtained from the RACGP Redbook for childhood:

- height
- weight.

The National Health and Medical Research Council guidelines recommend using repeated body mass index (BMI) measurements to assess a child's weight status (National Health and Medical Research Council 2003). These can identify children who are already overweight but also those who are crossing the percentile lines on the BMI percentile chart and are at risk of becoming overweight. To accurately measure a child's BMI there needs to be a fixed wall stadiometer and the measurement should be to the nearest millimetre. Weight should be measured on electronic scales and measured to the nearest 0.1 kg. As children grow, their amount of body fat changes and so will their BMI. For example, BMI usually decreases during the preschool years and then increases into adulthood. For this reason a BMI calculation for a child or an adolescent must be compared against age and gender percentile charts. The height and weight need to be measured for each child and then the BMI calculated. If a computer is not available to calculate BMI, the following formula can be used:

$$BMI = weight\ (kg) \div height\ (cm) \div height\ (cm) \times 10\,000$$

5. **Eyesight**

- includes a visual inspection
- parental concerns about vision, such as amblyopia—sometimes called 'lazy eye', squint, infection, injury
- family history of eyesight problems.

One of the charts that can be used to test a child's eyesight is the Lea (pronounced Lee-ah) Children's Chart. The Lea symbols chart is designed to eliminate problems associated with language barriers, so is ideal for use pre-literate and non-literate children. The chart uses symbols that are familiar to children, such as a circle, square, apple and house. The chart gives high sensitivity for measuring visual acuity in childhood (age four and above) with early and reliable detection of amblyopia (difference in vision between the two eyes). Following discussion with the GP, referral to an optometrist or ophthalmologist is recommended for any concerns in this area.

6. **Hearing**

- ear examination
- parental concerns about the child's listening, hearing or language

- history of ear infections, ear discharge, recurrent or chronic otitis media
- audiology assessment, if appropriate.

Concerns regarding a child's hearing may be identified using the Parents' Evaluation of Developmental Status (PEDS) screen but an examination of the ears should also be undertaken (Glascoe 1998; Irving 2008). Unless specifically trained, nurses are not expected to examine a child's ear. Asking the parent if there has been any history of ear infections, discharge or chronic otitis media may be all that is required. If there are any concerns the child will need to be referred to the GP for referral to an audiologist.

7. **Oral health**

- Has the child visited a dentist?
- How often does the child brush their teeth?

As soon as children have teeth, parents are being encouraged to check the teeth monthly. One program called 'Lift the Lip' program is ideal for this purpose (Centre for Oral Health Strategy 2009). The parent is encouraged to lift the lip and look at the teeth for signs of potential or existing tooth decay. Whitish lines along the edge of the gum may be early signs of tooth decay, and brown or yellow spots that don't brush off may indicate established decay. If either is present, the child should see a dentist as soon as possible. Good dental care in early years prevents decay and caring for primary teeth assists in the healthy development of secondary teeth.

8. **Toilet habits**

- Can the child use a toilet independently or do they need assistance?
- Is the child a bed wetter?

The Healthy Kids Check requires that toilet habits are discussed with the parent, whether the child needs assistance or can use a toilet independently, and whether the child is a bed wetter. Both of these issues can be identified during the PEDS screen under the self-help domain, or under 'any other concerns'. In some cases the parent may not consider that a four-year-old requiring help to use a toilet is cause for concern and so may need to be prompted for more information (Glascoe 1998; Irving 2008).

9. **Allergies**

- document known or suspected allergies.

10. **Recommended intervention and referrals**

Reflections

Are you competent to perform these assessments based on your existing education or do you need additional training?
What is your relationship with the local maternal and child care health nurse?

Other matters for consideration which are *not* mandatory to fulfil Medicare Benefits Schedule (MBS) criteria include the following:

1. **Eating habits**
   - child's appetite
   - variety of food eaten
   - frequency of processed food eaten.
2. **Physical activity**
   - time spent in active or energetic play
   - time spent in sedentary activities.
3. **Speech and language development**
   - concerns about the words the child uses
   - concerns about understanding directions
   - taking part in active conversation.
4. **Fine and gross motor skills**
   - ability to pick up small objects
   - walking, running, jumping, hopping, climbing stairs, riding a tricycle.
5. **Behaviour and mood**
   - sleeping
   - energy levels
   - social and emotional wellbeing
   - ability to separate from the main carer.

Based on the examination and history taken, a clinical judgment will determine which in any intervention is necessary and to whom the referrals need to be written. Providing health advice and information to the child's parents or guardian may all that is required. A range of resources may be used for this including publications from the Department of Health and Ageing and the printed version of the child health record. The *Get set 4 Life* book is now available in Arabic, Chinese, Italian, Spanish, Greek and Vietnamese. A useful website for information on normal growth and development of children is the Raising Children Network. It provides reliable, scientifically validated information and resources to support parents in the day-to-day work of raising children and looking after their needs.

Parents' Evaluation of Developmental Status (PEDS)

Historically, numerous clinical assessment tools have been used to assess a child's development, all requiring the child to complete specific tasks while being observed for a short time. There are many limitations to this type of assessment as the child may not want to 'perform for a stranger', or may just be having a bad day and not want to perform the task even though they are quite capable of doing so. Most states of Australia and New Zealand are now using PEDS as the initial screening tool for infants and children from four months until eight years of age. The tool was developed in the USA by Frances Page Glascoe in 1998 and has been validated in Australia by the Centre for Community Child Health, Royal Children's Hospital, Melbourne (Coghlan, Kiing & Wake 2003; Centre for Community Child Health 2006). The underlying principle for using PEDS is to ensure that development and behaviour problems in young children are detected and addressed. This is accomplished by carefully recognising parents' concerns, ascertaining the children's level of risk for developmental delay and identifying the best pathway for intervention (Glascoe 1998). There is much research that demonstrates the importance of identifying problems with a child's development early, before the problems become entrenched. Intervening early in the course of the condition or problem increases the chance of a positive outcome. The earlier any intervention is started, the more likely it is to be effective and the less expensive it will be (Irving 2008). The PEDS test is not diagnostic; it is a screening tool that identifies the children who require more specific assessment.

The PEDS tool recognises the parent as the expert in knowing their child and relies on their daily observations of their child. PEDS has been shown to be as accurate as any of the previously developed screening tests. However, PEDS has the distinct advantages of taking less time, needing no specialised equipment and having a strong emphasis on parental involvement (Irving 2008). Using the PEDS tool requires specific training as the validity of the screening relies on consistent use of the tool, as research has shown that altering the PEDS questions leads to substantial under-identification of children with problems (Glascoe 1998). Training is being conducted throughout Australasia for child health nurses and practice nurses.

The PEDS questionnaire covers eight domains of development:

1. Expressive language/articulation
2. Receptive language
3. Fine motor skills
4. Gross motor skills
5. Behaviour
6. Social-emotional
7. Self-help
8. Learning preschool skills.

The 10 items in the questionnaire have all been rated as predictive or non-predictive of developmental delay, and these change according to the child's age. The number of predictive and non-predictive items is totalled and the PEDS interpretation form directs the appropriate pathway for intervention. If there are two or more significant predictive concerns, the pathways suggest referral for audiological and speech or language testing. Professional judgment is used to decide if referrals are also needed for social work, occupational therapy, physiotherapy or mental health services. The child will need to be referred to the GP for further assessment or direct referral to the appropriate service.

PEDS also includes two open-ended questions where the parent can express any concerns about their child. The open-ended questions may elicit concerns relating to medical conditions such as asthma, abdominal pain or many other issues. If these concerns are raised the child should be referred to their GP for assessment.

The language used in the questions has been rigorously tested and standardised to ensure clarity for the parent and accurate in identification of problems for the child. The administration of PEDS usually takes about two minutes for the parent to complete. This can be done while waiting for their appointment in the clinic or if there are language or literacy problems, it can be completed with the practice nurse and an interpreter if necessary (Irving 2008).

The major focus of the PEDS is listening to the parents. Parents are much more likely to follow through with referrals, procedures or programs if they feel they are respected and have been involved in the process. PEDS comprises three components:

1. PEDS response form that the parent completes
2. PEDS score form
3. PEDS interpretation form for the health professional to complete, which identifies the appropriate intervention strategies.

It is reassuring that PEDS research shows that approximately 40–50% of parents will not have any concerns about their child's development (Glascoe 1998). There will be an occasional situation when the parent has no concerns but the nurse does have a concern about the child's development. Further discussion and questioning with the parent and likely referral to the GP will be required to tactfully raise the issue of a potential problem. Conversely, problems identified by the parent will need further discussion to ensure that parental expectations are aligned to normal developmental benchmarks.

Secondary screening

If there is one significant predictive concern, a secondary screening may be administered to improve the specificity of the process. Secondary screening reduces the number of children referred for detailed assessment who do not have a developmental delay or disability. A child who fails the secondary screen requires referral for assessment (Glascoe 1998). Depending on their level of experience, the practice nurse may choose to carry out the secondary screening, although referral to the M&CHC nurse or GP may be more appropriate.

Conclusion

As part of their role practice nurses are assessing, triaging and initiating management of sick children in collaboration with the general practitioner. They are also identifying those children in need of medical intervention, and supporting children and their families in accessing care that is required to manage those acute needs. As part of national policy directives, practice nurses are seen as an effective means to improve the preventative health measures available to children in those important preschool years. They can also forge the link between maternal and child health care services and the general practice in providing continuing care to young children as they enter their school and adolescent years.

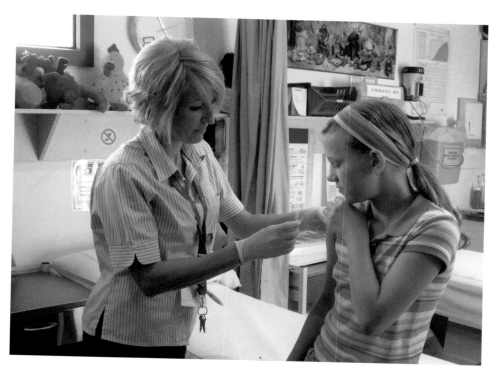

CASE STUDY

| Name of nurse |
| Karen Booth |

| Practice |
| Leichhardt General Practice, Sydney, NSW |

Tessa had been a patient at the Leichhardt General Practice but left the area at the age of one. Three years later Tessa presented to her former GP twice with childhood illnesses of respiratory tract infections and earache which responded rapidly to treatment. On the third occasion Tessa was referred to the practice nurse for her 'four-year-old' immunisations.

During the pre-vaccination assessment the nurse noted that Tessa was a smiling and happy child but was small for age small and speech was noted to be impeded. Tessa's older sister and cousins were in attendance at the consultation and it was noted that Tessa was smaller in comparison, and had small hands and mildly dysmorphic facial features. Due to time constraints, the parents were invited to bring Tessa back for the 'four-year-old healthy kids check'.

On further questioning it was noted that the family had been given a referral for a speech pathologist assessment by their previous GP but the assessment was very expensive and they could not afford it at that time. The parents were also concerned about Tessa's hearing and on examination Tessa was noted to have bilateral ear effusion with tense drums.

The mother was not concerned about Tessa's social skills, as Tessa had good relationships and enjoyed playing with her cousins. Diet was varied and other habits were age appropriate (toileting, dry at night and hygiene).

The findings of the four-year-old check were presented to Tessa's parents and she was referred to the GP for review of the assessment. Tessa was referred for a hearing assessment and was found to have a moderate hearing deficit. More active management was commenced for treating the sinuses and the child was referred to an ENT specialist for review. Tessa was also referred to a paediatrician who conducted extensive developmental and genetic testing. The findings were that Tessa's height was approximate of a three-year-old and, apart from the speech, her other developmental test were age appropriate.

After comprehensive specialist review a diagnosis was made of Turner syndrome, a chromosomal abnormality. The parents were expecting a normal assessment and that she would grow out of her speech problems when she started preschool. Although surprised they were accepting of the diagnosis, aware of the implications and the subsequent required follow-up, including cardiology review.

Having the diagnosis of a long-term condition made early in the child's development has ensured that problems are addressed early. Tessa has been able to commence school and has been given the assistance required to ensure optimal learning in the early stages of development. The vigilance and expertise of the practice nurse was crucial in identifying signs that made this diagnosis possible and has meant that Tessa was healthy, fit and ready to learn when she started school.

Key messages

Children with fever are a common presentation to general practice.

Foundations for good health in the long term are laid down in childhood.

Parents are experts in knowing their own children and recognising illness.

Practice nurses can play an important role in preventative health of children and the identification of issues affecting long-term health.

Useful resources

Care of sick children: a basic guide by Gerry Silk
Ausmed Publications, Melbourne.

Brigance screen
Hawker Brownlow Education
Telephone: 03 9555 1344 (1800 334 603)
http://www.hbe.com.au/

Ages and stages screening and questionnaires
Brookes Publishing Co.
Telephone: 02 9349 5811
http://www.pbrookes.com/

Lea eye chart
Design for Vision, PO Box 366, Abbotsford, VIC. 3067
Telephone: 03 9419 5599

Get set 4 life—habits for healthy kids
Department of Health and Ageing
http://www.health.gov.au/

Raising children
http://www.raisingchildren.net.au/

BMI charts
http://www.education.vic.gov.au/

Australian guide to healthy eating
http://www.health.gov.au/

Continued

Useful resources *continued*

MBS Online, Medicare Benefits Schedule
http://www.health.gov.au/internet/mbsonline/publishing.nsf/Content/
Medicare-Benefits-Schedule-MBS-1

Royal Australian College of General Practitioners, *Guidelines for preventive activities in general practice* (The Red Book), 7th edn, 2009
http://www.racgp.org.au/

Preventive activities over the lifecycle—children
http://www.racgp.org.au/Content/NavigationMenu/ClinicalResources/
RACGPGuidelines/TheRedBook/Red_book7_Child_Chart.pdf

Physical activity recommendations for 5–12 year olds
http://www.health.gov.au/internet/main/publishing.nsf/Content/phd-
physical-activity-kids-pdf-cnt.htm/$FILE/kids_phys.pdf

Australian Institute of Family Studies
http://www.aifs.gov.au/

Royal Children's Hospital Melbourne
http://www.rch.org.au/

Australian Breastfeeding Association
http://www.breastfeeding.asn.au/

References

1. Australian Bureau Statistics (ABS) 2006, *National Health Survey 2004–05: summary of results*, viewed 21 November 2009, <http://www.abs.gov.au/AUSSTATS/abs@.nsf/DetailsPage/4364.02004-05?/>.

2. Australian Institute of Health and Welfare (AIHW) 2008, *Australia's health 2008*, viewed 21 November 2009, <http://www.aihw.gov.au/>.

3. Australian Institute of Health and Welfare (AIHW) 2009, *A picture of Australia's children 2009*, viewed 30 August 2009, <http://www.aihw.gov.au/>.

4. Centre for Community Child Health 2006, 'Body Mass Index (BMI) for children', *Community Paediatric Review*, vol. 15, no. 1, pp. 1–4, viewed 21 January 2010, <http://www.rch.org.au/emplibrary/ccch/CPR_Vol15No1.pdf>.

5. Centre for Oral Health Strategy 2009, *Early childhood oral health guidelines or health professionals*, 2nd edn, NSW Health, viewed 21 November 2009, <http://www.health.nsw.gov.au/>.

6. Coghlan, D, Kiing, J & Wake, M 2003, 'Parents' evaluation of developmental status in the Australian day-care setting: developmental concerns of parents and carers', *Journal of Paediatrics and Child Health*, vol. 39, no. 1, pp. 49–54.

7. Colahan, A 2009, 'Maternal and Child Health Service', presentation at the Medicare '4-year-old health check' training session held in January 2009 at Nurses Memorial Centre, Melbourne.

8. Crocetti, M, Moghbeli, N & Serwint, J 2001, 'Fever phobia revisited: have parental misconceptions about fever changed in 20 years?', *Pediatrics*, vol. 107, no. 6, pp. 1241–6.

9.   Department of Health and Ageing 2009, *Enhanced Primary Care Program (EPC)*, viewed 21 January 2010, <http://www.health.gov.au/epc/>.

10. Glascoe, FP 1998, *Collaborating with parents: using parents' evaluation of developmental status to detect and address developmental and behavioral problems in children*, Ellsworth and Vandemeer Press, Nashville, TN.

11. Grattan-Smith, P 2006, 'Seizures and non-epileptic events', in P Cameron, G Jelenik, I Everitt, G Browne & J Raftos (eds), *Textbook of Paediatric Emergency Medicine*, Elsevier, London.

12. Great Ormond Street Hospital 2005, *Obstructive sleep apnoea and CPAP information sheet*, viewed 21 November 2009, <http://www.ich.ucl.ac.uk/>.

13. Hewson, PH & Oberklaid, F 1994, 'Recognition of serious illness in infants', *Modern Medicine of Australia*, July, pp. 89–96.

14. Irving, E 2008, 'Parents' Evaluation of Developmental Status (PEDS) trainer notes', Centre for Community Child Health, Royal Children's Hospital, Melbourne.

15. MBS Online, Medicare Benefits Schedule 2009, viewed 21 January 2010, <http://www.health.gov.au/internet/mbsonline/publishing.nsf/Content/Medicare-Benefits-Schedule-MBS-1>.

16. Mok, QQ 1999, 'Special needs of the critically ill child', in AJ McNab, DJ Macrae & R Henning (eds), *Care of the Critically Ill Child*, Churchill Livingstone, London.

17. Morley, CJ, Thornton, AJ, Cole, TJ, Fowler, MA & Hewson, PH 1991, 'Symptoms and signs in infants under 6 months of age correlated with the severity of their illness', *Pediatrics*, vol. 88, no. 6, pp. 1119–23.

18. Morley, CJ, Thornton, AJ, Fowler, MA, Cole, TJ & Hewson, PH 1990, 'Respiratory rate and severity of illness in babies under 6 months old', *Archives of Disease in Childhood*, vol. 65, no. 8, pp. 834–7.

19. National Health and Medical Research Council (NHMRC) 2003, *Clinical Practice Guidelines for the Management of Overweight and Obesity in Children and Adolescents*, Department of Health and Ageing, viewed 21 January 2010, <http://www.health.gov.au/>.

20. National Institute for Health and Clinical Excellence (NIHCE) 2007, *Feverish illness in children: assessment and initial management in children younger than 5 years*, RCOG Press, viewed 21 November 2009, <http://www.nice.org.uk/>.

21. Rogers, JS 1998, 'Respiratory system', in TE Soud & JS Rogers (eds), *Manual of Pediatric Emergency Nursing*, Mosby, St Louis.

22. The Royal Children's Hospital (RCH) 2008, *Clinical Practice Guideline. Febrile child under 3 years*, viewed 15 June 2009, <http://www.rch.org.au/>.

23. Russell, F, Shann, F, Curtis, N & Mulholland, K 2003, 'Evidence on the use of paracetamol in febrile children', *Bulletin of the World Health Organization*, vol. 81, no. 5, pp. 367–74.

24. Silk, G 2006, *Care of sick children: a basic guide*, Ausmed Publications, Melbourne.

25. Smith, J 1988, 'Big differences in little people', *American Journal of Nursing*, vol. 88, no. 4, pp. 458–62.

Chapter thirteen

Well women in general practice

by Cate Nagle
and Lynne Walker

Overview

This chapter will focus on three specific areas of women's health: the care of women in pregnancy, the care of woman relating to cervical cancer screening and breast health. Common to all three topics is the opportunity for the practice nurse to play an important role in risk assessment, health promotion and health education.

Objectives

At the completion of this chapter you should be able to:

· recognise the opportunities for the practice nurse to contribute to improved health outcomes for women;

· describe the features of contemporary pregnancy care in the Australian setting;

· discuss ways of promoting women's participation in pregnancy care;

· appreciate the dimensions of risk assessment, health education and health promotion in pregnancy care;

· recognise the role of the practice nurse in cervical screening; and

· be confident in promoting breast health.

Introduction

The Australian Government has recognised that health inequalities exist between groups of Australian women and there are differences in health outcomes related to gender (Department of Health and Ageing 2008). Women have been identified as the majority of health consumers, the majority of service providers and the majority of carers (Department of Health and Ageing 2008). The practice nurse is in the ideal position to impart health prevention messages to women as opportunities arise when women visit the general practice for emergency care, planned care and when accompanying other members of the family as carers.

National Women's Health Policy

The aim of the National Women's Health Policy is to respond to needs of women and actively promote their participation in making decisions about managing their health. Health promotion messages can be imparted in a variety of ways, from personal communication with patients, written reminders and health promotion material in the practice, to strategic marketing opportunities targeting women.

Reasons given for the development of the women's health policy include:

- Breast cancer is a major cause of burden of disease in the 15–74 age group.
- Antenatal and postnatal depression affects approximately 15% of women during pregnancy and early childhood.
- The incidence of chlamydia infection is increasing.
- Gestational diabetes is diagnosed in 5–12% of pregnant women, who then have a 50% risk of developing type 2 diabetes within five years.
- Symptoms of menopause can significantly impact on women's lives.
- Caesarean section rates have increased from 18% in 1991 to 30% in 2005.

Furthermore, Aboriginal and Torres Strait Islander women experience poorer health than non-Indigenous Australian women, with more than double the rate of cervical cancer in 2000–04 (Australian Institute of Health and Welfare (AIHW) 2009) and higher rates of chlamydia and hepatitis C. Significantly higher rates of cervical cancer are found in women in rural and remote areas compared to women living in cities, as women in remote areas participate less in cervical and bowel screening programs (AIHW 2008a; AIHW 2008b).

Pregnancy care

In order to achieve the highest levels in safety and quality of maternity care it is important that, at a minimum, women have access to the level of care that is appropriate to their clinical need. Providing pregnancy care in the general practice setting is an important strategy to improving access to primary and secondary levels of maternity care and presents nurses working in general practices, particularly those with midwifery qualifications, with the opportunity to complement the role of the general practitioner (GP). Underpinning safe quality care is the assumption that all health professionals providing pregnancy care are working within their respective scopes of practice with effective communication and collaboration between multidisciplinary team members.

A general practice is often the first contact women have with a health professional in pregnancy and this presents a valuable opportunity to discuss options of care, conduct a risk assessment and provide women with information.

Epidemiology

Information on all births occurring in Australian hospitals, birth centres and the community is collected annually by state and territory agencies and it provides details on pregnancies and the characteristics of women who gave birth and their babies and details of pregnancy outcomes. From this information we know that in terms of maternal mortality and morbidity and neonatal mortality it has never been a safer time in history to give birth or to be born in Australia (Laws & Hilder 2008). There are, however, particular groups of women such as Indigenous women and younger women who are over-represented in adverse outcomes. This has clear implications for the provision of pregnancy care.

There has been a continued increase in births since 2001 and in 2006, 277 436 women gave birth to 282 169 babies in Australia (Laws & Hilder 2008).

In 2006 the characteristics of women birthing were:

- 3.7% were of Aboriginal or Torres Strait Islander origin
- 41.6% gave birth for the first time
- 1.7% had a multiple pregnancy
- 25.1% had their labours induced
- 58.1% had a spontaneous vaginal birth, 30.8% gave birth by caesarean section, 0.4% had a vaginal breech birth and 10.7% had an assisted vaginal birth.

The characteristics of babies born in 2006 were:

- 8.2% were preterm (less than 37 weeks' gestation)
- 6.4% of babies were of low birth weight (less than 2500 grams)
- 14.9% of babies were admitted to a special care nursery or neonatal intensive care unit.

(Laws & Hilder 2008)

Aims of pregnancy care

The aim of pregnancy care is to optimise maternal and fetal wellbeing. To realise this aim health professionals should:

- develop a shared understanding with the woman to meet her individual needs;
- provide care that reflects the experience of pregnancy involving physical, emotional and social adjustments;
- promote information sharing and encourage women to be involved in decision making;
- identify any complications in pregnancy and treat/refer appropriately; and
- practice evidence-based care.

A number of factors have been associated with women's increased satisfaction with pregnancy care including: sufficient time in appointments; minimal waiting time; flexibility in scheduling appointments; friendly and supportive staff; consistent information and care; a good level of communication, attentive listening by staff and being involved in their care (Waldenstrom et al. 2000; Homer, Davis & Brodie 2000). These factors have clear implications for all providers of maternity care and models of care that involve continuity and are centred on the needs of the woman can provide many advantages.

Options of care

Women at low risk of complications can have their maternity care provided by primary care models involving midwives and/or GPs. Where complications exist but are assessed as moderate in nature, women can be cared for in a secondary level of care such as general practice with consultation with specialist medical care. Tertiary level care is required for complex cases and involves multidisciplinary specialist care. A variety of guidelines defining low-risk pregnancies have been developed (Australian College of Midwives 2008; The Royal Australian and New Zealand College of Obstetricians and Gynaecologists (RANZCOG) 2009) and are applied to guide referral, consultation and transfers of care between models on the basis of identified risk factors.

Maternity care can be classified on the basis of privately or publicly funded models. Privately funded models include private obstetric care or care shared by the obstetrician and GP. Publicly funded models generally involve care with a public hospital. There are numerous models of shared care in Australia available to women at low to moderate risk of complications. These models of care can be led by a GP, midwife and obstetrician or by a team approach.

Women's decisions regarding a model of care can be influenced by many factors, including whether or not they have health insurance, previous experience, advice of friends or family or wanting to give birth at a particular maternity service. Advice from health professionals can assist women's decision making.

Example 13.1

Enza is a 33-year-old woman in her first ongoing pregnancy and presents to your clinic for confirmation of her pregnancy. She has seen the GP and following a dating scan it is determined she is seven weeks' gestation. Enza is now consulting with you to decide on a model of care.

> What questions do you pose to Enza to assist her with her decision making?
> What are all the options available to Enza in your geographical location?
> What are the relative benefits of each?

Continuity of care

Where possible, models that feature continuity of care should be promoted. Continuity of care or carer, where care is provided by the same health professional or a small group of health professionals throughout pregnancy, during birth and in the postnatal period, is associated with positive outcomes for women (Biro, Waldenstrom & Pannifex 2000), maternity care clinicians (Turnbull et al. 1995) and organisations (Homer et al. 2001). A systematic review of continuity of care by midwives versus non-continuity of care by midwives and doctors (Hodnett 2000) involving more than 1000 women found that women were:

- more likely to discuss their pregnancy and postnatal concerns;
- more likely to attend pregnancy education classes;
- less likely to be admitted to hospital during pregnancy;
- more likely to feel prepared for childbirth; and
- more likely to be pleased with care in pregnancy, labour and postnatally.

One of the features of pregnancy care in the primary care setting is the extent to which GPs, midwives and practice nurses are able to get to know women and build on existing relationships with women.

Creating a supportive environment

Pregnancy is a normal physiological process and pregnant women are usually healthy with no risk factors for complications. However, complications both physical, pregnancy related and psychosocial can interrupt a woman's experience of pregnancy. Some situations require advanced communication skills on the part of the health professional because of the sensitive nature of the issue. In instances of communicating with women about issues such as depression, anxiety, domestic violence and substance use, GPs and midwives can benefit from professional development to improve their confidence and skills in communicating with women (Gunn et al. 2006) and creating the environment where women feel comfortable to disclose issues (Hegarty et al. 2007). Attentive listening, picking up on cues and the appropriate use of questioning are all required facets of communication.

The layout of the room can also be important in creating a comfortable environment so attention should be given to the position of chairs, table and computer in order to remove barriers between the health profession and the woman. The ambience of the room is also important to optimise engagement with the woman during the consultation.

Organisation of care

A pregnancy is often referred to in relation to trimesters, which are periods of approximately three months. The first trimester is 13 completed weeks, the second trimester extends from 13–25 weeks and the third trimester is from 26 weeks to birth. Historically, pregnancy care has been provided on a schedule of 14 visits across the three trimesters. However, studies have demonstrated that in women with low-risk pregnancies, a reduction in the number of visits to

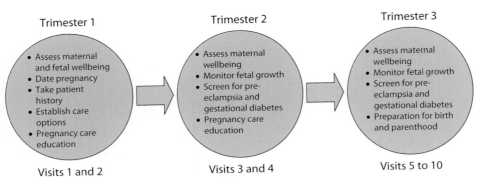

Figure 13.1 Scheduling of pregnancy care visits

between seven to ten does not adversely affect perinatal outcomes (Villar et al. 2001, Carroli et al. 2001) and contemporary maternity care is often organised around a schedule of visits similar to that shown in Figure 13.1 opposite.

Additional visits should be scheduled by the woman as required and it is likely that women who are having a baby for the first time will require more visits than a woman who has had children. GPs will recommend more visits when pregnant women have pre-existing conditions or when complications are suspected or confirmed.

The number and timing of the visits should be flexible to accommodate women's lifestyle (Mercy Hospital for Women, Southern Health Service & Women's & Children's Health Service 2001). One way of achieving this is to ensure that each visit should have a specific purpose and where possible tests and investigations should be arranged to coincide with these visits.

GP–midwife model of care

In the GP–midwife model of care, the GP provides most of the antenatal care, with assistance from a midwife. This is usually performed in private rooms or hospital clinics.

Ideally, women should be given information on the models of care available prior to their first visit as there is much to consider and many decisions to make, even in a normal healthy pregnancy.

Assessing risk factors

The initial visit in pregnancy is usually the longest, particularly if the woman is new to the practice. Risk factors need to be assessed through thorough history taking, physical examination and tests and investigation.

History taking

Ideally, risk factors have been assessed prior to pregnancy but, as many pregnancies are not planned, this is not always possible. Pregnancy-care records seek to identify risks that relate to a woman's state of general health, medical (see Table 13.1 overleaf), obstetric and social history as well as lifestyle factors. A thorough physical examination, accurate history taking and the results of tests and investigations form the basis of this risk assessment.

The age of women birthing in Australia is increasing and in 2006 the average age was 29.8 years with more than a fifth of women aged 35 years or older (Laws & Hilder 2008). Increased maternal age is associated with

Table 13.1 Assessment of risk in pregnancy

Risk factor	Examples
Cardio vascular disease	Hypertension
Renal disease	Recurrent urinary infections, autoimmune disease
Endocrine disease	Diabetes, thyroid disorders
Haematological disorder	Anaemia, clotting disorders
Neurological	Epilepsy
Respiratory	Asthma
Infectious disease	Hepatitis, HIV

Source: modified from Three Centres 2001

an increased risk of hypertensive disorders, multiple pregnancy, fibroids and diabetes (Van Katwijk & Peeters 1998; Berkowitz et al. 1990). The risk of having a pregnancy affected by a trisomic abnormality, such as Down syndrome, also increases with a woman's age (Resta 2005; Hook 1981). At the other end of the age continuum, younger pregnant women aged under 20 years are also at increased risk of selected fetal abnormalities. Abnormalities involving defects of the abdominal wall, exomphalos and gastroschisis, are more likely in younger women.

Ethnicity is an important consideration in taking an obstetric history due to the increased risk for some conditions that may warrant additional investigation. Conditions such as thalassemia or sickle cell anaemia are more prevalent in women from Mediterranean countries, the Middle East, Africa and India (O'Connor & Kovacs 2003). Some ethnic groups are over-represented in poor birth outcomes. Women of Aboriginal or Torres Strait Islander origin experience higher rates of low birth-weight babies than non-Indigenous women. Low-birth weight is associated with factors including socioeconomic status, number of babies previously born, mother's nutritional status, smoking and alcohol intake, and illness during pregnancy (Ashdown-Lambert 2005; Mohsin et al. 2003). Low birth-weight babies are more likely to require more hospitalisation and have a greater risk of ongoing health concerns (Goldenberg & Culhane 2007). Women born outside Australia, particularly those from developing countries, may not have had early childhood screening for cardiac abnormalities (Consultative Council on Obstetric and Paediatric

Mortality and Morbidity 2008). Considering ethnicity in the clinical picture may inform whether specific assessments or follow-up are warranted.

A GP or midwife will also assess a woman's risk in pregnancy by taking a genetic history to determine predisposition for genetic conditions or carrier status. Genetic conditions, such as cystic fibrosis or X-linked conditions, can be tested prior to or in the early stages of pregnancy. In certain cultures it is accepted that biological relatives partner and have children therefore genetic conditions are more likely to arise as a result. Some conditions are associated with the environment in which individuals live so taking a family history is also informative.

Obtaining an obstetric history is also an important component of the initial visit and reviewing the clinical summary of previous pregnancies should provide all necessary details. Obstetric risk factors include: history of severe pre-eclampsia, birth weight under 2500 grams or over 4500 grams, uterine surgery, antepartum haemorrhage or postpartum haemorrhage on more than two occasions; conditions detected in pregnancy such as pre-eclampsia, suspected fetal growth restriction, pre-labour rupture of membranes, multiple pregnancy, prolonged pregnancy and bleeding. Other risk factors include inadequate pregnancy care and a history of recurrent miscarriages, a mid-trimester fetal death, stillbirth or neonatal death, fetal abnormality, five or more births (Mercy Hospital for Women, Southern Health Service, Women's & Children's Health Service 2001). These factors are associated with poor outcomes and appropriate consultation, referral or transfer to specialist care is usually required.

Tests and investigations

It is important that women receive written information on the tests and investigations they are offered in pregnancy (National Collaborating Centre for Women's and Children's Health 2008) (see Table 13.2 overleaf) and that they have the opportunity to ask any questions or clarify any issues. Some tests such as a full blood examination will be recommended by the GP while others such as testing for Down syndrome will be offered. It is important that the woman understands the risks, benefits and consequences of the tests she is having. In particular, understanding the difference between screening and diagnostic tests in pregnancy is important and there are resources that can assist women to make decisions that are consistent with their values.

The resources section at the end of this chapter contains a selection of useful websites.

Table 13.2 Schedule of tests and investigations in pregnancy

Gestation (weeks)	Recommended tests to be discussed	Physical assessments
7–12	– Full blood examination – Blood group and antibodies – Mid-stream urine – Hepatitis B – Hepatitis C – Syphilis – Rubella – HIV – Down syndrome (T21) if first trimester testing – Ultrasound scan – Vitamin D – Ferritin – Thalassemia	– Review physical health – Calculate body mass index – Establish baseline blood pressure
12–20	– Down syndrome (T21) if second trimester testing – 18–20 week ultrasound scan for fetal abnormalities	– Blood pressure measurement – Fundal height measurement
18–22	– 18–20 week ultrasound scan for fetal abnormalities	– Blood pressure measurement – Fundal height measurement
26–28	– Gestational diabetes screening – FBE and if Rh negative, Rh antibodies and Anti D at 28 weeks	– Blood pressure measurement – Fundal height measurement – Abdominal palpation
30–32		– Blood pressure measurement – Fundal height measurement – Abdominal palpation
33–36	– FBE and if Rh negative, Rh antibodies and Anti D at 34 weeks	– Blood pressure measurement – Fundal height measurement – Abdominal palpation
36–38	– Group B Strepococcus screening	– Blood pressure measurement – Fundal height measurement – Abdominal palpation

Gestation (weeks)	Recommended tests to be discussed	Physical assessments
38–40		– Blood pressure measurement – Fundal height measurement – Abdominal palpation
40–42	– Cardiotocography – Amniotic Fluid Index	– Blood pressure measurement – Fundal height measurement – Abdominal palpation – Vaginal assessment

Physical assessment

Body mass index

A woman's weight and height should be measured at the initial visit in pregnancy to calculate a body mass index (BMI). Routine weighing is no longer indicated in low-risk women (National Collaborating Centre for Women's and Children's Health 2008) as maternal weight gain is deemed an unreliable predictor of low birth weight (Dawes & Grudzinskas 1991). Extremes in maternal BMI warrant referral to specialist multidisciplinary care.

Blood pressure measurement

Pre-eclampsia and eclampsia are hypertensive disorders of pregnancy accompanied by proteinuria that remain leading causes of maternal morbidity and mortality, and poor neonatal outcomes. Recording a woman's blood pressure measurement at each visit in pregnancy is the method of screening for pre-eclampsia. It is important that the correct technique is used including: ensuring the woman is in a supported position; selecting the correct-sized cuff and palpating the systolic blood pressure at the brachial artery. Hypertension in pregnancy can be defined as a systolic blood pressure 140 mmHg or more or 30 mmHg above the initial measurement and/or a diastolic measure equal to or higher than 90 mmHg or 15 mmHg above the initial measurement (Society of Obstetric Medicine of Australia and New Zealand 2008) warrants investigations for proteinuria. Elevated blood pressure measurements in pregnancy warrant immediate medical review.

Fundal height measurement

From 12 weeks' gestation, the top (fundus) of the uterus can be palpated above the pelvic brim and from 20 weeks the fundus is usually detected at the level of the umbilicus. Measurements from the fundus to the symphysis pubis assist in assessing fetal growth (Neilson 2000) and should be performed at each visit. It is important that the person performing the measurement is experienced and uses a consistent technique (Bailey et al. 1989) and that a non-elastic tape measure is used with the markings faced downwards (Mercy Hospital for Women, Southern Health Service & Women's & Children's Health Service 2001). From 20 weeks' gestation, each week approximates to a corresponding measurement in centimetres. For example, for a woman at 24 weeks' gestation the fundal height measurement would be expected to have a fundal height measurement of approximately 24 centimetres. A number of factors including maternal height and the lie of the fetus need to be considered in interpreting this measurement (Gardosi & Francis 1999) and it should not be interpreted in isolation (see also Figure 13.2 below). Any concerns regarding fetal growth warrant referral by the GP or midwife for an ultrasound scan. Although listening to the fetal heart rate does not inform clinical practice it is often performed and can be reassuring for the woman and clinician.

Abdominal palpation

From approximately 28 weeks how the fetus is lying in the uterus is assessed and documented and from 36 weeks the descent of the fetal head into the pelvis is measured.

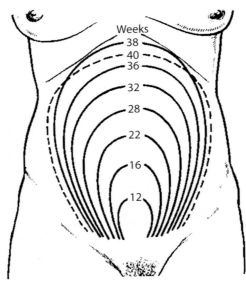

Figure 13.2 Fundal height measurement

Midwife- or nurse-led care

Midwife- or nurse-led care refers to the models where the midwives or nurse provides all or nearly all of the antenatal care. This can involve birth teams and birthing centres.

The midwife or nurse can play an integral role in to working in partnership with the woman during pregnancy particularly in the sharing of information and health education and health promotion. In a general practice setting the nurse/midwife can complement the explanations provided by the GP and acts as an advocate to ensure the woman has understood the information provided. Women may require encouragement to ask some of the following questions:

- Why do I need to have this test?
- What does the test involve?
- Will it hurt?
- What will happen next if the test shows something isn't quite right?
- Are there any potential risks, drawbacks or harm in having this test?
- What are the potential benefits or advantages of having this test?
- When will I get the results?
- How will I find out?
- Does my age or ethnic background impact the detection rate for this condition or the chance the result is wrong (that is, a false positive or false negative result)?

(Mercy Hospital for Women, Southern Health Service, Women's & Children's Health Service 2001)

Engaging the woman in her pregnancy care

In order to individualise a woman's care the midwife or nurse needs to understand the woman's past and present. One model of facilitating woman-centred care used effectively in pregnancy care consultations (Gunn et al. 2006; Hegarty et al. 2007) contains the following aspects:

- Introduction: greeting the woman, introducing yourself, explaining your role and addressing confidentiality.
- Understanding the woman as a person: asking the woman about her feelings, fears and concerns; picking up on spoken and non-verbal cues by listening attentively.
- Understanding the woman's experience of pregnancy: asking about life events, family and cultural issues; addressing the woman's expectations of pregnancy and her pregnancy care.

- Finding common ground: involving the woman in the planning of her pregnancy care; achieving a common understanding of any issues of concern.
- Information giving: assessing the woman's need for information; allowing her to ask questions; giving small amounts of information at a time; checking understanding; focusing on emotional and social health as well as physical health.
- Ending interview: summarising, drawing to a conclusion and preparing for next pregnancy visit.

Encouraging women to participate in their pregnancy care can be facilitated by providing written information (National Collaborating Centre for Women's and Children's Health 2008) and additional resources such as approved websites to complement verbal explanations. The amount of information women seek varies significantly so it is important to be able to refer women to resources that are appropriate to their needs. The resources should be informed by the best evidence base available and some examples of information from federal and state health departments are provided at the end of the chapter.

Decision aids

For decision support in more complex matters such as screening tests for fetal abnormalities or vaginal birth after caesarean birth, decision aids can assist women to make decision that are based on correct information and consistent with their values (O'Connor et al. 1999; Shorten et al. 2004; Nagle et al. 2008). Decision aids are different from simple informational resources as they provide women with information on the risks, benefits and consequences of all options involved in a decision as well as a level of decision support. Decision aids complement but should not replace a consultation with a health professional.

Another way of increasing a woman's satisfaction and sense of control during pregnancy is by using hand-held maternity records (Brown & Smith 2004). In some maternity services women are given their own case notes to look after and bring to each antenatal visit. Despite concerns that records may be lost, a systematic review has demonstrated that the use of paper-based records increased the availability of pregnancy records during hospital attendance (Brown & Smith 2004). Where a number of providers are involved in a woman's pregnancy care, paper-based records may aid communication between pregnancy care providers as well as encouraging consistency of information and care.

Health education and health promotion

Common symptoms of pregnancy, such as nausea and vomiting, heartburn, constipation and varicosities, can cause some women significant discomfort and require treatment, while other woman experience mild discomfort or are not affected. It is important that women receive advice that is informed by quality evidence. In some instances there is little high-level evidence available and suggested remedies may or may not be effective.

Lifestyle considerations are discussed at each visit in pregnancy. Early in pregnancy the amount of information women receive can be overwhelming so, as previously noted, it is important to supplement verbal explanations with written information. Information on physical, psychosocial and emotional changes in pregnancy is discussed, together with dietary advice on macro- and micronutrients, exercise, and prescribed and over-the-counter medication and illicit drug use.

In general the focus of dietary advice should be on a healthy balanced diet with regular exercise. Regarding dietary modifications in pregnancy, it is important that women are informed that folic acid supplementation before conception and up to 12 weeks' gestation reduces the risk of neural tube defects such as spina bifida. Other micronutrient intake that may be discussed are iron, and vitamins A and D. Listeriosis is a food-acquired infection that can lead to fetal death, stillbirth and severe neonatal infection, and women should receive information on reducing the risk of exposure by avoiding specific foods in pregnancy such as soft cheese, processed meats and many pre-prepared meals.

Two important health promotional messages in pregnancy concern the risks of smoking and alcohol consumption. All health professions play a pivotal role in smoking cessation interventions and these strategies are known to be effective in assisting individuals to quit smoking and stay quit (Lumley et al. 2009). In 2006 approximately 17% of Australian women reported that they smoked during pregnancy, and this rate has changed little over the previous four years. Smoking is associated with many health conditions in general and in pregnancy is associated with an increased risk of miscarriage, fetal growth restriction, preterm birth, placental abruption and placenta praevia. Children of parents who smoke are at an increased risk of sudden infant death syndrome and experience increased rates of respiratory conditions. It can be difficult to engage women who smoke about quitting and one framework that is used in pregnancy care consultations is called the '5 As model'. This is discussed further in Chapter 16 (see p. 388).

There is a large body of evidence linking maternal alcohol consumption during pregnancy with adverse effects on the developing fetus and child (Sokol, Delaney-Black & Nordstrom 2003). The evidence for harm is particularly strong with binge and heavy drinking, particularly for birth defects, if consumed in the first trimester (National Health and Medical Research Council 2009; Henderson, Gray & Brocklehurst 2007). The effects of low or moderate alcohol consumption are conflicting (Colvin et al. 2007; O'Leary et al. 2007) and in the absence of evidence to support a level of alcohol consumption that is safe, national guidelines recommend avoiding alcohol in pregnancy.

Parenting and breastfeeding information is an important aspect of pregnancy care so these are topics that are covered in more detail during childbirth education sessions. It is important to be aware of the options for childbirth education classes available in your local area. Most maternity hospitals and some community health centres provide classes. Classes can also be arranged privately in some areas, which may accommodate more flexible scheduling.

Cervical cancer

Internationally, cervical cancer is the second most common malignant tumour among women (Australian Institute of Health and Welfare 2009). In Australia, cervical cancer accounted for 329 deaths in 1991 and 212 deaths in 2004, making it the 18th most common cause of cancer mortality in Australian women (Australian Institute of Health and Welfare 2009). Cervical cancer is one of the most preventable cancers and one of the few where screening can be used to detect pre-cancerous cell changes. The Pap test has been available since 1949 and is the most widely used cancer screening test in the world (Monsonego et al. 2003).

National Cervical Screening Program

Screening to detect abnormalities of the cervix has been available on an ad hoc basis to women in Australia since the 1960s. The National Cervical Screening Program was introduced as a structured program in 1991 as a joint Australian and state governments initiative. Its aim was to reduce the incidence and mortality of cervical cancer in females and provide standardised guidelines for the interval and the target age group for screening. As a test used for population screening, the Pap test involves the systematic testing of asymptomatic individuals who have unrecognised disease and who will benefit from further intervention to reduce the incidence and mortality of cervical cancer. The Pap test is not a diagnostic test but it does identify those women who require further testing for the presence of disease.

Currently the National Cervical Screening Program has an overall screening rate of approximately 61% of the eligible population, however, this rate varies according to the age group. In 2004, the screening rates varied from 47.7% in the 20–24 year age group to 66.9% in the 50–59 year age group (AIHW 2009). Importantly, these figures reveal several age groups where the screening rates are noticeably lower than the average: 57.8% in the 25–29 year age group, 47.7% in the 60–64 and 49.7% in the 65–69 year age group.

Pap tests are provided as part of mainstream health services available to all Australians and 70–80% are performed by GPs (AIHW 2009; Girgis et al. 1999). Incentives have been provided to general practice to increase cervical screening rates via the cervical screening Practice Incentives Program (PIP). Having a structured approach to cervical screening will help to reach set targets for cervical screening rates. PIP is discussed in more detail in Chapter 2.

Increasingly, practice nurses have undergone education which prepares them to be able to identify, screen and follow up women with both normal and abnormal Pap test results. In Victoria, 21 668 Pap tests (3.8%) were collected by nurses in 2008. This number has more than doubled in the last 10 years (Victorian Cervical Cytology Registry 2008). Furthermore, Pap tests collected by nurses are more likely to have an endocervical component which is considered to be a reflection of the smear quality (Victorian Cervical Cytology Registry 2008). This supports the practice nurse as an alternative provider for women undertaking cervical screening and, as a Medical Benefits Schedule item number is now available to support funding of this service, can contribute to practice income.

Recommendations

Currently the National Cervical Screening Program recommends:

1. Routine screening with Pap tests should be carried out every two years for women who have no symptoms.

2. All women who have ever been sexually active should start having Pap tests between the ages of 18 and 20 years, or one or two years after beginning sex, whichever is later.

3. Pap tests may cease at the age of 70 years for women who have had two normal Pap tests within the last five years. Women over 70 years who have never had a Pap test, or who request a Pap test should be screened (The Cancer Council Australia 2007).

As part of the National Cervical Screening Program, each state operates a cervical screening registry. The objectives of the registry are to:

- remind females to attend for screening;
- ensure the follow-up of females with abnormal Pap tests;
- provide cervical screening histories to laboratories and clinicians to aid reporting management; and
- monitor the effects of initiatives to improve participation by females in screening.

Although a national program has simplified the collection of data and works towards increasing screening rates, there are many reasons that women do not present for screening. Barriers identified by Girgis and others to women presenting for Pap tests include:

- lack of time (7%)
- other commitments (19%)
- difficulty getting to the surgery (5%)
- unsuitable appointment times (22%)
- a male provider (31–35%).

(Girgis et al. 1999; Walsh 2006)

The more barriers the women in this study perceived, the less likely they were to attend for a Pap test. An appropriately trained female practice nurse with a flexible appointment system can overcome several of these barriers to Pap testing and could potentially remove barriers for more than 50% of these women.

For Indigenous women the lack of availability of a female provider has also been identified as a major barrier to accessing cervical screening (Commonwealth of Australia 2004).

The role of the practice nurse is increasingly encompassing cervical screening, as funding initiatives support this. At the time of screening, opportunities also arise for the delivery of other key health messages by the practice nurse. These include breast health, lifestyle issues, identification of risk factors, smoking cessation information and general health and wellbeing advice.

If practice nurses choose not to undertake education in this area, the opportunity to promote cervical screening to those women coming into general practice still exists and should become part of their routine health promotion messages.

> **Reflections**
>
> *How does your clinic offer well women the choice of providers and appointments for cervical screening?*

Breast cancer

The biggest risk factor for developing breast cancer is age and by the age of 85 years, a woman has a 1 in 8 chance of being diagnosed with breast cancer (The Cancer Council Australia 2007). Of all breast cancer cases in females in 2006, 6% occurred in females younger than 40 years of age, 69% in those aged 40 to 69 years and 25% in women aged 70 years and over (Australian Institute of Health and Welfare & National Breast and Ovarian Cancer Centre 2009). Following non-melanoma skin cancer, breast cancer was the most common cancer affecting women in 2006 (The Cancer Council Australia 2007). Given that 85% of the population visit their GP at least once a year (AIHW 2008a) the practice nurse has a variety of ways to promote breast health messages to all women visiting their general practice. Recent research has indicated that practice nurses play a significant role in providing education to patients (Phillips et al. 2008) and breast health messages can be part of that education.

Breast screening

As did the National Cervical Screening Program, BreastScreen Australia commenced in 1991. It is a structured Australian and state governments funded program which aims to reduce morbidity and mortality from breast cancer by early detection. This dedicated screening and assessment service uses mammographic screening at both fixed and mobile centres throughout the country and access is available with no doctor's referral needed.

The target group for mammographic screening is 50–69 years as this is the group for which screening is most beneficial on a population basis. In this age group routine mammographic screening reduces the risk of dying of breast cancer by 25% (The Cancer Council Australia 2007). However, the program can be accessed by women between the ages of 40–49 years and over 70 years.

Recommendations

Women between 50–69 years of age should have breast screening every two years through BreastScreen Australia.

Breast awareness

More than half of breast cancers are found by the woman or her doctor after noticing a change in the breast (The Cancer Council Australia 2007). The National Breast and Ovarian Cancer Centre and the Cancer Council Australia now advocate a 'breast awareness' approach which encourages all women to report new or unusual breast changes. Rather than breast self-examination (BSE) or clinical breast examination (CBE) the message has been updated. Women are now encouraged to become familiar with the look and feel of their breasts so that they are able to recognise any changes that may occur in the breasts and report these changes to their doctor. Used in conjunction with mammographic screening for women in the target age group, breast awareness is now seen as the preferred method of detection of early breast cancer.

Recommendations

All women should be familiar with the normal look and feel of their breasts. Unusual changes should be checked by a GP immediately. Possible symptoms of breast cancer may include:

- a lump, lumpiness or thickening in the breast or armpit;
- changes in the skin, such as puckering, dimpling or a rash;
- persistent or unusual breast pain;
- a change in the shape or size of the breast;
- any area that feels different from the rest; or
- discharge from a nipple, a nipple rash or a change in its shape.

(The Cancer Council Australia 2007)

The delivery of these key health messages in general practice can be accomplished by many strategies. Not only can nurses speak directly to women during a consultation, they can promote cervical screening and breast health messages in the waiting room, by direct mailouts, nurse-led clinics, reminder letters and to local community groups.

Reflections

What opportunities do you have in your practice to promote breast health messages to women?

Conclusion

Women are a major consumer of health services and many opportunities arise for practice nurses to impart key health message which directly affect women's state of health and wellbeing. Many women visit a general practice at some point during pregnancy. Women electing to receive all or part of their ongoing pregnancy care in the primary care setting have the opportunity to develop relationships with their care providers and to benefit from this continuity. It is important that the care provided is based on contemporary quality evidence both in terms of the organisation of care as well as the clinical aspects. Midwife- or nurse-led pregnancy care must be predicated on individuals working within their scope of practice.

As the continuity of care covers the entire life cycle of women, practice nurses can continue their care in other significant areas of women's health, that being cervical screening and breast health. The many opportunities to speak with women of all ages afford practice nurses the privilege of influencing health behaviours by delivering preventive health messages in a confident manner at opportune times.

CASE STUDY

Name of nurse
Rachel Sargeant
Practice
Draper Street Family Medical, Cairns, Qld

Cairns is an area in which there are many young couples and families who have moved away from established family support. Within this community, I identified a need for quality coordinated midwifery support in all stages of conception, pregnancy and postnatal care. I observed new parents struggle for information and guidance, and many of these new parents and prospective parents become extremely anxious. Without family support they were unable to find a source of information, assistance and continuity of care that they could trust and rely on. Furthermore, access to a suitable provider for cervical screening was identified as a need.

We aimed to provide a service which addressed the need for support prior to conception, and continuing for as long as the parents felt they needed the service. The nurses became involved from very early in a parents' decision to have a family by offering conception and fertility advice. Thus we commenced a relationship so that once pregnant, mothers chose to become involved in our antenatal care program. A shared care program was established with GPs providing medical support as required and there is now a comprehensive shared care program in place with both the private and public hospitals in Cairns.

The midwives are able to offer conditional postnatal home visits following delivery, and this support continues with the normal range of child health services including lactation support, growth checks, health assessments and childhood immunisations.

Both practice nurses in the practice are Pap test accredited and the uptake of patients choosing to request Pap tests has been fantastic, due mainly to issues of access. Pap tests can be offered in a timely manner and we also found that reduced time pressures allowed the practice nurse to spend a little more time with patients than the GPs may otherwise be able to.

Providing complete midwifery support and continuity of care for women—conception, pregnancy, lactation advice, childhood immunisations, Pap smears and ongoing health maintenance—has enabled relationships to be built with women that would be more difficult in an ad hoc approach. These relationships allow patients to feel comfortable discussing details of their pregnancy or relationships that they may not have otherwise been happy divulging. This also allows for very rewarding practice; it is fulfilling and the nurse knows how to try to make a difference. We were also able to develop a pregnancy information folder where we liaised with other allied health providers and hospitals so that women had written options for all their care, empowering them to make informed choices.

From an economic point of view, the Pap smear provision bought its share of income to the surgery but it was with the introduction of the 16400 Medicare item numbers that really showed a financial contribution. Statistics showed that our small surgery alone claimed 3.98% of these services for the whole of Queensland in 2008, amounting to $8500 towards the running costs of the surgery.

Though a difficult decision, I have left this position to become the Maternal and Child Health Educator at Apunipima, which is part of the Cape York Health Council based in Cairns. I have been lucky enough to become involved with a community-controlled health organisation whose aim is to provide culturally appropriate health services to Cape York communities and improve access, availability, quality and sustainability of these services.

Testimonial

As an independent provider with an appointment system, billing structure and autonomy, I was very valued within the team setting where my decisions were respected and my opinions valued—it was a great working environment which I thoroughly enjoyed.

Key messages

Practice nurses can contribute to care of pregnant women by assisting in physical, emotional and social care.

Antenatal care can be provided safely by the GP and practice nurse working as a team.

Promoting preventive health messages regarding cervical screening and breast health are practice nurse roles which can increase access for women, increase screening rates and build capacity of practices.

A nurse-led cervical screening service can overcome barriers to women accessing cervical screening.

Useful resources

Australian College of Midwives
'Guidelines for Midwifery Practice'
http://www.midwives.org.au/scripts/cgiip.exe/WService=MIDW/ccms.r?Pagel
d=10037

The Cancer Council Australia
http://www.cancer.org.au/

National Breast and Ovarian Cancer Centre
http://nbocc.org.au/

National Institute for Health and Clinical Effectiveness Clinical Practice Guidelines
http://guidance.nice.org.uk/CG62/

New South Wales Health Department
'Having a baby'
http://www.nsw.gov.au/Baby_results.asp?area=PREGNANCY_BABY_LIFE_
SNSW&parent=BABY_LIFE_SNSW

Queensland Health Department
'Pregnancy and Childbirth'
http://access.health.qld.gov.au/hid/WomensHealth/
PregnancyandChildbirth/index.asp

Royal Australian and New Zealand College of Obstetricians and Gynaecologists
http://www.ranzcog.edu.au/

Royal College of Obstetricians and Gynaecologists
http://www.rcog.org.uk/

Royal Women's Hospital Clinical Practice Guidelines
http://www.thewomens.org.au/MaternityClinicalPracticeGuidelines

South Australian Health Department
'Pregnancy'
http://www.cyh.sa.gov.au/SubDefault.aspx?p=432

Tasmanian Health Department
'Pregnancy, Parenting and Your Health'
http://www.dhhs.tas.gov.au/health__and__wellbeing/life_stages/related_
topics/having_a_baby

Victorian Health Department
'Having a baby in Victoria'
http://www.health.vic.gov.au/maternity/

'A guide to tests and investigations for uncomplicated pregnancies'
http://www.health.vic.gov.au/maternitycare/tests.pdf

Western Australian Health Department
'Pregnancy'
http://www.health.wa.gov.au/health_index/p/pregnancy.cfm

References

1. Ashdown-Lambert, JR 2005, 'A review of low birth weight: predictors, precursors and morbidity outcomes', *Journal of the Royal Society for the Promotion of Health*, vol. 125, no. 2, pp. 76–83.

2. Australian College of Midwives (ACM) 2008, *Australian midwifery guidelines for consultation and referral*, ACM, Canberra.

3. Australian Institute of Health and Welfare (AIHW) 2008a, *Australia's health 2008*, AIHW, viewed 23 January 2010, <http://www.aihw.gov.au/>.

4. Australian Institute of Health and Welfare (AIHW) 2008b, *National Bowel Cancer Screening Program monitoring report*, AIHW, viewed 22 January 2010, <http://www.aihw.gov.au/>.

5. Australian Institute of Health and Welfare (AIHW) 2009, 'Cervical screening in Australia 2006–2007', AIHW, Canberra, viewed 22 January 2010, <http://www.aihw.gov.au/>.

6. Australian Institute of Health and Welfare & National Breast and Ovarian Cancer Centre (AIHW & NBOCC) 2009, *Breast cancer in Australia: an overview, 2009*, Cancer series, no. 50, cat. no. CAN 46, AIHW, Canberra.

7. Bailey, SM, Sarmandal, P & Grant, JM 1989, 'A comparison of three methods of assessing interobserver variation applied to measurement of the symphysis-fundal height', *British Journal of Obstetrics and Gynaecology*, vol. 96, no. 11, pp. 1266–71, viewed 23 January 2010, <http://www.bjog.org/>.

8. Berkowitz, GS, Skovron, ML, Lapinski, RH & Berkowitz, RL 1990, 'Delayed childbearing and the outcome of pregnancy', *New England Journal of Medicine*, vol. 322, no. 10, pp. 659–64, viewed 23 January 2010, <http://content.nejm.org/cgi/content/abstract/322/10/659>.

9. Biro, M, Waldenstrom, U & Pannifex, J 2000, 'Team midwifery care in a tertiary level obstetric service: a randomized controlled trial', *Birth*, vol. 27, no. 3, pp. 168–73, viewed 22 January 2010, <http://www.ingentaconnect.com/>.

10. Brown, H & Smith, H 2004, 'Giving women their own case notes to carry during pregnancy', *Cochrane Database of Systematic Reviews*, issue 2, art. no. CD002856, doi: 10.1002/14651858.CD002856.pub2.

11. The Cancer Council Australia (TCCA) 2007, *National Cancer Prevention Policy 2007–09*, TCCA, NSW, viewed 23 January 2010, <http://www.cancer.org.au/>.

12. Carroli, G, Villar, J, Piaggio, G, Khan-Neelofur, D, Gülmezoglu, M, Mugford, M, Lumbiganon, P, Farnot, U & Bersgjø, P 2001, 'WHO systematic review

of randomised controlled trials of routine antenatal care', *Lancet*, vol. 357, no. 9268, pp. 1565–70, viewed 22 January 2010, <http://www.thelancet.com/>.

13. Colvin, L, Payne, J, Parsons, D, Kurinczuk, JJ & Bower, C 2007, 'Alcohol consumption during pregnancy in nonindigenous West Australian women', *Alcoholism, Clinical and Experimental Research*, vol. 31, no. 2, pp. 276–84.

14. Commonwealth of Australia 2004, 'Principles of practice, standards and guidelines for providers of cervical screening services for Indigenous women', viewed 23 January 2010, <http://www.cancerscreening.gov.au/internet/ screening/publishing.nsf/Content/73772661560D0A81CA2574EB007F73AD/ $File/indi-women.pdf>.

15. Consultative Council on Obstetric and Paediatric Mortality and Morbidity (CCOPMM) 2008, *Annual Report for the Year 2006 incorporating the 45th Survey of Perinatal Deaths in Victoria*, CCOPMM, Melbourne.

16. Dawes, M & Grudzinskas, J 1991, 'Patterns of maternal weight gain in pregnancy', *British Journal of Obstetrics and Gynaecology*, vol. 98, no. 2, pp. 195–201.

17. Department of Health & Ageing 2008, *Developing a women's health policy for Australia—setting the scene*, viewed 21 January 2010, <http://www.health.gov. au/>.

18. Gardosi, J & Francis, A 1999, 'Controlled trial of fundal height measurement plotted on customised antenatal growth charts', *British Journal of Obstetrics and Gynaecology*, vol. 106, no. 4, pp. 309–17.

19. Girgis, A, Bonevski, B, Perkins, J & Sanson-Fisher, R 1999, 'Self-reported cervical screening practices and beliefs of woman from urban, rural and remote regions,' *Journal of Obstetrics and Gynaecology*, vol. 19, no. 2, pp. 172–9.

20. Goldenberg, RL & Culhane, JF 2007, 'Low birth weight in the United States', *American Journal of Clinical Nutrition*, vol. 85, no. 2, pp. 584S–90S.

21. Gunn, J, Hegarty, K , Nagle, C, Forster, D, Brown, S & Lumley, J 2006, 'Putting women centred care into practice: (ANEW) A new approach to psychosocial risk assessment during pregnancy', *Birth*, vol. 33, no. 1, pp. 46–55.

22. Hegarty, KS, Brown, S, Gunn, J, Forster, D, Nagle, C, Grant, B & Lumley, J 2007, 'Women's views and outcomes of an educational intervention designed to enhance psychosocial support for women during pregnancy. A new approach to psychosocial risk assessment during pregnancy', *Birth*, vol. 34, no. 2, pp. 155–63, viewed 22 January 2010, <http://www3.interscience.wiley.com/ journal/118533603/abstract>.

23. Henderson, J, Gray, R & Brocklehurst, P 2007, 'Systematic review of effects of low-moderate prenatal alcohol exposure on pregnancy outcome', *British Journal of Obstetrics and Gynaecology*, vol. 114, no. 3, pp. 243–52.

24. Hodnett, ED 2000, 'Continuity of caregivers for care during pregnancy and childbirth', *Cochrane Database of Systematic Reviews* (Online)(2): CD000062.

25. Homer, C, Davis, G & Brodie, P 2000, 'What do women feel about community-based antenatal care?', *Australian and New Zealand Journal of Public Health*, vol. 24, no. 6, pp. 590–5.

26. Homer, C, Matha, D, Jordan, L, Wills, J & Davis, G 2001, 'Community-based continuity of midwifery care versus standard hospital care: a cost analysis',

Australian health review: a publication of the Australian Hospital Association, vol. 24, no. 1, pp. 85–93.

27. Hook, EB 1981, 'Rates of chromosome abnormalities at different maternal ages', *Obstetrics and Gynaecology*, vol. 58, no. 3, pp. 282–5.

28. Laws, P & Hilder, L 2008, *Australia's mothers and babies 2006*, cat. no. PER 46, Perinatal statistics series, no. 22, AIHW National Perinatal Statistics Unit, Sydney.

29. Lumley, J, Chamberlain, C, Dowswell, T, Oliver, S, Oakley, L & Watson, L 2009, 'Interventions for promoting smoking cessation during pregnancy', *Cochrane Database of Systematic Reviews*, issue 3, art. no. CD001055, doi: 10.1002/14651858.CD001055.pub3.

30. Mercy Hospital for Women, Southern Health Service & Women's & Children's Health Service 2001, *Three Centres Consensus Guidelines on Antenatal Care*, Mercy Hospital for Women, Southern Health Service and Women's & Children's Health Service, Melbourne, viewed 22 January 2010, <http://www.health.vic.gov.au/>.

31. Mohsin, M, Wong, F, Bauman, A & Bai, J 2003, 'Maternal and neonatal factors influencing premature birth and low birth weight in Australia', *Journal of Biosocial Science*, vol. 35, no. 2, pp. 161–74.

32. Monsonego, J, Bosch, FX, Coursaget, P, Cox, JT, Franco, E, Frazer, I, Sankaranarayanan, R, Schiller, J, Singer, A, Wright, T, Kinney, W, Meijer, C & Linder, J 2003, 'Cervical cancer control, priorities and new directions', *International Journal of Cancer*, vol. 108, pp. 329–33.

33. Nagle, C, Gunn, J, Bell, R, Lewis, S, Meiser, B, Metcalfe, S, Ukomunne, OC & Halliday, J 2008, 'Use of a decision aid for prenatal testing of fetal abnormalities to improve women's informed decision making: a cluster randomised controlled trial [ISRCTN22532458]', *British Journal of Obstetrics and Gynaecology*, vol. 115, no. 3, pp. 339–47.

34. National Collaborating Centre for Women's and Children's Health 2008, *Antenatal care: routine care for the healthy pregnant woman*, National Institute for Health and Clinical Excellence, Dorchester, viewed 22 January 2010, <http://www.nice.org.uk/>.

35. National Health and Medical Research Council (NHMRC) 2009, *Australian guidelines to reduce health risks from drinking alcohol*, NHMRC, Canberra.

36. Neilson, J 2000, 'Symphysis–fundal height measurement in pregnancy', *Cochrane Database of Systematic Reviews*.

37. O'Connor, AM, Rostom, A, Fiset, V, Tetroe, J, Entwistle, V, Llewellyn-Thomas, H, Holmes-Rovner, M, Barry, M, & Jones, J 1999, 'Decision aids for patients facing health treatment or screening decisions: systematic review', *British Medical Journal*, vol. 319, no. 7212, pp. 731–4.

38. O'Connor, V & Kovacs, G 2003, *Obstetrics, Gynaecology and Women's Health*, Cambridge University Press, Cambridge.

39. O'Leary, CM, Heuzenroeder, L, Elliot, EJ & Bower, C 2007, 'A review of policies on alcohol use during pregnancy in Australia and other English-speaking countries', *Medical Journal of Australia*, vol. 186, no. 9, pp. 466–71.

40. Phillips, C, Pearce, C, Dwan, K, Hall, S, Porritt, J, Yates, J, Kljakovic, M & Sibbald, B 2008, 'Charting new roles for Australian general practice nurses',

abridged report, Australian General Practice Network, viewed 23 January 2010, <http://www.anu.edu.au/aphcri/Domain/PracticeNursing/index.php>.

41. Resta, R 2005, 'Changing demographics of advanced maternal age (AMA) and the impact on the predicted incidence of Down syndrome in the United States: implications for prenatal screening and genetic counseling', *American Journal of Medical Genetics*, vol. 133A, no. 1, pp. 31–6.

42. The Royal Australian and New Zealand College of Obstetricians and Gynaecologists (RANZCOG) 2009, *RANZCOG Guideline: Suitability criteria for models of care and indications for referral within & between models of care*, RANZCOG, Melbourne.

43. Shorten, A, Chamberlain, M, Shorten, B & Kariminia, A 2004, 'Making choices for childbirth: development and testing of a decision-aid for women who have experienced previous caesarean', *Patient Education and Counseling*, vol. 52, no. 3, pp. 307–13.

44. Society of Obstetric Medicine of Australia and New Zealand (SOMANZ) 2008, *Guidelines for the management of hypertensive disorders of pregnancy*, SOMANZ, Sydney.

45. Sokol, R, Delaney-Black, V & Nordstrom, B 2003, 'Fetal alcohol spectrum disorder', *Journal of the American Medical Association*, vol. 290, no. 22, pp. 2996–9.

46. Turnbull, D, Reid, M, McGinley, M & Shields, N 1995, 'Changes in midwives' attitudes to their professional role following the implementation of the midwifery development unit', *Midwifery*, vol. 11, no. 3, pp. 110–119.

47. Van Katwijk & C, Peeters, LLH 1998, 'Clinical aspects of pregnancy after the age of 35 years: a review of the literature', *Human Reproduction Update*, vol. 4, no. 2, pp. 185–94.

48. Victorian Cervical Cytology Registry (VCCR) 2008, 'Statistical Report 2008', VCCR, viewed 23 January 2010, <http://www.vccr.org/>.

49. Villar, J, Carroli, G, Khan-Neelofur, D, Piaggio, G & Gulmezoglu, A 2001, 'Patterns of routine antenatal care for low-risk pregnancy', *Cochrane Database of Systematic Reviews (Online)*, issue 4, art. no. CD000934, doi: 10.1002/14651858.CD000934.

50. Waldenstrom, U, Brown, S, McLachlan, H, Forster, D & Brennecke, S 2000, 'Does team midwife care increase satisfaction with antenatal, intrapartum, and postpartum care? A randomized controlled trial', *Birth*, vol. 27, no. 3, pp. 156–67.

51. Walsh, J 2006, 'The impact of knowledge, perceived barriers and perceptions of risk on attendance for a routine cervical smear,' *The European Journal of Contraception and Reproductive Health Care*, vol. 11, no. 4, pp. 291–6.

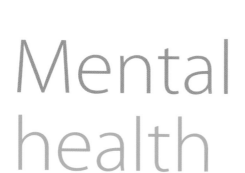

Chapter fourteen

Mental health

by Natisha Sands

Overview

A survey of general practice activity has found that 11.1% of GP encounters involved the management of psychological problems, with depression the fourth most commonly managed problem in general practice (Britt et al. 2007). As practice nurses play an important role in triaging patients, having an understanding of mental illness presentations and subsequent care is beneficial for providing initial assessment and observation. Caring for people undergoing changes in behaviour as a result of mental illness, or psychiatric disorder, can be challenging. This chapter will provide basic information to assist nurses to make appropriate decisions regarding triage, ongoing care and referral.

Objectives

At the completion of this chapter you should be able to:

- have an understanding of the incidence and significance of mental health problems in Australia;

- become familiar with the signs and symptoms of common mental illnesses;

- have an understanding of mental health assessment across the lifespan, including risk assessment;

- develop your knowledge in assessing and managing psychiatric crises; and

- identify the ongoing roles and responsibilities of primary health nurses in caring for people with mental illness.

Introduction

Mental illness is highly prevalent in Australia; with one in five people expected to experience a mental health problem at some stage during their lives (Australian Institute of Health and Welfare (AIHW) 2008). Mental illness is the leading cause of non-fatal burden of disease and injury in Australia (Begg et al. 2007). Globally, the incidence of mental illness is estimated to be in the hundreds of millions (World Health Organisation (WHO) 2001). Depression is highly represented in these figures, with 154 million people worldwide currently suffering the illness, and approximately 877 000 suicides every year (WHO 2005a). The World Health Organisation (2005b) predicts that by 2020, mental illness will account for 15% of the global disease and injury burden.

Primary health is the first point of contact for many Australians seeking assistance with mental health problems, and thus it has an important role in the early identification, prevention and treatment of mental illness (Australian General Practice Network 2005). Embedded in the Australian Government's *National Action Plan on Mental Health* (Council of Australian Governments (COAG) 2006) is the aim of reducing the stigma of mental illness and improving access to quality mental health care in the community. One of the strategies the government employed to meet this aim was the introduction of general practice mental health care items into the Medicare Benefits Schedule (MBS). This scheme was part of the *Better Access to Mental Health Care Initiative* (COAG 2006) which was underpinned by the goal of improving access to mental health services provided by primary health. The mental health care items provide a framework for assessment, treatment and referral of people with mental illness.

The inclusion of these items in the MBS has led to a stronger focus on mental health in primary health care settings, which will inevitably lead to greater involvement by practice nurses in providing care for people with mental illness, as has been the case in other countries (Gray et al. 2001). While practice nurses currently do not write mental health care plans, as part of the multidisciplinary team, they may be involved in contributing assessment information and carrying out components of the plan in conjunction with general practitioners. The discussion in this chapter presents information on holistic biological, psychological and social assessment and care planning for people with mental illness, and is aimed at supporting practice nurses in their clinical practice.

Mental health and illness

Mental health is a state of emotional and psychological wellbeing whereby the individual can cope with life's stressors, achieve their goals and live a satisfying life.

Mental illness can be defined as a range of cognitive, behavioural and emotional disorders that can significantly interfere with the individual's level of functioning and quality of life. These disorders affect the way a person thinks, feels and behaves, and may impact on the individual's ability to effectively communicate with others. Mental illness can cause major impairment to functioning in all areas of life such as relationships (social functioning), work–school life (occupational functioning), and physical and emotional health (personal functioning) (Kaplan & Sadock 2007).

Mental illnesses range in severity from mild or moderate conditions to major mental illnesses (referred to as serious mental illness). The incidence of anxiety disorders and depression in the general population is high, and these conditions are therefore referred to as 'high prevalence' disorders (VicHealth 2007). High prevalence disorders are predominantly treated in primary health settings. Major mental illnesses such as bipolar disorder and schizophrenia, on the other hand, affect only 1% of the population and are referred to as 'low prevalence' disorders (VicHealth 2007). In the past, people with serious mental illness were treated principally by public mental health services but more recently primary health has increased its service provision to include major mental illnesses (COAG 2006).

Some groups within the community are more vulnerable to mental health problems than others due to a complex range of social, psychological and physiological factors. Refugees (WHO 1996), Indigenous people, and those who have been victims of trauma, violence and/or sexual assault are examples of vulnerable groups (WHO 2005). Women who have been or are victims of interpersonal violence also commonly experience mental health problems such as anxiety, depression and post-traumatic stress disorder (Hegarty et al.

2004). In addition, young people (generally categorised as those aged 12 to 25 years) are also a vulnerable group, as evidenced by the relatively high rates of youth suicide in Australia (Sawyer et al. 2000).

Identifying mental illness

Mental illnesses are diagnosed according to criteria outlined in formal diagnostic classification systems. In Australia, two main classification systems are used for psychiatric diagnosis: the Diagnostic and Statistical Manual of Mental Disorders (DSM-IV-TR) (American Psychiatric Association 2000), and the International Statistical Classification of Diseases and Related Health Problems (ICD-10) (WHO 2007). Please refer to these manuals for more in-depth information on the range of mental disorders and their diagnostic criteria.

Psychiatric disorders can be broadly categorised into two groups: psychotic and non-psychotic disorders.

Psychotic disorders

Psychotic disorders, for example, schizophrenia, are psychiatric conditions that feature signs and symptoms of psychosis, such as impaired reality testing, hallucinations, delusions and thought disorder (severe thinking disturbances). In the acute phase of the illness, mood disorders, such as bipolar disorder (manic phase) and psychotic depression, may also feature psychosis. Acute psychosis may be caused by known pathophysiology, such as drug intoxication or infection; however, the aetiology of conditions such as schizophrenia remains unclear (Kaplan & Sadock 2007).

Schizophrenia

Schizophrenia is a common psychotic disorder involving delusions (fixed false beliefs), hallucinations (perceptual disturbance of any of the five senses) and thought disorder (disorganised, disturbed thinking). The most common type of hallucinations experienced by people with schizophrenia is auditory hallucinations (hearing voices), and frequently delusions are paranoid in nature whereby the individual believes they are being persecuted. People with schizophrenia may also exhibit unusual or bizarre behaviour, particularly in the acute phase of the illness. The age of onset for schizophrenia is often in the late teens, which can impact on normal social, occupational and personal development, resulting in reduced social functioning. Some examples of psychotic disorders include schizophrenia, schizoaffective disorder, postpartum psychosis and drug-induced psychosis (Kaplan & Sadock 2007; American Psychiatric Association 2000; WHO 2007).

Non-psychotic disorders

Non-psychotic disorders are psychiatric conditions that do not involve psychosis. Conditions, such as anxiety disorders, eating disorders and personality disorder, are examples of non-psychotic disorders. Non-psychotic disorders can be just as debilitating as psychotic disorders, in that they too affect social, occupational and personal functioning (Kaplan & Sadock 2007).

Anxiety disorders

Anxiety disorders are very common across the lifespan, and vary considerably in severity and associated disability. The main symptoms of anxiety disorders include: persistent worrying; feelings of dread; irrational fears; palpitations; hyperventilation; insomnia; feelings of panic; poor concentration; and changes to appetite. The symptoms of anxiety are persistent and pervasive, and many people experience a severe loss of confidence in their ability to cope with the normal activities of daily life. There are a number of types of anxiety disorders, however, the most common disorders include: generalised anxiety disorder; panic disorder; obsessive–compulsive disorder; phobic disorder; and post-traumatic stress disorder (Kaplan & Sadock 2007).

Mood disorders

Mood disorders are characterised by extreme disturbances in mood. In order for a diagnosis to be made, the mood disturbance must be continuously present for a period of two weeks. The most common mood disorder is depression, which ranges from mildly to severely disabling (Kaplan & Sadock 2007).

Major depression

The symptoms of major depression include: a persistent low mood; insomnia; feelings of hopelessness and helplessness; loss of interest in usual activities; lowered libido; inertia; guilty feelings; agitation; rumination; poor concentration; constipation; anorexia; and in severe cases, suicidal ideation and behaviours. Depressed patients require ongoing monitoring of their mental state assessment (including risk assessment) to ensure early identification of suicidal thoughts and prevention of self-harm (Kaplan & Sadock 2007; American Psychiatric Association 2000; WHO 2007).

Bipolar disorder

Bipolar disorder is mood disorder characterised by extreme mood swings. Previously known as 'manic depression', it is characterised by episodes of both mania and depression. In the manic phase of the illness the patient typically experiences euphoria, hyperactivity, insomnia, grandiose delusions, disinhibition, irritability, pressured speech, poor concentration and impaired judgment. Manic patients may engage in overspending, promiscuousness and other risky behaviours arising from impaired reality testing. In the depressed phase of the illness, the symptoms are consistent with major depression, as described earlier. Bipolar disorder carries a relatively high risk for suicide as compared with other mental illnesses, so thorough, ongoing assessment is vital to ensure the patient's safety. The most common mood disorders include major depression, bipolar disorder, dysthymia and postnatal depression (Kaplan & Sadock 2007; American Psychiatric Association 2000; WHO 2007).

Personality disorders

People with personality disorders exhibit enduring and pervasive patterns of behaviour that are inconsistent with society's expectations and norms. Typically, people with a personality disorder have difficulty regulating their emotions and behaviours, which commonly manifests as instability of mood and emotional intensity. Personality disordered people experience significant distress as a result of these symptoms, as well as impairment in social and occupational functioning. Comorbidity of substance abuse and other mental illnesses is also common (Kaplan & Sadock 2007; American Psychiatric Association 2000; WHO 2007).

Borderline personality disorder

The type of personality disorder most commonly seen in health care settings is borderline personality disorder (BPD). The symptoms of BPD include: self-harm; destructive relationships; poor coping skills, high levels of distress; 'black and white' (dyadic) thinking; and impulsiveness. BPD is more frequent in females than males, and many BPD sufferers have a childhood history of sexual or physical abuse or trauma, which is thought to contribute to the development of the disorder (Kaplan & Sadock 2007; American Psychiatric Association 2000; WHO 2007).

Antisocial personality disorder

Antisocial personality disorder (APD) is relatively common personality disorder seen more often in males than females. In some senses it is similar to BPD, in that the individual commonly reports a history of trauma, neglect, or physical and/or sexual abuse. The signs of APD are also similar to BPD and include: dyadic thinking; impulsiveness; risky behaviour; destructive relationships; and instability of mood. In addition to these symptoms, people with APD commonly exhibit 'acting out' behaviours such as violence and public nuisance, and usually have a history of criminality stretching back to adolescence. Those with APD often appear shallow emotionally and may show little remorse for their behaviour (Kaplan & Sadock 2007; American Psychiatric Association 2000; WHO 2007).

Cognitive disorders

Cognitive disorders are mental disorders that affect cognitive functions, such as memory processing, language processing, perception and problem solving. One of the key observable signs of cognitive disorder is confusion whereby the individual is disoriented in time, place and person. Cognitive disorders such as delirium (sometimes called acute confusional states) are acute and usually caused by serious illness or drug toxicity, and respond to treatment; however, cognitive disorders such as dementia have a slow onset and are progressive, incurable neurodegenerative diseases. Both delirium and dementia are common cognitive disorders seen frequently in primary health care, and it is important to be able to differentiate between the two. In both illnesses, cognition is impaired; however, dementia affects mainly memory, while delirium affects mainly attention (Kaplan & Sadock 2007; American Psychiatric Association 2000; WHO 2007).

Alzheimer's disease

The most common type of dementia is Alzheimer's disease, in which the age of onset is usually over 65, but it has been diagnosed in people as young as 40. The signs and symptoms of Alzheimer's disease include severe short-term and long-term memory loss, as well as impairment to most other areas of an individual's cognitive functioning, such as aphasia,

Reflections

What tools do you use to assess memory when performing an 'over 75s' health assessment?

apraxia, agnosia and impaired executive functioning (Kaplan & Sadock 2007; American Psychiatric Association 2000; WHO 2007).

Psychiatric disorders in children

Mental disorders in children encompass a broad range of emotional and behavioural disorders of various degrees of severity. The incidence of mental illness in Australian school-age children and adolescents is estimated to be approximately 14%, with nearly one in five children and adolescents aged 4 to 16 years experiencing mental health problems (Sawyer et al. 2000). The increasing rates of depression and self-harming behaviours in children (Lacey 1999) underscore the importance of early identification of mental health issues in primary health. Risk factors for mental illness in children include: exposure to family violence, sexual abuse, poverty, neglect and having a parent with a substance abuse disorder and/or mental illness (Lacey 1999).

Anxiety and depression

High prevalence disorders, such as depression and anxiety, are common in children (Commonwealth Department of Health and Family Services 1997), and without treatment can impact negatively on normal development, for example, in school performance and peer relationships (Commonwealth Department of Health and Family Services 1997). Children suffering from depression may describe the same symptoms as adults; however, symptoms are also commonly expressed in behaviours such as school refusal, nightmares, somatic complaints and behavioural disturbances. In extreme cases, children with depression may also develop suicidal ideas and behaviour (Commonwealth Department of Health and Family Services 1997).

Attention deficit hyperactivity disorder

Attention deficit hyperactivity disorder (ADHD) is a common childhood disorder characterised by hyperactivity (overactivity), difficulty maintaining attention and concentration, and behavioural problems. Without treatment ADHD can extend into late adolescence and adulthood, and impact significantly on social relationships, and on school and work performance (Kaplan & Sadock 2007).

Behavioural disorders, such as oppositional defiant disorder in children, feature a range of challenging behavioural problems which include fighting, running away, disobedience and temper tantrums (Kaplan & Sadock 2007). In adolescence this disorder is referred to as conduct disorder (Kaplan & Sadock 2007) and behavioural problems, such as those listed above, and others such as stealing, vandalism, destructiveness and delinquency, may be present. These problems cause significant disruption to family life and the child's functioning at school. In the longer term, children with conduct disorder have increased risk of criminality, substance abuse, and mental health issues in late adolescence and adulthood (Kaplan & Sadock 2007).

Pervasive developmental disorders

Pervasive developmental disorders (PDD) are childhood mental disorders characterised by delays in the development of communication and socialisation (Lord et al. 2000). Children with PDD may exhibit limited social skills, repetitive play/actions and an inability to empathise or relate to others. The most common types of PDD are autism, Asperger syndrome and pervasive developmental disorder not otherwise specified—conditions commonly referred to as the autism spectrum disorders (Anderson et al. 1987). The onset of these illnesses is usually before the age of three, but parents commonly report observing symptoms in infancy. The level of impairment in children with PDD varies widely from gross language impairment (for example, mute) to relatively normal language development (Lord et al. 2000).

Reflections

What questions do you ask children and their parents about mental health when seeing them for other reasons, for example, the 'Healthy Kids Check'?

Eating disorders

Eating disorders, such as anorexia nervosa and bulimia nervosa, are characterised by behaviours aimed at reducing body weight by self-starvation, binging and purging. Typically sufferers have a distorted view of their body image and see themselves as grossly overweight. Eating disorders are potentially life threatening and require assertive intervention by specialist mental health services (Kaplan & Sadock 2007).

Women's mental health

Pregnancy and childbirth are risk factors for mental illness in some women. Women require careful monitoring of their mental health in the perinatal period to ensure that any problems are identified early and can be treated to prevent more complex conditions developing. In particular, any changes reported by women regarding their mood, sleep, behaviour and feeling of psychological wellbeing should be investigated without delay.

Perinatal depression

Ten per cent of Australian women experience an episode of depression during pregnancy (beyondblue & St John of God Health Care 2008)—antenatal depression—and approximately 16% of women develop depression in the period following the birth of a child—postnatal depression. The symptoms of these conditions are consistent with major depression, however, the loss of energy, motivation and depressed mood can have a serious impact on child and maternal bonding, and in some cases children may be at risk of harm and neglect. The symptoms may be short lived, but in some cases, can persist for many months. All women require stringent screening for perinatal mood disorders, as early identification and treatment of problems can prevent longer-term mental health complications from developing, and ensure that children are safe and well cared for.

> ### Reflections
>
> *What is your practice policy on screening women for perinatal depression?*

Postpartum psychosis

Another significant mental illness associated with pregnancy is postpartum psychosis, which affects approximately one in 1000 mothers (Brockington 1996). The condition features severe psychotic symptoms comparable to those seen in schizophrenia and mania. The onset of postpartum psychosis is usually occurs soon after birth, with symptoms rapidly escalating to extreme disturbances of behaviour and thinking. Symptoms typically include: mania; euphoria; overactivity; insomnia; irritability; auditory hallucinations; disorganised behaviour; and delusions which are commonly grandiose, religious or paranoid in content. Postpartum psychosis is a very serious condition that requires immediate and assertive intervention from specialist mental health services as the risk of harm to both mother and child is high due to the unpredictable behaviour that arises from severe psychosis.

Conducting a mental health assessment

Mental health assessment involves taking a detailed history from the patient that explores current mental health problems (or symptoms), recent significant events or stressors, past psychiatric history, current treatment, social circumstances and potential risks (beyondblue & St John of God Health Care 2008). A thorough assessment requires the nurse to view the patient holistically, that is, to take into account the biological, psychological and social factors that may be influencing the current presentation, including the person's age, gender and specific cultural issues (Brockington 1996).

The key to gaining assessment information is to engage with the patient. This involves forming a trusting relationship that is based on mutual respect. Establishing a rapport with the patient will facilitate the assessment process. It is helpful to forming a rapport with the patient if the nurse is able to demonstrate empathy and compassion, in addition to holding an open-minded non-judgmental attitude (Brockington 1996).

Methods of assessment: the psychiatric interview

Psychiatric assessment should include a structured interview process with the patient and, where appropriate and practicable, families and/or carers. The psychiatric interview is conducted face to face, with the interviewer directing the process (beyondblue & St John of God Health Care 2008). When conducting psychiatric interviews the nurse should take into consideration what the patient states in conversation in addition to observable behaviours. It is important to note incongruities between statements made by patients, and information given by informants such as carers and significant others (Brockington 1996).

Assessment begins from the moment of the first observation. The client communicates many signs and symptoms that the nurse may observe non-verbally. Body language, facial expressions, manner of dress and gestures are all examples of non-verbal cues (Brockington 1996).

Many psychiatric disorders and treatments can produce physical symptoms in the individual: weight loss and dehydration in the depressed patient; tachycardia, perspiration and tremors in the anxious client; and many potential body system effects from pharmacological treatments. It is essential for the nurse to firstly complete a thorough past and present health status assessment (Brockington 1996). Basic physiological functions to review include: nutrition, hydration, elimination, activity, and rest and sleep. A key question to consider is: *Are there any physical problems impacting on the patient's current presentation?*

Once the physical assessment is completed, proceed to the mental health assessment. A simplified 'ABC approach' to mental health assessment is outlined below.

Mental status examination: an ABC approach

The mental status examination (MSE) (beyondblue & St John of God Health Care 2008) is a tool designed to obtain information about specific aspects of the individual's mental state and behaviour at the time of interview. The main areas of assessment in the MSE include: appearance; behaviour; speech; thought process; perception; mood; appetite/sleep; insight; judgment; orientation; memory; social status; previous psychiatric and medical history; substance use history; and current or past risks.

The following ABC approach (Trzepacz & Baker 1993) has been adapted from the mental status examination to provide a streamlined approach to assessment.

A

Appearance

What does the patient look like?

Dishevelled, unkempt, clothing inappropriate for the weather, bizarrely dressed, underweight, dehydrated, well presented.

Affect or emotional tone—*What impression do you get about the patient's current emotional state?*

Tearful, guarded, suspicious, smiling/laughing inappropriately, elated, sad, depressed, fearful, anxious, blank, unresponsive, warm and reactive, inappropriate (for example, incongruent with circumstances).

B

Behaviour

How is the patient behaving?

Calm, agitated, restless, hostile, angry, withdrawn, bizarre posturing and/or facial grimacing, intimidating, aggressive, yelling out, hostile, hypervigilant, suspicious, unusual gait, hyperventilating, talking to self.

Agitation—*Is the patient distressed?*

Motor restlessness, tearfulness, anxiousness and fearfulness. Severe, moderate, mild.

C

Conversation

Self-report—*What is the patient telling you?*

Recent stressors, recent losses such as job/partner, relationship breakdown, recent humiliation such as gambling loss, frightened, being persecuted, hearing voices, hearing voices commanding them to act in some way, feeling suicidal, feeling things are hopeless, wanting to hurt somebody, getting messages from television or radio, experiencing racing thoughts, recent substance use, cannot cope with circumstances, poor sleep, poor appetite, has taken an overdose, has stopped taking prescribed medication, has low mood, feeling depressed, suspicious and paranoid (for example, expressing irrational thoughts about being poisoned).

Speech—*How does the patient's speech sound?*

Rapid rate, racing sentences, very slow, very softly spoken, slurred, yelling, incoherent.

Thought—*Does the patient make sense?*

Thought flow—sentence structure clear, jumbled, rambling, disconnected sentences, losing the thread of discussion, disjointed, fragmented.

Thought content—bizarre or frightening, preoccupied with an event, religious themes, paranoia, irrational, illogical, nonsensical, patient describes receiving messages from TV, radio, computer equipment (ideas of reference), suicidal thoughts, thoughts of harming others.

Perception—*Does the patient report any perceptual disturbance?*

Hearing voices, unusual smells/tastes, seeing things (illusions), tactile disturbances (feeling bugs, bites, insects on or under the skin), parts of body missing or diseased.

Cognition—*Is the person orientated?*

Is the person aware of the time of day, year, the environment and how they came to be at the doctor's surgery? Confusion, disorientation, memory disturbance, poor attention and concentration.

Social circumstance—*What social supports does the patient have?*

Living alone, with parents/family, with partner, with friends, with carer, with children. Is the patient employed, on disability pension, at school?

Cultural aspects—*What is the language spoken?*

Is an interpreter needed? Religious or cultural practices impacting on the assessment, such as gender related issues.

Substance use—*Is there a history of substance use/abuse?*

Substance type, amount, frequency of use, current intoxication.

Risk assessment

Risk assessment is a core component of mental health assessment that aims to ensure the patient is safe. Early detection of risk optimises the potential for interventions to be put in place to safeguard the patient's safety (Stuart & Laria 2001). Risk assessment involves making observations of the client's current presentation, including their appearance, conversation and behaviour. In addition, risk must also be assessed in the context of the patient's history as people with a history of self-harm, suicide attempt or violence may have an increased risk of future risky behaviours (Stuart & Laria 2001). Where possible, clinicians should seek collateral information to inform risk assessment, ideally, from several sources. The information must then be evaluated to ascertain which risk factors are present and the extent to which these risks, combined with situational and environmental factors, may indicate potential for harms (Stuart & Laria 2001).

Although it can be challenging to ask patients directly about past history of violence or current suicidal thoughts, a direct enquiry can yield important assessment data that is critical to clinical decision making about risk (Gerdtz et al. 2008). Nurses also require access to information, such as case histories, to evaluate the history of, or potential for, high risk behaviours (Stuart & Laria 2001).

Risk assessment is undertaken to determine whether a care plan should include interventions for the management of risks such as self-harm, suicide and violence. Ideally, multidisciplinary input into risk assessment from the areas of psychiatry, medicine and social work should be available. The outcomes of the risk assessment must be carefully documented and communicated to all relevant stakeholders within the bounds of service-user confidentiality (Stuart & Laria 2001).

Reflections

What is your practice policy and referral pathway for patients who present and are deemed to be at risk of harming themselves?

Risk of suicide   The following variables place the patient at higher risk of suicide (Sands, Gerdtz & Elsom 2009):

- previous suicide attempts
- alcohol/substance use
- history of mental illness
- feelings of hopelessness
- male aged 15–30
- expressing suicidal ideation
- has the means to commit suicide (for example, firearm)
- has a plan to commit suicide
- recent relationship break-up.

Risk of harm to others   The following variables place the patient at higher risk of harm to others (Stuart & Laria 2001):

- uncooperativeness
- suspiciousness
- hostility
- history of aggression
- alcohol/substance intoxication
- verbal abuse or threats
- thought disorder
- persecutory delusions.

Psychiatric emergencies

A psychiatric emergency is a situation in which, as a result of impaired mental state, the patient is presenting with significant risks that places them or others at risk of harm. Examples of psychiatric emergencies include suicidal crisis, risk of violence, or risk of harm or exploitation due to compromised mental state (for example, confusional states, delirium or mania) (Sands, Gerdtz & Elsom 2009).

Reflections

What is the process that occurs when patients present or telephone your practice in crisis?

Mental health legislation

At times, people experiencing a psychiatric emergency as a part of acute mental illness may require involuntary admission to a psychiatric hospital. All Australian states and territories provide a legislative framework for the care, treatment and protection of people with mental illness who do not or cannot consent to that care, treatment or protection. The respective *Mental Health Act* will outline procedures for initiating involuntary treatment and making involuntary treatment orders (Sands 2007).

Referral to mental health services

Knowing how to make an effective referral to mental health services is essential in ensuring a timely and appropriate response for patients in psychiatric crisis. Access to public mental health services in Australia is regulated through triage systems, which provide a 24-hour service. Referrals to triage are subject to a screening assessment to determine the type and level of service provision required (Hillard & Zitek 2004). An accurate and well-documented mental health referral is more likely to be accepted and acted upon in a timely manner. Important referral information includes the outcomes of mental state assessment, with an emphasis on current risks.

Reflections

What mental health services are available in your community?

Care planning

Mental health plans are developed for patients following comprehensive mental health assessment (Brockington 1996). Ideally, the plan should be developed in collaboration with the patient, and the goals planned with, and agreed to, by the patient. The patient should be given a copy of the plan to keep. The following essential information (Australian General Practice Network 2005) should be contained within the plan:

- demographic information
- outcomes of MSE
- diagnosis
- current and future risks

- previous history
- comorbidities
- substance use patterns
- co-workers involved in care (for example, mental health team, practice nurse)
- goals to improve mental health problems
- strategies for achieving the goals (for example, treatments)
- indicators of improvement–outcome measures
- person or persons responsible for implementing strategies
- family/carer/partner supports
- evidence of patient education
- allergies
- medications
- date of review.

Ongoing care and support

Practice nurses have an important role in the ongoing care and support of patients with mental health problems. Through the ongoing therapeutic relationship, nurses can get to know their patients well and assist them in achieving optimal states of wellness (Brockington 1996).

Becoming familiar with the signs of relapse in the patient and providing interventions to prevent a more complex deterioration of mental state is essential in helping the patient remain well (Brockington 1996; Sands 2004). In particular, nurses can assist the patient in preventing relapse by helping them to become aware of their own symptoms of relapse, helping them to remain adherent to medications (enquiring as to where prescriptions are current/need filling), and providing them with information about after-hours support (for example, phone numbers for triage). It is also important to help the patient become familiar with their medications, including explaining typical side effects and steps to take in case of adverse reactions (Brockington 1996; Sands 2004).

In addition, the nurse can assist the patient in developing an Advance Directive (Victorian Government 1986) that can articulate what will happen if the client is in crisis, who to contact and preferred treatment. It is helpful to be familiar with the social services available in the area, such as support groups and charitable organisations that provide psychosocial rehabilitation, which the patient can be referred to for further support (Brockington 1996; Sands 2004).

Reflections

Are all clinical staff in your practice familiar with Advanced Directives?

Example 14.1

Andrew is a 17-year-old Aboriginal boy brought to the (remote) clinic by his uncle. He has a seven-day history of talking to himself, insomnia and expressing ideas that his house is under surveillance by police helicopters. He has a history of cannabis and alcohol abuse, and was expelled from school following several episodes of violence to other students. On assessment he is fearful, agitated and reluctant to talk to the duty nurse.

> What are the potential diagnoses for this presentation?
> What are the potential risks?

Example 14.2

Marion is a 78-year-old woman who was brought to the clinic by her neighbour. Up until two days ago she had been very well, but last night her neighbour became concerned for her when she was seen wandering around in the backyard in a state of semi-undress. She presents as somewhat agitated with difficulty remaining focused and is confused about the time of day.

> What are the potential diagnoses for this presentation?
> What are the potential risks?

Conclusion

In summary, mental health problems are highly prevalent in Australia, and in the past decade there has been an increased focus on managing mental illness in primary health settings. Practice nurses have an increasingly important role in caring for people with mental health problems as they work together with general practitioners and the multidisciplinary team to assess, plan and implement mental health care for people across their lifespan.

Key messages

One in five people is expected to experience a mental health problem at some stage during their lives.

Children may also be at risk of mental illness.

Practice nurses play a role in assessment of mental health status, especially in a crisis situation.

Useful resources

beyondblue—the national depression initiative
'beyondblue guide to the management of depression in primary care: a guide for health professionals'
http://www.beyondblue.org.au/index.aspx?link_id=7.102&tmp=FileDownload&fid=1335

Post and Antenatal Depression Association (PANDA)
http://www.panda.org.au

Mental Health Emergency Triage Education Kit Mental Health Triage Tool
http://www.health.gov.au

References

1. American Psychiatric Association 2000, *Diagnostic and statistical manual of mental disorders*, 4th edn (text revision) (DSM-IV-TR), Arlington, VA.

2. Anderson, JC, Williams, S, McGee, R & Silva, PA 1987, 'DSM-III disorders in preadolescent children: Prevalence in a large sample from the general population', *Archives of General Psychiatry*, vol. 44, pp. 69–76.

3. Australian General Practice Network 2005, Primary Mental Health Care, viewed 5 August 2009, <http://www.agpn.com.au/programs/mental_health>.

4. Australian Institute of Health and Welfare (AIHW) 2008, *Australia's health 2008*, AIHW cat. no. AUS 99, AIHW, Canberra, viewed 1 December 2009, <http://www.aihw.gov.au/>.

5. Begg, S, Vos, T, Barker, B, Stevenson, C, Stanley, L & Lopez, A 2007, *The burden of disease and injury in Australia 2003*, AIHW cat. no. PHE 82, AIHW, Canberra, viewed 1 December 2009, <http://www.aihw.gov.au/>.

6. beyondblue & St John of God Health Care 2008, *Perinatal mental health national action plan 2008–2010*, beyondblue—national depression initiative.

7. Britt, H, Miller, GC, Charles, J, Pan, Y, Valenti, L, Henderson, J, Bayram, C, O'Halloran, J & Knox, S 2007, 'General practice activity in Australia 2005–06', General practice series no. 19, Australian Institute of Health and Welfare, Canberra, viewed 1 November 2009, <http://www.aihw.gov.au/>.

8. Brockington, IF 1996, *Motherhood and Mental Health*, Oxford University Press, UK.

9. Commonwealth Department of Health and Family Services, 1997, *Youth suicide in Australia: the national youth prevention strategy*, Commonwealth Department of Health and Ageing.

10. Council of Australian Governments (COAG) 2006, *National Action Plan on Mental Health 2006–2011*, viewed 1 December 2009, <http://www.coag.gov.au/coag_meeting_outcomes/2006-07-14/docs/nap_mental_health.pdf>.

11. Gerdtz, MF, Considine, J, Crellin, D, Sands, N, Pollock, W & Stewart, C 2008, Emergency Triage Education Kit, Australian Commonwealth Department of Health and Ageing.

12. Gray, R, Parr, A, Plummer, S, Sandford, T, Ritter, S, Mundt-Leach, R, Goldberg, D & Gournay, K 2001, 'A national survey of practice nurse involvement in mental health interventions', *Journal of Advanced Nursing*, vol. 30, no. 4, pp. 901–6.

13. Hegarty, K, Gunn, J, Chondros, P & Small, R 2004, 'Association between depression and abuse by partners of women attending general practice: descriptive, cross sectional survey', *BMJ*, no. 328, pp. 621–4.

14. Hillard, R & Zitek, R 2004, *Emergency Psychiatry*, McGraw-Hill, New York.

15. Kaplan, H & Sadock, BJ 2007, *Kaplan and Sadock's Synopsis of Psychiatry: behavioral sciences, clinical psychiatry*, 10th edn, Lippincott, Williams & Wilkins, Baltimore.

16. Lacey, I 1999, 'The role of the child primary health worker', *Journal of Advanced Nursing*, vol. 30, no. 1, pp. 220–8.

17. Lord, C, Cook, EH, Leventhal, BL & Amaral, DG 2000, 'Autism spectrum disorders', *Neuron*, vol. 28, no. 2, pp. 355–63.

18. Sands, N 2004, 'Mental health triage nursing: an Australian perspective', *Journal of Psychiatric and Mental Health Nursing*, vol. 11, issue 2, pp. 150–5.

19. Sands, N 2007, 'Assessing the risk of suicide at triage', *Australasian Emergency Nursing Journal*, vol. 10, issue 4, pp. 161–3.

20. Sands, N, Gerdtz, M & Elsom, S 2009, *Final Report, Clinical Practice Guideline: violence risk assessment at triage*, University of Melbourne and Nurses Board of Victoria.

21. Sawyer, MG, Arney, FM, Baghurst, PA, Clark, JJ, Graetz, BW, Kosky, RJ, Nurcombe, B, Patton, GC, Prior, MR, Raphael, B, Roy, J, Whaites, LC & Zubrick, SR 2000, *The Mental Health of Young People in Australia*, Mental Health and Special Programs Branch, Commonwealth Department of Health and Aged Care.

22. Stuart, GW & Laria, M 2001, *Principles and practice of psychiatric nursing*, 5th edn, Mosby, St. Louis.

23. Trzepacz, PT & Baker, R 1993, *The Psychiatric Mental Status Examination*, Oxford University Press, UK.

24. VicHealth 2007, *Burden of disease due to mental illness & mental health problems 2007*, viewed August 2009, <http://www.vichealth.vic.gov.au/>.

25. Victorian Government, *The Mental Health Act (1986)*, Victorian Government Printers.

26. World Health Organisation (WHO) 1996, *Mental health of refugees*, ISBN 92: 41544844, World Health Organisation, Geneva.

27. World Health Organisation (WHO) 2001, *World Health Report 2001: Mental Health: new understanding, new hope*, World Health Organisation, Geneva.

28. World Health Organisation (WHO) 2005a, *Mental health policy, plans and programme*, (updated version), Mental Health Policy and Service Guidance Package, Geneva.

29. World Health Organisation (WHO) 2005b, *Revised global burden of disease (GBD) 2002 estimates*, viewed 1 December 2009, <http://www.who.int/>.

30. World Health Organisation (WHO) 2007, *International statistical classification of disease and related health problems*, 10th revision, WHO, Geneva.

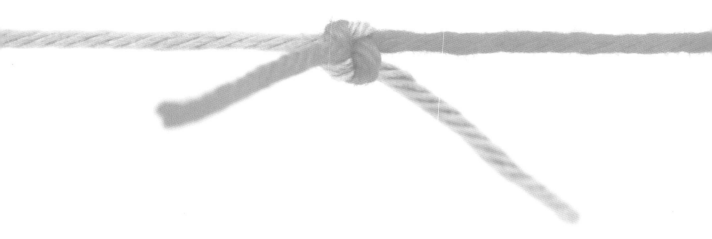

Chapter fifteen

Chronic disease management

by Lynne Walker and
Doris Young

Overview

Chronic diseases require continuous, comprehensive and coordinated care involving a range of providers from the primary, secondary and tertiary sectors. With a high cost of managing chronic disease and limited resources, it has become a national priority to develop cost-effective systems to manage these conditions, especially in the primary care sector. This chapter will focus on chronic disease management, particularly those elements which facilitate cost-effective, coordinated and systematic strategies.

Objectives

At the completion of this chapter you should be able to:

- list the components necessary for successful chronic disease management (CDM);

- recognise the barriers to chronic disease management;

- describe the chronic care model;

- identify ways that you can improve CDM in your work environment; and

- list the generic skills needed by all health professionals to care for patients with a chronic disease or condition.

Introduction

Chronic diseases are conditions that are prolonged, do not resolve spontaneously and are rarely cured completely (Forbes & While 2009). Their treatment places a major burden on health care systems worldwide. The prevalence of chronic disease is escalating and is fuelled by issues such as obesity, physical inactivity, smoking and increased longevity. Chronic diseases have been labelled 'diseases of urbanisation' by the World Health Organisation as more people move to the urban areas and there is an increase in advertising and marketing of unhealthy products such as tobacco, alcohol and fast food.

Nurses currently make up the greater proportion of professionals in our health care workforce and so it is vital that any system designed to manage patients in the community will involve nursing care. In 2007–08, Australians made 5.2 visits per head of population to general practitioners (GPs); approximately 52% of those encounters were for chronic conditions (Britt et al. 2004). Therefore, as part of the primary health care team, nurses working in general practice are in a prime position to contribute to the care of patients with chronic diseases.

Chronic disease management (CDM) is a term that is used frequently and often the practice nurse is perceived to be the most appropriate member of the team to undertake this role. Chronic diseases such as heart failure, diabetes, asthma, hypertension, cancer and depression have all been identified as being suitable for a structured approach to management (Norris et al. 2003) and yet very often the practice approach to managing these conditions is still very ad hoc and opportunistic.

This chapter will focus on the components necessary in a changing, patient-centred, resource-limited environment to be able to manage any chronic disease. It is envisaged that practice nurses, as part of the health care team, will be able to understand the principles and apply this knowledge so that all patients suffering from any chronic condition will be able to access safe and effective care. Ultimately, nurses will provide care to patients individually as well as part of a systems approach and this chapter will challenge nurses to critically analyse the way care is provided to patients with chronic conditions in the general practice environment.

Epidemiology

Chronic diseases are traditionally thought of as those that originate from non-communicable conditions such as heart disease, diabetes and asthma, but this term also encompasses communicable diseases such as HIV and AIDS, mental disorders such as depression and schizophrenia, and physical disabilities including blindness, deafness, persistent pain and amputations. The World Health Organisation (WHO 2002) highlights the fact that by the year 2020 depression will only be surpassed by heart disease in terms of the disability it causes. WHO also claims that chronic diseases are increasing globally with no distinction between social class or region. It is of particular significance in developing countries where, by the year 2020, chronic conditions including injuries and mental disorders will be responsible for 78% of the global disease burden (WHO 2002).

Chronic diseases are common among the Australian population. The Australian Institute of Health and Welfare (AIHW) published a report titled *Chronic Diseases and Associated Risk Factors in Australia, 2006* (AIHW 2006) which outlined the population groups most affected by chronic disease. It is important for practice nurses to understand the incidence as well as the prevalence of risk factors which may lead to chronic disease and the population groups most affected. With this information nurses can identify these groups within their own practice population and target specific interventions to reduce the impact and severity of those risk factors which inevitably lead to complications. The main findings from this report were:

- Chronic diseases are common: in 2004–05, 77% of Australians had at least one long-term condition; common were asthma (10.0% of the total population), osteoarthritis (7.9%), depression (5.3%) and diabetes (3.5%).

- Chronic diseases can be a problem at all ages: almost 10% of children aged 0 to 14 years had three or more long-term conditions; this figure increased to more than 80% for those aged 65 years and over.

- Some people are affected much more than others: for example, compared with other Australians, Aboriginal and Torres Strait Islander persons have higher mortality from diabetes (14 times higher), chronic kidney disease (8 times) and heart disease (5 times).

- Many people are at risk of developing chronic diseases: for example, 54% of adult Australians are either overweight or obese.

- Chronic diseases are a drain on the health system: in 2000–01 they accounted for nearly 70% of the total health expenditure that can be allocated to diseases.

Some diseases, such as diabetes and arthritis, have a range of severity with most patients at the less severe end of the range. These patients are generally

Reflections

Are you able to determine how many patients in your practice suffer from one or more long-term conditions? Do you know which patients in your practice are of Aboriginal or Torres Strait Islander origin?

able to be managed in primary care while those at the more severe end of the spectrum may require specialist care and be referred to secondary and tertiary agencies.

Acute versus chronic health care

The health care system in Australia has historically been focused on acute episodic care provided by a single provider (often the general practitioner) in a standard environment (often the general practice). Acute care focuses on triage of the patient, patient flow-through, symptomology, laboratory results and prescriptions; patient education is brief and follow-up is usually initiated by the patient (Glasgow, Sibthorpe & Gear 2005). It has been funded by a fee-for-service system which encourages rapid, repetitive consultations to address diseases and their complications; this system no longer meets the needs of those patients with chronic and complex conditions. This type of payment offers little incentive to modify patient risk factors or address the other determinants of health as described in earlier chapters. As a result, care has been fragmented, disorganised, duplicated and focused on managing established disease and complications (Norris et al. 2003).

Long-term illness occurs across the entire spectrum of diseases including mental health, communicable and non-communicable diseases, and may affect people at any age. The AIHW (2006) describes features common to most chronic diseases:

- complex causality, with multiple factors leading to their onset
- long development period, some of which may have no symptoms
- prolonged course of illness, perhaps leading to other health complications
- associated functional impairment or disability.

Thus it is evident the care provided to people with chronic disease needs to be quite different from the care provided for acute episodic illness. The Flinders Human Behaviour and Health Research Unit as cited by Lambert (2005) summarises the differences in Table 15.1 overleaf.

Patients as well as health professionals must recognise that effective chronic disease care requires a change in the system so that limited resources can be maximised to increase returns and improve patient outcomes; hence, the need for the development of a new national strategy for chronic disease.

Table 15.1 Differences in care of acute and chronic illnesses

Acute care	Chronic care
Episodic	Ongoing
Cure expected	Incurable
Quality of life highly dependent on professional care of the patient	Quality of life highly dependent on self-management and decision making
Quality of life dependent on short-term services	Quality of life highly dependent on ongoing support services
Health professional generally the expert	Patient often has more knowledge
Short-term goals	Short-term goals meet long-term outcomes
Compliance expected	Compliance and self-reliance expected

Source: Flinders Human Behaviour and Health Research Unit 2003

National Chronic Disease Strategy

The National Chronic Disease Strategy (NCDS) has been developed to provide national policy directions which will improve chronic disease care and prevention for all Australians (National Health Priority Action Council (NHPAC) 2006). The objectives of NCDS are to:

- prevent and/or delay the onset of chronic disease for individuals and population groups;
- reduce the progression and complications of chronic disease;
- maximise the wellbeing and quality of life of individuals with chronic disease and their families and carers;
- reduce avoidable hospital admissions and health care procedures;
- implement best practice in the prevention, detection and management of chronic disease; and
- enhance the capacity of the health workforce to meet population demand for chronic disease prevention and care into the future.

It recognises that the health system must achieve significant change which is sustainable and that managing chronic disease requires more than input from the health system, that it should include input from sectors that influence social and environmental factors. Furthermore, the NCDS recognises that successful chronic disease management requires a whole of government as well as a whole of community response if the health system is going to be able to effectively treat patients with a chronic condition.

Action areas that have been identified in the NCDS are:

Prevention across the continuum   This focuses on the risk and protective factors that influence the development and progression of chronic disease and includes interventions from before birth to preschool and childhood interventions. Prevention is discussed in greater detail in Chapter 10.

Early detection and treatment   This can result in reductions in mortality complications and comorbidities. Effective early treatment can improve the quality of life and provide savings to the health system. Early detection and treatment can be achieved by improved screening and early detection with follow-up of patients deemed to have identified risk factors. Examples of interventions include establishment of recall and reminder systems and disease registers.

Integration and continuity of prevention and care   This provides a challenge as care needs to be provided over time and at different stages of chronic disease progression. It requires integration between different conditions, across different services with different providers and recognises the contribution of patients and their carers. Examples of actions to support this include improved discharge procedures from hospital, multidisciplinary care planning and team-based approaches, information management systems, and care coordination across multiple health providers.

Self-management   This has been identified as being fundamental to the success of the partnership between patients and their health care professionals in managing and monitoring chronic illnesses. Self-management is discussed in detail in Chapter 16.

Because it is a complex area, there are many opportunities at many levels for the practice nurse to be involved in managing chronic disease from the time of initial diagnosis, through self-management support to complex case management and palliative care.

Figure 15.1 below illustrates some of the core elements in chronic disease management (NHPAC 2006).

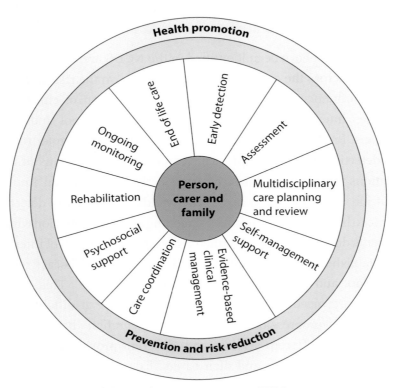

Figure 15.1 Core elements of chronic disease management (CDM)
Source: National Chronic Disease Strategy 2006, p. 8

Thus, practice nurses will be able to contribute significantly to almost all of these core elements in the continuum of disease. This gives enormous scope to the practice nurse to be able to contribute to patient care in a variety of ways at an individual level, practice level and community level.

The evidence–management gap

If we examine and compare the evidence for best practice and actual care delivered by health professionals for the management of chronic disease, it is clear that a large gap exists (National Health and Medical Research Council 2008; Nolte & McKee 2008; Bodenheimer et al. 2002). In the UK, a recent national audit revealed that 60% of people with diabetes were not receiving recommended care (NHS 2009) and in Australia similar deficiencies have been identified. The National Heart Foundation has reported that only 30% of patients with hypertension are treated optimally and less than 20% of patients with cardiovascular disease have ideal lipid levels (National Heart Foundation 2009).

With expanding numbers of people with chronic disease, it is likely that this gap will widen if we continue to use the current method of health care delivery with the current health workforce. It is therefore necessary to examine new ways of addressing a complex problem and practice nurses have been identified as a means to improve management of patients with chronic disease in an integrated general practice and primary care system (Royal College of Nursing, Australia 2005; Zwar et al. 2006).

The systematic approach

Generally, a patient with a chronic illness requires a variety of interventions as the condition is often complex. In recent years, innovation in health care delivery has seen attempts to develop strategies that will manage both the numbers and the complexity of patients with chronic conditions. Norris et al. (2003) have identified a number of themes that have arisen in an attempt to develop these strategies. They are:

- coordinated approaches to care delivery within organisations;
- an intensified focus on populations at high risk of poor outcomes in addition to individual care;
- delivery of preventive services, proactive patient management, and outreach;
- an increasing role for the patient in defining their needs and directing their care;
- greater emphasis on quality of life and other patient-oriented organisation and outcomes;
- a demand for minimisation of medical errors;
- evidence-based medicine;
- an emphasis on cost; and
- cost effectiveness of intervention.

In order to provide the best care to individual patients, it is necessary to look at the systems we use to do this and to look at how individual care fits into the population approach to health care. After all, it is individuals who comprise our communities and our population.

In a review of the evidence, Glasgow, Sibthorpe and Gear (2005) identified the main ingredients for success in organisational delivery of chronic care and included:

- central registry of particular disease types;
- clinical guidelines and physician education;

- collaboration, better communication, delegation of tasks to other team members;

- decision support for primary care workers;

- patient self-management education and support;

- patient-centred organisation;

- regular assessments/follow up; and

- system delivery design and stakeholder involvement.

A systems approach differs significantly from an ad hoc individual approach to the management of chronic care and requires staff, including nurses, to have resources and support to enable this to happen. Within a systems approach, there may be a variety of approaches including GP mini-clinics or case management. Glasgow, Sibthorpe and Gear (2005) concluded that multifaceted strategies that draw on the main ingredients identified above and are supported by well-designed systems are more likely to lead to enhanced outcomes. In other words, whatever approach a practice chooses, it should include the above ingredients.

The chronic care model

Although there are several models of care for the management of chronic illness, perhaps the one that has been seen as most effective is the chronic care model (see Figure 15.2 opposite). This model was first developed by Dr Edward Wagner from the McColl Institute for Healthcare Innovation and is a multidimensional solution, with components that have been described by Norris et al. (2003). Recognition is made within this model that most management of patients with chronic disease occurs in primary care but it is important to remember that chronic care takes place within the entire community, the health care system and the provider organisation—in this case, general practice. All three areas are important components in the chronic care model.

Components of the chronic care model

Six essential elements of the chronic care model have been described by Bodenheimer, Wagner and Grumbach (2002). These are not separate but rather interlinked and build upon each other. It is unlikely that a general practice will excel in all six elements, but with effective leadership and quality improvement processes, this framework can be used to attain excellence in chronic care.

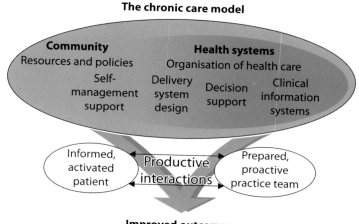

The chronic care model

Community
Resources and policies

Health systems
Organisation of health care

Self-management support

Delivery system design

Decision support

Clinical information systems

Informed, activated patient

Productive interactions

Prepared, proactive practice team

Improved outcomes

Figure 15.2 The chronic care model
Source: Wagner 1998.
Developed by the MacColl Institute © ACP-ASIM Journals and Books

Of the six elements both community resources and self-management are patient centred. The six elements are:

1. **Community resources and policies**   Links to these services are necessary so that organisations providing chronic care can refer patients to community-based programs such as exercise groups, self-support groups, hospital-based programs such as hospital in the home, Hospital Admission Risk program and district nursing services. Forming community partnerships with organisations will support and develop interventions that fill gaps in services required by patients and these partnerships may be especially important for low socioeconomic, indigenous, refugee or other marginalised groups within our communities. It is essential that the practice nurse has a good knowledge of community resources and incorporates them into any plans for patient care.

2. **Self-management support**   This involves assisting patients to be actively involved in their own care, including medication use. They can gain skills to use glucometers and sphygmomanometers as well as gaining the confidence necessary to assess their own needs and make decisions based on these needs. Support strategies may include assessment of their own condition, goal setting, action planning, problem solving and follow up.

3. **Health care organisation**   Chronic care needs to be a focus and a priority for organisations providing chronic care. This allows for innovation and the development of new ways of approaching chronic disease management. This may include appointment changes and rescheduling, patient reminders and group visits. Above all, leaders within the organisation should develop a culture which visibly supports continuous improvement and promotes strategies aimed

at systems change. Incentives based on quality of care may be provided. On a national level, the Commonwealth Government has introduced Enhanced Primary Care item numbers to assist general practitioners in providing longer, more comprehensive consultations.

4. **Delivery system design**   The way in which care is delivered needs to be structured so that the right person with the appropriate skills is working with clear expectations of the services that they will provide in conjunction with other health professionals. For example, the traditional GP-led model of care could be changed to a practice nurse-led model of care for patients with stable conditions. Planned visits rather than an *ad hoc* approach are important and this may involve separation of acute care from planned care for the management of patients with chronic disease. Planned consultations may require significant practice redesign as will group activities which are funded for certain health professionals under the Medicare Benefits Schedule (MBS). With the expansion of practice nurse numbers and role and the growth of multidisciplinary teamwork, it is essential that patients see these initiatives as adding value and quality to their care rather than viewing nurses as substitutes for existing providers. It may also be that the range of health care professionals that are able to deliver care is expanded.

5. **Decision support**   Support in the form of clinical practice guidelines based on the best available evidence should ideally be integrated into everyday practice and if necessary shared with patients to encourage their participation. Additional access to telephone consultation may be obtained from specialists when a full referral, often involving a long wait, is not needed. Web-based information can be developed for patients to access.

6. **Clinical information systems**   Systems, often electronic, are used for a variety of reasons including recall and reminders as well as developing disease registries. These systems allow population-based health care and facilitate practices to identify subgroups which may require specialised care, monitoring or interventions. In order to improve practice performance data must be collected on individuals as well as the practice population and information systems are essential for this reason. They will also assist in monitoring practice performance of practice teams. Clinical software can be used as reminder systems for both practice staff and patient benefit but may prove to be expensive and require training to use effectively. Often this training is not provided and practice staff are unable to use clinical systems to their full potential. Therefore it is important to ensure that the introduction of new technologies is accompanied by access to training and ongoing support.

Many studies, including those examined in a systematic review related to diabetes care, reinforce these elements and demonstrate that the most effective

Reflections

Can you draw any similarities between what has been identified in the Australian National Chronic Disease Strategy and the chronic care model?

interventions for improving care involved changes to at least the organisation of practice, information systems enhancements and programs to support patients (Rothman & Wagner 2003).

Chronic disease management

To date a variety of definitions have been used to describe chronic disease management (CDM) resulting in the lack of clarity for clinicians in understanding the term and the expected outcomes. A more recognised definition will also help researchers evaluate programs designed to examine the effectiveness of different models of CDM. One simple definition from the Royal College of Physicians, London (NHS Alliance 2004, p. 1) is:

a system of coordinated healthcare interventions and communications for populations with long term conditions in which patient self-care is significant.

Another longer and more comprehensive definition is given below, but note that both definitions make reference to population management rather than just individual management of patients. The following definition of chronic disease management, based on the chronic care model, comes from Norris et al. (2003, p. 8) and attempts to encompass all the factors needed to manage patients with chronic and ongoing illness:

Chronic disease management is an organized, proactive, multi-component patient-centered approach to healthcare delivery that involves all members of a defined population who have a specific chronic disease, or a subpopulation with specific characteristics.

Care is focused on and integrated across the entire spectrum of the disease and its complications, the prevention of comorbid conditions and the relevant aspects of the health care delivery system. Ultimately, the ideal chronic care model consists of an informed patient interacting with a well-prepared practice team (Wagner et al. 1999).

Components of chronic disease management

In order to manage any chronic disease, Norris et al. (2003) describe five necessary components of CDM. They are:

1. identification of patients with a specific disease;
2. implementation of guidelines or performance standards for management of the identified patients;
3. implementation of one or more interventions;
4. clinical information systems for tracking and monitoring interventions and outcomes; and
5. measurement and management of patient and population outcomes.

One of these elements, interventions, is discussed in further detail below.

Interventions for chronic disease management

The interventions needed to manage patients with chronic disease may be patient or population focused, provider and practice focused or processes that revolve around the health system infrastructure and processes. The following points from Norris et al. (2003) summarise the components and some of the interventions that may be implemented.

1. **Patient- or population-focused interventions**
   - patient-centred care strategies with mutual understanding of roles and responsibilities, and shared goals
   - self-management education of the patient and support persons
   - patient reminder/recall
   - patient feedback
   - telephone call outreach
   - electronic patient decision support
   - stratification of the population
   - patient-provider communication training.

2. **Provider- and practice-focused interventions**
   - role specification
   - provider reminders
   - provider education
   - provider monitoring, feedback
   - care by non-physician, non-nursing staff with development of potential new roles

- decision support: flow charts, specialist consultation
- case management.

3. **Health care system infrastructure and processes**
    - practice redesign: appointment scheduling, role delineation
    - models of care, such as mini-clinics
    - patient group or cluster visits
    - electronic information systems: registries, other patient-centred databases, electronic medical records, automated reminder systems
    - support from upper management, such as practice principles.

Reflections

What interventions for the management of chronic illness have you tried to implement in your practice? What were the results?

Benefits of planned care

Although widespread improved clinical outcomes from care planning are yet to be shown, it is thought that there are some benefits in care planning to both the patient and the practice. For patients, a structured approach such as a care plan will increase their knowledge and participation in their care, and for the practice, it will assist with service delivery. The following list of exemplary benefits is based on those that have been promoted by the Department of Health and Ageing (NHPAC 2006) as a way of improving the uptake of General Practitioner Management Plans (GPMPs) for those patients who have a chronic medical condition.

- Care planning helps to coordinate the services and treatment that a patient requires and can be used as a tool for organising the care a patient needs.
- Care planning enables a proactive role managing the health care requirements of patients. A care plan is a useful mechanism for recording comprehensive, accurate and up-to-date information about the patient's condition and all of the treatment they are receiving.
- Development of a care plan can also help encourage the patient to participate in being actively involved in their care and to take some responsibility for their care.
- Effective care of chronic conditions requires an evolution from episodic, acute models towards a comprehensive system involving continuity of care across patient conditions, health care providers and settings over time. Key supports for this are structured information systems and multidisciplinary teamwork.

- Structured care planning is designed to support teamwork both within general practice and between it and other services and health professionals especially allied health professionals.
- Positive research is emerging which shows that multidisciplinary care plans improve the quality of care and clinical outcomes for people with chronic disease (for example, improved total cholesterol and blood pressure outcome measures for people with diabetes).

Note that a care plan is described as a tool for organising patient needs and as such does not take the place of ongoing dialogue and discussion with the patient about their needs. Frequent review of this plan is fundamental to its success and this review is also supported by the availability of MBS item numbers designed for this purpose.

Reflections

What other benefits do you see in planning care?

A care plan

A care plan is a 'structured, comprehensive plan developed by the patient and their significant others, carers and health professional(s)' (Battersby et al. 2007).

The care plan should be developed in conjunction with health professionals involved in the care of the patient as well as other supports and includes both medical management and self-management. The purpose of the care plan is to inform the patient of issues relating to their health, to engage them in their own health care and treatment, and to give them the confidence to be able to effectively make changes to achieve improved self-management and better health outcomes.

The care plan should include:

- patient-defined problems;
- patient-defined goals;
- medical management;
- a prioritised action plan based on self-management needs of the patient and their carer;
- community education programs or resources; and
- time for review and follow up.

(Flinders Human Behaviour and Health Research Unit 2009, p. 20)

In today's general practice environment, these care plans are usually called General Practitioner Management Plans (GPMPs) and can be combined with a Team Care Arrangement (TCA). In practice many are written by practice nurses in conjunction with the patient's general practitioner. GPMPs and TCAs should be comprehensive documents that set out and enable evidence-based management of the patient's health and care needs. These are available to patients who will benefit from a structured approach to management of their chronic or terminal medical condition and care needs (MBS 2009). Care plans have been described by GPs as clinical tools to organise and facilitate clinical care delivery and engage patients in their own care. Care plans were primarily developed as templates for accessing allied health services. Unfortunately, patients who were the recipients of these care plans recalled very little about their care plans and none of them were using the written plan in their day-to-day self-management (Shortus et al. 2007).

In a retrospective audit by Vagholkar et al. (2007) on multidisciplinary care plans prepared for patients with type 2 diabetes, they found that although the content was relevant to diabetes the striking feature was the limited information documented. This was despite all of the GPs in the study using templates provided by divisions of general practice or the Royal Australian College of General Practitioners. The study highlighted the need to reflect on the thinking behind care plans and whether they are meeting the needs of patients with chronic diseases. What this study did show, however, is that when a diabetes care plan is followed, the care provided to patients adhered significantly more closely to process guidelines in relation to weight, foot and microalbumin examinations. Metabolic control and cardiovascular risk factors have been shown to have improved in those patients receiving multidisciplinary care (Zwar et al. 2007) but whether this is related to the care plan is not clear. Until more evidence is produced regarding the value of multidisciplinary care planning, it is difficult to say whether they are of great benefit to health outcomes of patients.

Several factors have been identified by Martin (2008) as being necessary for effective care planning. Martin describes four domains which have an impact on effectiveness—the patient, the GP, the practice and the health system. These reinforce the elements of the chronic care model which include these as components of a successful model to manage chronic disease and reinforce the notion that it is not possible for one provider, such as a practice nurse or general practitioner, to be able to singlehandedly manage patients with chronic illness.

Steps in planned care

The steps involved in preparation of a GPMP are clearly articulated by the MBS and include:

1. assessing the patient to identify and/or confirm all of the patient's health care needs, problems and relevant conditions;
2. collaborating with the patient to set management goals to achieve desired changes;
3. identifying any actions to be taken by the patient;
4. identifying treatment and services that the patient is likely to need and making arrangements for provision of these services and ongoing management; and
5. documenting the patient needs, goals, patient actions, treatment, services and a review date.

Redefining roles to manage chronic illness

Workforce issues such as the lack of general practitioners and nursing staff are well documented and have contributed to policy changes in recent times. In order to deliver effective health care there must be suitable health care professionals to deliver the right care to the patient at the right time. The introduction and expansion of multidisciplinary teams, patient-focused care, population-based approaches and the emphasis on improving quality of care will all have an impact on health care professionals delivering the care.

Patients with a chronic and complex illness are likely to benefit from multiple providers ranging from specialists to volunteers over time but this requires care to be more integrated rather than task orientated. Health care workers need to have a broad understanding of each others's roles as care will be provided by a variety of disciplines and each member will have different skills, knowledge and experience. In order to develop new ways of providing comprehensive care, conventional structures and boundaries need to be challenged. Research by Richardson et al. (1998), cited in Nolte and McKee (2008, p. 147), suggests that 'many medical professionals . . . spend a large proportion of their time performing tasks that do not necessarily require their particular professional expertise'.

In general, many doctors and nurses feel threatened by the thought that other less skilled health professionals may take over some of their work. It is necessary

Reflections

Identify parts of the nursing role which do not actually require your level of expertise. Who could do this work?

to acknowledge that the workforce will change and needs to be adaptable and flexible to manage the numbers and complexities of patients (and their carers) presenting with chronic and complex care requirements. Being able to involve patients and their carers as part of the decision making in care requirements is often a far cry from the traditional model of care that prevails for the management of acute illness and requires a change in thinking for many health professionals.

Generic competency

Given that a variety of disciplines deliver care to patients with chronic and ongoing disease, it would seem logical that there are some generic skills that all health care providers in this situation should possess. The World Health Organisation (2005), with support from the International Council of Nurses and other peak bodies, has identified five basic competencies that apply to all health care staff caring for patients with chronic health problems. They are:

1. **Patient-centred care**—which allows the patient's values, needs and preferences to be considered in addition to any clinical factors when formulating a plan and making decisions about care. This will strengthen the patient's ability to manage their own illness and they become expert in their own care. In patient-centred care, patients move from being passive recipients to being actively involved in their own care. Self-management is discussed further in Chapter 16.

2. **Partnering**—with other health care providers, which is fundamental to providing a consistent and coordinated approach to chronic care. Care must be coordinated across different settings, multiple providers and over a long period. Partnerships have the ability to provide care which is not available in any one institution and allow resources including other providers and the community to be fully utilised. In order to partner effectively, health care workers must be able to communicate effectively with the patient. The skills needed involve the ability to:

   - negotiate;
   - share decisions;
   - collectively solve problems;
   - establish goals;
   - implement action;
   - identify strengths and weaknesses;
   - clarify roles and responsibilities; and
   - evaluate progress.

3. **Quality improvement**—which underpins health care in all dimensions and is an approach and an attitude that should accompany everything that those providing

services to patients do. Emphasis is now applied to improve services, reduce errors, avoid duplications, implement changes to improve outcomes and to evaluate the outcomes of those interventions. Nurses need to have a basic understanding of how to design and test interventions with the intent of improving quality, safety and efficiency. Because of the rapid changes in technology and health care systems, health care workers need to be able to accept change, embrace it and capitalise on it. This is especially the case for nurses looking to expand their role and be innovative in the care they deliver and the way they deliver it. Being able to ask questions, look for evidence and translate this evidence into patient care will be required for all health care workers, including practice nurses.

4. **Information and communication technology**—which may range from traditional paper-based systems to increasingly sophisticated computerised technology. This allows for access to evidence and education on line; the creation of sophisticated databases and disease registers; send text messages and emails; the development of websites; the transmission of telemedicine, and the efficient flow of information to all providers in a safe and timely manner. It is likely that we will see the development of a shared electronic health record in Australia in the near future and this will mean all health care professionals have access to, and the ability to use, technology. Increasingly health messages are being delivered by electronic methods to reach maximum numbers of people using fewer resources.

5. **Public health perspective**—when added to the traditional perspectives by health care workers will improve health outcomes. Population care will require practice nurses to think of care not only for individuals but also across a defined population of their clinics, practices and communities. Addressing health care on a population basis adds another dimension as individuals benefit from the information developed for the populations to which they belong and interventions are targeted towards those most likely to benefit. This may mean expanding practice nurse roles to develop new skills in health promotion, screening, coaching, motivational interviewing and management of other staff. Systems for providing alternative consultation arrangements, such as group visits and follow-up by telephone, may also be required. Evaluation of programs and interventions will be necessary to ascertain where resources should be directed and avoid focusing on individuals but rather assess success on a practice level. Importantly, health care providers are recognised as role models within their communities and have the opportunity to influence the attitudes and behaviours of patients.

Reflections

How many of these core competencies do you have knowledge about and feel confident in?

Role of the practice nurse

Nurses working in general practice have been called upon to define and clarify their roles—a task which has proven to be very complex and influenced by many factors (see Chapter 1). Being involved in caring for patients with chronic illness is an inevitable part of working in the general practice environment and the way in which this is done will vary from one patient to another, one practitioner to another and from one practice to another.

Nurses have been described as being able to contribute to chronic disease care on both an individual level and a systems level (Forbes & While 2009). Nursing contribution has been described as:

- nurse-led care (independent nursing practice where the nurse identifies the need and then organises and/or refers to others);

- nurse-led and nurse-delivered care (independent nursing practice where the nurse identifies the need and manages the problem); and

- nurse-delivered care (the nurse provides care under the direction of others, such as the GP or advanced nurse—dependent-nursing practice).

There is considerable evidence which suggests that nurses, including those nurses working in primary care, can contribute to effective care and achieve positive health outcomes (Chiarella 2008; Halcomb et al. 2008; Keleher et al. 2009). There is little doubt that nurses as part of the primary

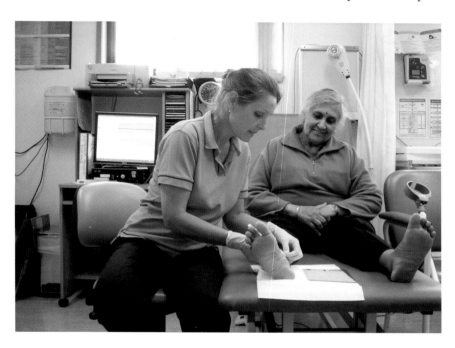

health care team are well placed to contribute in a meaningful way to patients with chronic and complex needs. The challenge remains for practice nurses and organisations to determine how this can best be achieved with the structure, staffing and culture in which they are employed.

Reflections

Given your practice structure and culture, how can you contribute to the care of patients with a chronic illness?

Factors that indicate successful management of chronic disease

It is acknowledged that no single factor determines the success of a program, and when examining some exemplary models of CDM in the UK (NHS Alliance 2004), several factors are identifiable as being critical in the success of CDM programs. They include:

- clinical leadership—redesigning care delivery with innovative solutions to reduce the frustrations experienced by many clinicians when using ineffective systems;
- clinicians and managers working together—identifying problems in both clinical and administrative areas and focusing on redesigning the system to improve the patient experience;
- building trust—developing good working relationships fundamental to a cohesive approach; building trust between primary care clinicians, secondary care clinicians, managers and patients themselves;
- team working—eradicating dysfunctional professional barriers, involving each participant in the patient care journey, and contributing according to knowledge and ability.

The key to effective care is the right person, in the right place, at the right time, doing the right thing.

(NHS Alliance 2004, p. 7)

- complex patient needs—recognising that patients with comorbidity present a particular challenge;
- patient involvement—helping patients and carers to become the managers of their own chronic conditions and trusting them to make appropriate decisions

regarding their health care; sharing information and knowledge to plan services to allow innovation and change;

- resources—such as time, people and money are necessary for developing effective care; investing in infrastructure to develop new models of care; and

- solutions—developing a systematic approach to implementing solutions.

Conclusion

As the population ages and the prevalence of chronic disease increases, examining the way we provide care to those chronically ill patients will be fundamental to the success of reducing any gaps in care to any populations and individuals in any country. Innovative ways of providing comprehensive care requires a paradigm shift for nurses. Looking at new roles, concentrating on remaining patient focused and working within a business model present challenges, not only at a clinical and individual level but also at a professional and population level. Practice nurses will need to embrace this if they are to become an essential member of the multidisciplinary team in the 21st century.

CASE STUDY

Name of nurse
Heather Scott
Practice
Breed Street Clinic, Traralgon, Vic.

After identifying that patients were having difficulty accessing appointments for routine reviews, and subsequently presenting with complications of their illnesses, the Breed Street Clinic initiated a service into their practice with the aim to provide proactive care and reduce the risk of complications in patients with chronic diseases. The practice determined that a coordinated system was needed with a designated leader responsible for implementing change; the nurse coordinator, Heather, was appointed leader and coordinator of the project.

Her role was to streamline and coordinate processes. The first step was to send the patient an explanatory letter and a pathology request form. The patient was requested to have the pathology test and visit the optometrist before attending a 45-minute assessment with a practice nurse. If patients did not complete the pathology, a reminder phone call was made to encourage patients to have the tests and the complete assessment.

The assessment included collection of information such as height, weight, blood pressure and urinalysis, and an ECG and ABPI were performed in the clinic. In addition to this the patient file was updated, patient medications checked for accuracy and allergies documented. The patient was then seen by their usual GP to complete the assessment. The GPs see this as a worthwhile process as it has made the consultation more effective, with time spent discussing the real issues and options rather than data collection and taking anthropometric measurements.

As leaders of the team, the practice nurse and GP facilitated fortnightly team meetings to maintain the focus on CDM. Reception staff provided support in making patients' appointments, being familiar with billing processes and offering clerical assistance, while other practice nurses assisted in the assessment process.

Local nursing students were included in the assessment as part of their clinical placement and many of them used these opportunities as their clinical assessment.

Prior to the employment of Heather, the diabetes SIP payment rate was 25% and has now increased to 68%, indicating that over two-thirds of the practice population of patients with diabetes have had a cycle of care completed.

The income generated from chronic disease management funds the employment of practice nurses. Furthermore, their wages have increased and incentives are offered to attract and retain quality staff. Streamlined processes have resulted in fewer appointments for an individual patient, enabling increased access for others.

Primarily through following the targets set by the National Primary Care Collaborative (of which Breed Street Clinic was a leading participant), the clinic has been able to reduce complications in their patients and increase the number of patients achieving national targets. For example: HbA1c <7% has increased from 8% to 55% (national average = 42%), and those with BP <130/80 has increased from 14% to 37% (equal to national average). An outstanding example of an improved patient outcome involves a patient whose HbA1c was 17.7% in November 2006, reduced to 6.5% in June 2008. The clinic has also been involved in the development of a simpler referral process to allied health providers locally (dieticians and diabetes educators) through the Better Health Outcomes in Gippsland project.

Testimonial

Appointing Heather to lead the team in managing chronic disease has been one of the most proactive and valuable decisions that Breed Street Clinic has made. A significant reason for the demonstrated patient improvements has been the systematic processes underpinning the excellent clinical care that is provided to the patient by the whole team. (Dr Paul Brougham, Breed Street Clinic, Traralgon.)

Key messages

There are multiple opportunities for practice nurses to be involved in the management of patients with chronic diseases in the general practice and primary care setting.

Teamwork is necessary for effective management of chronic disease.

Proactive, comprehensive and coordinated primary care is the foundation of effective CDM.

Useful resources

Australian Institute of Health and Welfare
> http://www.aihw.gov.au/

Australian Primary Health Care Research Institute—a systematic review of chronic disease management
> http://www.anu.edu.au

References

1. Australian Institute of Health and Welfare (AIHW) 2006, *Chronic diseases and associated risk factors in Australia, 2006,* AIHW, viewed 10 March 2010, <http://www.aihw.gov.au/>.

2. Battersby, M, Harvey, P, Mills, PD, Kalucy, E, Pols, RG, Frith, PA, McDonald, P, Esterman, A, Tsourtos, G, Donato, R, Pearce, C & McGowan, C 2007, 'SA Health Plus: a controlled trial of a generic model of chronic illness care', *The Millbank Quarterly*, vol. 85, no. 1, pp. 37–67, as cited in Commonwealth of Australia 2009, 'Capabilities for supporting prevention and chronic condition self-management: a resource for educators of primary health care professionals'.

3. Bodenheimer, T, Wagner, E & Grumbach, K 2002, 'Improving primary care for patients with chronic illness', *Journal of the American Medical Association*, vol. 288, pp. 1775–9.

4. Britt, H, Miller, G, Knox, S, Charles, J, Valenti, L, Pan, Y, Henderson, J, O'Halloran, J & Ng, A 2004, *General Practice Activity in Australia 2003–2004*, Canberra, Australian Institute of Health and Welfare, viewed October 2009, <http://www.aihw.gov.au/publications/index.cfm/title/10079>.

5. Chiarella, M 2008, 'Discussion paper: New and emerging nurse led models of primary health care', Australian Government Health and Hospitals Reform Commission.

6. Flinders Human Behaviour and Health Research Unit 2009, 'Capabilities for supporting prevention and chronic condition self-management: a resource for educators of primary health care professionals', Commonwealth of Australia.

7. Flinders Human Behaviour and Health Research Unit 2003, 'Chronic condition self management education module', Commonwealth of Australia.

8. Forbes, A & While, A 2009, 'The nursing contribution to chronic disease management: a discussion paper', *International Journal of Nursing Studies*, vol. 46, issue 1, pp. 120–31.

9. Glasgow, N, Sibthorpe, B & Gear, A 2005, 'Primary health care position statement: a scoping of the evidence', The Australian Primary Health Care Research Institute, Canberra, viewed June 2009, <http://www.agpn.com.au/site/index.cfm?module=DOCUMENTS&leca=16>.

10. Halcomb, EJ, Davidson, PM, Salamonson, Y & Ollerton, R 2008, 'Nursing in Australian general practice: implications for chronic disease management', *Journal of Nursing and Healthcare of Chronic Illness*, 17(5a), pp. 6–15.

11. Huang, N, Daddo, M & Clune, E 2008, 'Heart health CHD management gaps in general practice', *Australian Family Physician*, vol. 38, no. 4, April 2008, viewed 31 July 2009, <http://www.heartfoundation.org.au/SiteCollectionDocuments/A_CHD_TreatmentGaps_AFPArticle_April2009.pdf.pdf>.

12. Institute of Medicine 2001, *Crossing the quality chasm: a new health system for the 21st century*, National Academy Press, viewed June 2009, <http://www.nap.edu/openbook.php?record_id=10027&page=1>.

13. Keleher, H, Parker, R, Abdulwadud, O & Francis, K 2009, 'Systematic review of the effectiveness of primary care nursing', *International Journal of Nursing Practice*, vol. 15, pp. 16–24.

14. Lambert, S 2005, 'Chronic condition self-management: a primary health care change management problem', *Australian Journal of Primary Health*, vol. 11, no. 2, pp. 70–7.

15. Martin, C 2008, 'Improving chronic illness care—revisiting the role of care planning', *Australian Family Physician*, vol. 37, no. 3, pp. 161–4.

16. Medicare Benefits Schedule (MBS) 2009, viewed July 2009, <http://www9.health.gov.au/mbs/fullDisplay.cfm?type=note&qt=NoteID&q=A33>.

17. National Health & Medical Research Council 2008, *Evidence–Practice Gaps Report, Volume 1: a review of developments 2004–2007*, Canberra.

18. National Heart Foundation 2009, 'Snapshot of coronary heart disease management gaps and key messages', viewed 26 October 2009, <http://www.heartfoundation.org.au/SiteCollectionDocuments/A_CHD_TreatmentGaps_ISP_March2009_FINAL.pdf>.

19. National Health Priority Action Council (NHPAC) 2006, *National chronic disease strategy*, Australian Government Department of Health & Ageing Canberra, viewed 26 October 2009, <http://www.health.gov.au/internet/main/publishing.nsf/Content/pq-ncds-strat>.

20. NHS Alliance 2004, *Clinicians, services and commissioning in chronic disease management in the NHS: the need for coordinated management programmes*, Royal College of Physicians, London.

21. NHS 2009, The Information Centre, viewed 25 February 2010, <http://www.ic.nhs.uk/news-and-events/press-office/press-releases/audit-shows-sixty-percent-of-people-with-diabetes-in-england-not-receiving-recommended-care>.

22. Nolte, E & McKee, M (eds) 2008, *Caring for people with chronic conditions: a health system perspective*, Open University Press, Birkshire, viewed 11 March 2010, <http://www.euro.who.int/document/E91878.pdf>.

23. Norris, S, Glasgow, R, Engelgau, M, O'Connor, P & McCulloch, D 2003, 'Chronic disease management: a definition and systematic approach to component interventions', *Dis Management Health Outcomes*, vol. 11, pp. 477–88.

24. Richardson, G, Maynard, A, Cullum, N & Kindig, D 1998, 'Skill mix changes: substitution or service development?' *Health Policy*, vol. 45, pp. 119–32.

25. Rothman, A & Wagner, E 2003, 'Chronic illness management: what is the role of primary care?', *Annals of Internal Medicine*, vol. 138, no. 3, pp. 356–61.

26. Royal College of Nursing, Australia (RCNA) 2005, *Nursing in General Practice: a guide for the general practice team*, Canberra, viewed June 2009, <http://www.rcna.org.au/Default.aspx?PageID=1216914&A=SearchResult&SearchID=674068&ObjectID=1216914&ObjectType=1>.

27. Shortus, T, McKenzie, S, Kemp, L, Proudfoot, J & Harris, M 2007, 'Multidisciplinary care plans for diabetes: how are they used?', *Medical Journal of Australia*, vol. 187, no. 2, pp. 78–81.

28. Vagholkar, S, Hermiz, O, Zwar N, Shortus, T, Comino, E & Harris, M 2007, 'Multidisciplinary care plans for diabetic patients: what do they contain?', *Australian Family Physician*, vol. 36, no. 3, pp. 279–82.

29. Wagner, EH 1998, 'Chronic disease management: what will it take to improve care for chronic illness?', *Effective Clinical Practice*, vol. 1, no. 1, pp. 2–4.

30. Wagner, E, Davis, C, Schaefer, J, Von Korff, M & Austin, B 1999, 'A survey of leading chronic disease management programs: are they consistent with the literature?', *Managed Care Quarterly*, vol. 7, pp. 56–66.

31. World Health Organisation (WHO) 2002, *Innovative care for chronic conditions: building blocks for action—global report*.

32. World Health Organisation (WHO) 2005, 'Preparing a health care workforce for the 21st century: the challenge of chronic conditions', viewed August 2009, <http://www.who.int/chp/knowledge/publications/workforce_report/en>.

33. Zwar, N, Hermiz, O, Comino, E, Shortus, T, Burns, J & Harris, M 2007, 'Do multidisciplinary care plans result in better care for patients with type 2 diabetes?', *Australian Family Physician*, vol. 36, no 1/2, viewed July 2009, <http://www.racgp.org.au/afp/200701/14845>.

34. Zwar, N, Harris, M, Griffiths, R, Roland, M, Dennis, S, Powell Davies, G & Hasan, I 2006, 'A systematic review of chronic disease management,' *Research Centre for Primary Health Care and Equity*, School of Public Health and Community Medicine, UNSW, viewed October 2009, <http://www.anu.edu.au/aphcri>.

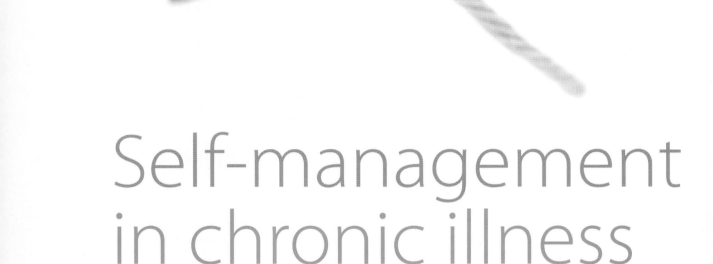

Chapter sixteen

Self-management in chronic illness

by Christine Walker

Overview

One of the most important elements of the chronic care model in managing chronic diseases is the concept of self-management. In this chapter we employ the term 'chronic illness' rather than chronic disease as the term 'illness' takes into account that a physical disease or condition has subjective and social dimensions as well as biomedical dimensions. Recognising this complexity is particularly important in working with people who have chronic or long-term illnesses as all these dimensions play a part in how people respond to and how they will live with those illnesses.

Objectives

At the completion of this chapter you should be able to:

- understand the growing role of self-management in the care of people with chronic illnesses;

- recognise the types of self-management strategies that are available to health professionals working in the community;

- appreciate the role of a practice nurse in implementing, supporting and sustaining self-management support strategies for patients; and

- understand the current evidence base for chronic disease self-management.

Introduction

In the last decades of the 20th century, chronic illnesses emerged as the most significant forms of ill-health among Western populations, including Australians. Coronary heart disease (CHD) was the leading cause of death for both Australian men and women in 2005, while cardiovascular disease and lung cancer were also significant causes of death in men. During this time women were more likely to die of cardiovascular disease, heart failure and chronic obstructive pulmonary disease (COPD); cancers and diabetes were among the top 10 causes of death for both men and women (Australian Institute of Health and Welfare 2008a).

These diseases contribute to premature mortality which means deaths occurring before the age of 75. Men are more likely to die of cardiovascular diseases and women of breast cancer before the age of 75. Lung cancer contributes to the premature deaths of both men and women. Deaths at these earlier ages from these diseases are generally avoidable and deaths from CHD, stroke and diabetes are all considered to be preventable through combinations of prevention and treatment.

Cardiovascular disease, diabetes, cancers and other chronic illnesses, such as asthma and musculoskeletal diseases, are all associated with high usage of health care services from general practitioners (GPs) and specialist visits through to hospital admissions, as well as high use of Pharmaceutical Benefits Scheme (PBS) medicines and home care (Australian Institute of Health and Welfare 2008b). This high usage can be greatly diminished when people adopt strategies to either prevent the onset of such chronic illnesses or they use strategies to care for themselves to prevent further deterioration after they are diagnosed with a chronic illness.

For people with long-term illnesses, self-management programs assist them to learn healthy behaviours and to sustain them over long periods of time. This can be challenging in a society that favours car travel to walking; eating fast foods and sweets to eating salad; and celebrating with alcohol and working very long hours. It can also be personally challenging depending on a person's life stage. Working women with young children, for instance, have little time to care for themselves, while some recently widowed men must learn the basics of caring for themselves, such as shopping and cooking. Sometimes, it is much easier to 'to stick with routines' than to step outside of them and adopt new behaviours.

Reflections

To understand how difficult it can be to change behaviour to cope with a chronic illness, think of the times when you needed to change your routines, for example, adopting a healthier diet or increasing your own physical activity.

The chronic care model

In Chapter 15, the chronic care model (CCM) was discussed to assist health professionals in managing their patients with chronic illness. This model was developed in the United States by Ed Wagner and associates in 1996 (Wagner et al. 1996) and has been refined since then. This model was developed to demonstrate that the care of chronic illnesses required a far broader approach than just medical care. It includes the roles for the community, health systems and self-management support, as well as an effective health delivery system, decision support and clinical information systems that are designed to meet the long-term needs of people with chronic illnesses. When such models are applied to the care of any chronic illness, Wagner argues the outcomes of such applications are better-informed patients who are actively engaged in their own healthcare that is, self-management (Wagner et al. 2001).

Definitions of self-management

Below are two well-known definitions of self-management, however, it is important to remember that self-management is a process that includes a set of attitudes, behaviours and skills.

Gruman and Von Korff (1996) define self-management as:

involving people with chronic diseases in the activities that protect and promote health, monitoring and managing of symptoms and signs of illness, managing the impacts of illness on functioning, emotions and interpersonal relationships and adhering to treatment regimes.

Redman (2004, p. 4) defines it as:

training that people with chronic health conditions need in order to be able to deal with taking medicine and maintaining therapeutic regimes, maintaining everyday life such as employment and family, and dealing with the future, including changing life plans and the frustration, anger and depression.

Self-management is based on people being actively involved in their own care although it is acknowledged that this may differ from one person to another at different stages of an illness and at different times across the lifespan. It is underpinned by the person being at the centre of their own health care and involves the skills and resources that a person needs to negotiate the health system and maximise their quality of life across the continuum of prevention and care (National Health Priority Action Council (NHPAC) 2006).

By embedding the principles of self-management into the health care system, the person with a chronic illness will be able to:

- understand the nature of their illness including risk factors and comorbidities;
- have knowledge of their treatment options and be able to make informed choices regarding treatments;
- actively participate in decision making with health professionals, family, and carers and other supports in terms of continuing care;
- follow a treatment or care plan that has been negotiated and agreed with their health care providers, family and carers and other supports;
- monitor signs and symptoms of change in their health condition and have an action plan to respond to identified changes;
- manage the impact of the disease on their physical, emotional and social life and have better mental health and wellbeing as a result;
- adopt a lifestyle that reduces risks and promotes health through prevention and early intervention; and
- have confidence in their ability to use support services and make decisions regarding their health and quality of life.

(NHPAC 2006)

Reflections

How does the chronic illness care in your practice contribute to the above points?

National and state policy on chronic disease self-management

In 1999 self-management became formally integrated into chronic disease management in Australia when the federal government set aside $14.4 million for the Sharing Health Care Initiative which included developing self-management programs (Alwell et al. 2004). Prior to this, self-management programs had been offered on an ad hoc basis by foundations such as the Cancer Council and the Arthritis Foundation. They were offered as a means of providing support and information. After 1999, self-management programs became part of the treatment regime in chronic disease.

Self-management programs are favoured by Australian governments because they lead to improved health behaviours, improved health status and reduced health service utilisation such as unplanned hospital admissions

(Battersby et al. 2003). This may also be described as secondary disease prevention. So far, as part of the National Chronic Disease Strategy (Department of Health and Ageing 2007), self-management programs are mainly funded for people with asthma, cancer, diabetes, cardiovascular diseases, musculoskeletal diseases, injury prevention and mental health.

The chronic care model has had an increasing influence on Australian health care policymakers and service providers with self-management being seen as an integral part of the need to develop health care systems that are responsive to chronic illnesses. For example, in 2004 a forum in Canberra on heart failure discussed the need for early intervention into heart failure in order to improve health outcomes and reduce hospital admissions. In both New South Wales and Victoria there were programs using the principles of the CCM to reduce hospital admissions (Phillips et al. 2004).

However, it was the establishment of the Australian Better Health Initiative (ABHI) by the Council of Australian Governments (COAG) in 2006 that formally introduced similar dimensions of the CCM into Australian health policy and practice at both state and federal levels (Department of Health and Ageing 2008). The aim of ABHI is to refocus the health system to promote good health for the overall population and to reduce the risks related to the burden of chronic disease to both the community and the health system. The initiative will support activities to improve health outcomes along the care continuum, from the well population to those with advanced chronic conditions.

There are five priority areas of action:

1. Promoting healthy lifestyles
2. Supporting early detection of risk factors and chronic disease
3. Supporting lifestyle and risk modification
4. Encouraging active patient self-management of chronic conditions
5. Improving the communication and coordination between care services.

These priority areas are similar to the elements of the CCM and demonstrate that self-management is now an integral part of a new approach in Australia to managing chronic illnesses. General practice has a vital role to play in all of these priority areas. The Australian General Practice Network (AGPN) and its state-based organisations are coordinating and resourcing general practices to participate in these system changes.

For example, the general practice network in South Australia (General Practice South Australia (GPSA) 2008) has received funding from the federal

Department of Health and Ageing for the priority area to encourage active patient self-management. The aim of the project is to strengthen the capacity of the existing and future primary care workforce to support chronic disease self-management (CDSM).

The GPSA Chronic Disease Self-Management Program aims to:

- provide the Divisions network with a stronger focus on CDSM and CDSM support;
- increase primary care providers awareness and understanding of what is meant by CDSM support;
- provide opportunities for discussion and promotion of CDSM and CDSM support;
- facilitate wide dissemination of new and existing CDSM support training, resources and information;
- increase systematic adoption and promotion of self-management programs;
- increase integration between South Australia's CDSM Network initiatives and other state and territory CDSM programs; and
- promote linkages to primary care programs, other ABHI initiatives, state and territory governments and consumer groups.

At the same time Western Australia has adopted a chronic disease self-management strategy where the GP networks in Western Australia are delivering Living Well programs based on the Stanford model of self-management to community members who are living with chronic illnesses (Western Australian Department of Health 2009).

The Australian Better Health Initiative is thus driving change in the way that general practice delivers services to people with chronic illnesses. It is further supported by the new Chronic Disease Management items on the Medicare Benefits Schedule, being the General Practice Management Plans (GPMPs) and Team Care Arrangements (TCAs) which aim to coordinate the care of people with chronic illnesses across the community and provide access to the allied health services they require. Self-management support and coordination of all the services people with chronic illness require is now seen as the role of the practice nurse (Harris et al. 2008; MacDonald et al. 2008), with practice nurses assisting in the drawing up of care plans in consultation with the patients' GPs.

Reflections

What type of CDSM support is available to your practice and have you been able to access it?

Chronic disease self-management programs

Given the complex environment in which people with chronic illnesses must manage their illnesses there are a range of ways a practice nurse can support them and incorporate self-management support strategies into planned patient care. Self-management is more than educating the person and providing information. For example, compliance with a medication regime is only one component of self-management. Having an understanding of the various models of chronic disease self-management support will provide the practice nurse with the basics from which strategies can be chosen to work effectively with people with chronic illnesses in their daily practice. Alternatively, practice nurses may choose to refer people on to appropriate self-management programs with allied health professionals within their local communities. Based on the chronic care model supported by educational, behavioural and motivational theories and methodologies, a number of CDSM programs have been developed to assist people in self-managing their chronic illness. The following highlights some of the recognised models which practice nurses may choose to assist patients in understanding and self-managing their ongoing illnesses.

Stanford (Lorig) Chronic Disease Self-Management Program (CDSMP)

The Stanford Model was the original CDSM program, which used peers to educate patients about disease to change health behaviours. It was developed as a generic program in the US by Dr Kate Lorig and is mainly used as part of the services provided by health maintenance organisations (HMOs) (Lorig et al. 2001). Both Arthritis Self-Management Programs and its generic counterpart Chronic Disease Self-Management Program (CDSMP) have been offered in Australia by the state-based arthritis foundations. This program is delivered in group sessions and is delivered weekly over a period of six weeks. Each session is heavily scripted and delivered by a health professional preferably accompanied by a peer educator. Goal setting and planning are central features of the program. Participants also learn to manage stress, fatigue and changed circumstances by adopting new behaviours and practicing them in the week between sessions. The UK-based Expert Patient Program is a variation of the Stanford program (Kennedy et al. 2005; Kennedy et al. 2007).

In 1999 the CDSMP was heavily promoted by the Australian Government on the basis that it provided a strong evidence base. Kate Lorig and her colleagues published a number of peer-reviewed articles in the US showing how the program made long-term improvements in exercise and adherence to health regimes (Lorig et al. 1999).

In Australia, however, randomised controlled trials of the CDSMP have not produced hugely significant results. The Peer Led Self-Management of Chronic Illness Project was a randomised controlled trial of the program among people from culturally and linguistically diverse backgrounds that showed small improvements in exercise and other health-related behaviours (Swerissen et al. 2006). These improvements were not likely to be sustained after the trial finished and did not justify large-scale government investment.

The CDSMP is still being delivered by the Arthritis Foundation as well as some community health centres and private practitioners in all states. It is now firmly established as one of the large suite of self-management strategies.

The Flinders model

The **Flinders model** includes structured self-management assessment, goal setting and care planning for chronic disease. Preliminary research suggests the program resulted in increased knowledge of the disease and its management, but this did not translate into a significant impact in physiological indicators at 12-month follow up. Partly based on the Stages of Change model, the Flinders Human Behaviour and Health Research Unit has developed a set of tools for clients and their health professionals to jointly undertake an assessment of the person's readiness to self-manage, to set goals and explore barriers to self-management. This produces a collaborative care plan for each individual. The tools include the Partners in Health Scale, Cue and Response Interview Schedule and Problem and Goals Assessment Tool (Flinders Human Behaviour and Health Research Unit 2009b).

These tools provide the basis for a practice nurse in collaboration with the client to assess the appropriate point to commence exploring self-management. There are regular workshops run by the Flinders Human Behaviour and Health Research Unit for health professionals either as individuals or through their organisations to learn more about the tools and developing care plans.

Health coaching programs

Health coaching programs have similarities to the Flinders model. It is 'structured guidance for health professionals to help patients to adhere to medical and health recommendations and to make health enhancing lifestyle changes' (Health Coaching Australia 2008).

Like the Flinders model, health coaching focuses and builds on activities patients can do to improve their health and promotes patient responsibility for their own health management. Health coaching health professionals combine their usual assessment, recommendations and patient education with assistance to change health behaviours. Health coaches may use their skills in conjunction with telephone coaching, internet-based coaching programs or they may conduct face-to-face consultations. In some instances health coaching is accompanied by active interventions, such as walking with a person or a group of people, to demonstrate to them that they can do this activity.

Telephone coaching

Providing regular contact to patients by telephone calls may be very appropriate for certain types of patients in assisting them to manage their illness. In the same way that consulting with patients on a face-to-face level can provide a valuable service, so too can a telephone approach. Telephone appointments can monitor patients' status, deliver education, provide appointment reminders and facilitate peer support and referrals. For some patients the ability to attend appointments and outpatients is difficult because of inflexible appointment times, work schedules, limited transportation, financial pressures and language barriers. By allowing health professionals and patients to communicate by telephone, care can be delivered in a timely manner with patients being in their homes or workplaces.

However, it has been shown that in order to be beneficial, telephone care must be structured and have specific goals in mind. It probably offers the greatest support to those patients who need reminders, monitoring, self-management and coaching (Piette 2005). Additional self-management support may be beneficial to those patients needing support after initial diagnosis (such as diabetes) or those experiencing significant changes to treatment regimes (such as insulin initiation).

One well-evaluated telephone coaching program, the COACH program (Coaching patients On Achieving Cardiovascular Health) (Vale et al. 2003) is a secondary prevention program that coaches people who have been hospitalised with coronary heart disease to reduce their coronary risk factors. Coaches work in partnership with the patient's GP post hospital discharge. The coach, who may be a nurse, dietician or other health professional, telephones patients on a regular basis to provide structured, individualised information, education and support on medications adherence, lifestyle changes and to engage with their GPs to effect change. This 'coaching' approach empowers the patients to engage with their GPs to make step wise changes until the risk factor reduction targets are achieved.

The COACH program is now being trialled in Victoria using practice nurses as telephone 'coaches' to engage their patients with poorly controlled type 2 diabetes to improve their diabetes care (Young et al. 2007). The intervention, if effective, will be implemented widely to practice nurses working in general practices to deliver chronic disease self-management to patients with type 2 diabetes.

The 5 As model

The 5 As is an application of the Stages of Change model (Prochaska & DiClemente 1986) to reduce tobacco smoking. Quit Victoria (2005) recognises that stopping smoking is not a single event and involves a number of stages before an individual reaches the point of attempting to give up. Even then, there may be many attempts before a person is successful.

The Quit Victoria (2005) program has identified that health professionals can use the 5 As to encourage more quit attempts and to increase success rates among their patients who still smoke. Recognising that general practitioners have limited time to work with smoking cessation, the 5 As provide them with a brief intervention (some three minutes) which can be part of the routine consultation. It is particularly relevant to the work undertaken by practice nurses.

The 5 As are to:

1. **Ask** about smoking at each visit.
2. **Assess** the patient's willingness and confidence to quit and note the stage they are at with their smoking and quitting.
3. **Advise** the smoker to quit based on the health effects, as well as the benefits to be gained from quitting.
4. **Assist** the patient with quitting according to which stage they are at with their smoking.
5. **Ask again** at a subsequent visit. Ask smokers if they have reconsidered quitting or check progress of patients who have quit or are trying to quit. If an attempt to quit has not been made, the 5 As are used again.

Given its simplicity this is an intervention that practice nurses can do quickly and opportunistically to smokers presenting to general practice for a variety of reasons.

Core skills for self-management support

In order to support patients in self-management of their chronic illness, it is necessary for health professionals working in general practice to have knowledge, attitudes and skills to be able to do this. Following extensive research and consultation with training organisations, the Flinders Human Behaviour and Health Research Unit has produced a toolkit which outlines 19 core capabilities which were defined and deemed as necessary for health professionals in the primary care sector to successfully manage patients within the self-management continuum. Table 16.1 overleaf summarises the knowledge, attitudes and skills needed by staff and practice nurses to be able to assist patients in managing their chronic illness. These skills include maintaining wellness, detecting risk factors and self-managing existing illness.

The practice nurse role

The role of the practice nurse in supporting people in self-management is varied and influenced by many factors. The nurses have multiple tasks for each day and these tasks reflect both the clientele of the general practices in which they work as well as the way the practice delivers its services. At the same time many of the estimated 5000 practice nurses in Australia currently work part-time (Australian Practice Nurses Association 2008), which impacts on the continuity of care provided to patients in their care.

The emphasis on tasks, such as immunisation and wound management, as well as predominately part-time work structure creates barriers to undertaking self-management support which requires a level of nurse–patient continuity. Conversely, seeing patients frequently for episodic care, such as wound management and immunisations, can create opportunities to reinforce patient behaviours as part of CDSM support, albeit in short but frequent consultations. Other barriers include the costs of training in self-management

Table 16.1 Core skills for the primary health care workforce

General patient-centred capabilities	Behaviour change capabilities	Organisational/systems capabilities
1. Health promotion approaches 2. Assessment of health risk factors 3. Communication skills 4. Assessment of self-management capacity (understanding strengths and barriers) 5. Collaborative care planning 6. Use of peer support 7. Cultural awareness 8. Psychosocial assessment and support skills	9. Models of health behaviour change 10. Motivational interviewing 11. Collaborative problem definition 12. Goal setting and goal achievement 13. Structured problem solving and action planning	14. Working in multidisciplinary teams/interprofessional learning and practice 15. Information, assessment and communication management systems 16. Organisational change techniques 17. Evidence-based knowledge 18. Conducting practice-based research/quality improvement framework 19. Awareness of community resources

Source: Flinders Human Behaviour and Health Research Unit 2009a, p. 12

strategies such as the Flinders model, the lack of support by practice management to undertake such training as well as the lack of inclination on the part of some practice nurses to undertake self-management support. Because of the relationship to the Medicare Benefits Schedule and the possibility to generate income for the practice, for some practices and some nurses, education in wound management for instance might be seen as a greater priority than education in self-management strategies.

There is then the problem of which model of self-management support should a practice nurse adopt. Not only will some strategies be unattractive to the practice nurse but not all strategies will suit all the patients that the nurse identifies as benefiting from self-management support. Often the choice comes down to personal preference. Some people simply don't like talking on phones and most prefer personal contact. Some people want individualised help from a health professional while others will blossom in a group situation. People who are working or who are caring for someone else have too much to do to commit to a six-week course and prefer the telephone help.

A practice nurse may decide it will be a greater benefit to the patient with a chronic illness to refer them to another service where self-management support can be provided by skilled facilitators. Whether the practice nurse chooses to refer someone on or decides to undertake the training or even just chooses to apply some principles of self-management support in their daily work without actually undertaking any formal training, there are some central premises of good self-management that should be a feature of any self-management support.

The first premise is that support should assist the person with a chronic illness to gain or regain personal control in their lives. A program must work to provide or restore a person's **self-efficacy**; that is, a person must feel that they are gaining or regaining control over their lives by adopting such behaviours. This sense of self-efficacy may be developed through goal setting. Bandura (1997) who explored the concept of self-efficacy saw it as the central tenet of self-management programs. A simple means to measure if a person's sense of their own self-efficacy is improving is to check they are experiencing a sense of achievement or they express a level of improved self-esteem. (For example, 'I never thought I'd ever be able to walk as far as that! It was a real thrill to achieve it! I'm going to try to walk a little further each day!')

The second premise is that all goals must be **achievable**. For example, when a person who rarely exercises decides to exercise more it will not be realistic for them to decide to run a marathon. Achievable goals are realistic ones. A practice nurse might encourage such a person to walk around the block briskly to start with and build up to more exacting exercise over a period of time. The sense of achievement the person experiences is part of self-efficacy.

The following characteristics from the Flinders model could therefore be seen to summarise a 'good' self-manager (Flinders Human Behaviour and Health Research Unit 2009b). They are individuals who:

1. Have knowledge of their condition
2. Follow a treatment plan (care plan) agreed with their health professionals
3. Actively share in decision making with health professionals
4. Monitor and manage signs and symptoms of their condition
5. Manage the impact of the condition on their physical, emotional and social life
6. Adopt lifestyles that promote health.

In self-management, the role of the health professional is to move beyond education and information to achieve compliance as an outcome, to achieving sustained behaviour change. The practice nurse does not have to be skilled in all the self-management strategies but they can assist the person to undertake and sustain many changes in their lives. One of the core skills which form the basis of behavioural change is to conduct motivational interviewing and assess the person's stages of change.

Reflections

How would you describe your role in self-management support? How can your practice integrate self-management support into the existing delivery of patient care?

Motivational interviewing as a core skill

Motivational interviewing is a skill for all health professionals including practice nurses to apply in their work with patients as it sets the supportive environment for the person to make their own behaviour changes. The Australian Institute for Professionals Counsellors (2009) points out that motivational interviewing does not provide practical solutions towards change and therefore it should be used together with other therapies such as cognitive or behaviour therapy. It requires that health professionals:

- understand and apply the techniques of motivational interviewing in partnership with the client;

- adopt core communication skills, particularly open and reflective strategies; and

- acknowledge that motivation levels fluctuate as the client's circumstances and commitment changes and that not all behaviour change may be permanent.

The skills in motivational interviewing relate to developing a relationship with the patient in order to understand the issues from the perspective of the patient and their family. Any goals adopted in this relationship must be those belonging to the patient, which the health professional supports. Within this relationship the health professional must assist the person to try out strategies for change and find the strategy that suits them best. Health professionals need to develop non-judgmental attitudes towards any resistance to change by their patients while pointing out that current behaviour is not allowing the person to reach the goals they have set themselves.

One of the most important skills for health professionals who wish to effect behavioural changes in their patients is to acquire motivational interviewing skills training. Prochaska and DiClemente (1986) developed the

Transtheoretical model of behaviour change, proposing that behaviour change does not take place in a linear process. Instead, they argue, people move back and forth between old behaviours and new ones. However, there are five distinct stages as follows:

1. First stage is **pre-contemplation** where the person does not recognise they have a problem and is not prepared to make any changes.

2. Second stage is **contemplation** where the person has recognised the need to change their behaviour and is seriously thinking about it.

3. Third stage relates to **preparation** where the person is reviewing their behaviour and may try some new strategies for a limited time.

4. Fourth stage is where the person **modifies** their behaviour and is aware of the difference it makes in their lives.

5. Final stage relates to **integrating** that new behaviour pattern into their lives.

Locating where a person is in this change process means the practice nurse can provide activities and advice that assist the person to progress. For example, it is of little value suggesting to someone they should exercise more when they don't think there is any need to do so. However, if a person is contemplating more exercise then it is timely to make suggestions about appropriate exercise regimes but not to insist they adhere to them. This approach can actually save a lot of time and frustration. It also means that when a person is ready to change they are more likely to return for advice and help as they don't feel they will be judged if they fail.

> ### Reflections
>
> How can you incorporate motivational interviewing into what are often very short consultations with patients who have a chronic illness, such as diabetes or who are overweight?

Current evidence supporting self-management programs

The evidence that self-management works is growing. Lorig et al. (1999; 2001) suggest that the CDSMP produces sustained behaviour change in individuals. Swerissen et al. (2006) found that the changes were small and dependent on the culture of the participants. Chodosh et al. (2005) undertook a meta-analysis and found that self-management programs for hypertension and diabetes mellitus probably produce clinically measurable benefits. A recent systematic review (Foster et al. 2007) queried the benefits of peer-led self-management programs. The authors argue that lay-led self-management education programs may lead to small, short-term improvements in participants' self-efficacy, self-rated health, cognitive symptom management and frequency of aerobic exercise, but there is no evidence that such programs improve psychological health, symptoms or health-related quality of life, or that they significantly alter health care use. The authors comment that in the future, research should explore longer term outcomes, their effect on clinical measures of disease and their potential role in children and adolescents, suggesting that it is not lay-led self-management programs that do not deliver the outcomes but that they could be better evaluated.

In Australia Zwar et al. (2006) carried out a systematic review which found that self-management support was effective across a range of chronic illnesses, particularly in diabetes, heart disease and hypertension. While Harris et al. (2008) agree that self-management programs do not reduce demand for health services, they consider the benefits from such programs as the Expert Patient Program in the UK as well as the benefits in diabetes and hypertension management to be important.

In many instances the lack of evidence relates to poor quality evaluations of programs rather than the results of the programs themselves. Improved individual evaluations will lead to more conclusive evidence.

Conclusion

General practices are the 'frontline' for the management of chronic illnesses. Self-management is now generally accepted as an integral part of the management of all chronic illnesses. As the role of the practice nurse in planning the care of people with chronic illness develops, the nurse may choose to adopt some of the approaches of self-management support to assist in these activities. Some practice nurses may choose to become skilled in delivering self-management programs. This may not be appropriate in every practice setting but all practice nurses require some familiarity with the concept of self-management and self-management support in order to make appropriate referrals of people with chronic illnesses to self-management programs run by other agencies in the community. The benefit to the practice nurse will be seeing patients improve their self-management skills while the benefit to the patients will be learning new self-management strategies.

Name of nurse
Henny Schrama

Practice
Broadford Medical Clinic, Broadford, Vic.

Broadford Medical Clinic was approached by the University of Melbourne to take part in a research project titled the PEACH study. The practice was part of the research looking to evaluate the effectiveness of practice nurses supporting patients to self-manage their type 2 diabetes using telephone coaching. It was hoped that this would be achieved by regular telephone coaching and face-to-face assessments. The patient was encouraged to take ownership of their diabetes condition. They were encouraged to follow the PEACH project guidelines and improve their lifestyle habits, for example: quit smoking, reduce alcohol intake, improve nutrition and participate in physical activity.

With the support of the PEACH project guidelines, and by working in a team with the GP, I hoped to achieve improvements in the patients' diabetes condition and thus reduce the risk of complications or minimise the progression of complications. The role of the practice nurse was to perform an initial assessment with the patients and collect baseline data. This was repeated at 12 months and 18 months. Between these assessments the patient was contacted regularly by telephone and offered support and encouragement. Advice was given on ways to improve blood sugar levels and their social and environmental circumstances taken into consideration. Where appropriate, referrals were made to community providers and the GP continued the medical management of the diabetes, referring to a specialist where necessary. By having the flexibility of telephone sessions rather than visits to the practice, patients were able to express their concerns regularly and at their convenience.

The entire practice team became committed to the project, and the reception staff followed up appointments and relayed patient concerns to the nurse. The GP was kept fully informed of the patients' progress both verbally and in writing.

Good working relationships and communication between the patient, nurse and GP resulted from the project and the practice has used the project guidelines to target other patients with diabetes.

The experience of being involved in this PEACH study research project was very exciting and stimulating; it allowed me to be involved in trialling a new model of care in general practice for the management of diabetes. It gave me extra autonomy in the practice of diabetes management. The coaching sessions allowed me to extend the rapport with the patient and the GP and develop another facet of their practice.

The coaching sessions were a time of learning for the nurse as well as the patient. One of the conclusions from this project was the realisation that health professionals need to accept the patient's decision as to the level of intervention they wish to have in managing their disease.

The benefits to the practice were the increased satisfaction of a job well done, improved outcomes for the patients and an increase in the diabetes cycles of care completed.

Key messages

There is more than one type of self-management strategy which may suit the patient.

Self-management is underpinned by the patient being the centre of their own health care.

The practice nurse can contribute to patient self-management in a variety of ways.

Useful resources

Flinders Human Behaviour and Health Research Unit
    http://som.flinders.edu.au/FUSA/CCTU/self_management.htm

Chronic Illness Alliance
    http://www.chronicillness.org.au/sig/

Smoking Cessation Guidelines for Australian General Practice
    http://www.quitnow.info.au/

References

1. Alwell, L, Spink, J & Robinson, S 2004, 'Consumer participation in the Sharing Health Care Initiative Demonstration Projects', *Health Issues*, no. 78, pp. 28–32.

2. Australian Institute of Health and Welfare 2008a, *Australia's health 2008*, Chapter 2, AIHW, Canberra, viewed 23 May 2009, <http://www.aihw.gov.au/>.

3. Australian Institute of Health and Welfare 2008b, *Australia's health 2008*, Chapter 5, AIHW, Canberra, viewed 23 May 2009, <http://www.aihw.gov.au/>.

4. Australian Institute of Professional Counsellors 2009, *Motivational interviewing: principles and techniques*, viewed 30 October 2009, <http://www.aipc.net.au/>.

5. Australian Practice Nurses Association 2008, *About practice nursing*, viewed 3 June 2009, <http://www.apna.asn.au/displaycommon.cfm?an=2.>

6. Bandura, A 1997, *The exercise of control*, WH Freeman and Company, New York.

7. Battersby, M, Ask, A, Reece, M, Markwick, M & Collins, J 2003, 'The partners in health scale: the development of a generic assessment scale for chronic condition self-management', *Australian Journal of Primary Care*, vol. 19, nos .2 & 3: pp. 41–52.

8. Chodosh, J, Morton, S, Mojica, W, Maglione, M, Suttorp, M, Hilton L, Rhodes, S & Shekelle, P 2005, 'Meta-analysis: chronic disease self-management programs for older adults', *Annals of Internal Medicine*, vol. 143, no. 6, pp. 427–38.

9. Department of Health and Ageing (DoHA) 2007, *National Chronic Disease Strategy*, DoHA, Canberra, viewed 24 May 2009, <http://www.health.gov.au/>.

10. Department of Health and Ageing (DoHA) 2008, *Australian Better Health Initiatives*, fact sheet, DoHA, Canberra, viewed 24 May 2009b, <http://www.measureup.gov.au/internet/abhi/publishing.nsf/Content/factsheet-abhi/>.

11. Flinders Human Behaviour and Health Research Unit 2009a, *Capabilities for supporting prevention and chronic condition self-management: a resource for educators of primary health care professionals,* viewed 11 March 2010, <http://som.flinders.edu.au/FUSA/CCTU/pdf/What%27s%20New/Capabilities%20Self-Management%20Resource.pdf>.

12. Flinders Human Behaviour and Health Research Unit 2009b, *Flinders Model*, Flinders University South Australia, viewed 23 May 2009, <http://som.flinders.edu.au/FUSA/CCTU/self_management.htm#Flinders_Model>.

13. Foster, G, Taylor, SJC, Eldridge, S, Ramsay, J & Griffiths, CJ 2007, 'Self-management education programmes by lay leaders for people with chronic conditions', *Cochrane Database of Systematic Reviews*, issue 4. art. no. CD005108, doi: 10.1002/14651858.CD005108.pub2, viewed 23 May 2009, <http://www.mrw.interscience.wiley.com/cochrane/clsysrev/articles/CD005108/frame.html>.

14. General Practice South Australia (GPSA) 2008, *Chronic disease self-management strategy 2008*, South Australia, viewed 29 May 2009, <http://www.gpsa.org.au/programs/chronic-disease/>.

15. Gruman, J & Von Korff, M 1996, *Indexed bibliography on self-management for people with chronic disease,* Centre for Advancement in Health, Washington DC.

16. Harris, M, Williams, A, Dennis, S, Zwar, N & Powell-Davies, G 2008, 'Chronic disease self-management: implementation with and within Australian general practice', *Medical Journal of Australia*, vol. 189, no. 10 (supplement), pp. S17–S20, viewed 24 May 2009, <http://www.mja.com.au/public/issues/189_10_171108/har10522_fm.html>.

17. Health Coaching Australia 2008, *About Health coaching*, viewed 29 May 2009, <http://www.healthcoachingaustralia.com/health-coaching/about-health-coaching.htm>.

18. Kennedy, A, Rogers, A & Gately, C 2005, 'Assessing the introduction of the expert patients programme into the NHS: a realistic evaluation of recruitment to a lay-led self-care initiative', *Primary Health Care Research and Development*, vol. 6, no. 2, pp.137–48.

19. Kennedy, A, Reeves, D, Bower, P, Lee, V, Middletone, E, Richardson, G, Gardner, C, Gately, C & Rogers, A 2007, 'The effectiveness and cost effectiveness of a national lay-led self care support programme for patients with long-term conditions: a pragmatic randomized controlled trial', *Journal of Epidemiology and Community Health*, vol. 61, pp. 254–61.

20. Lorig, K, Sobel, D, Stewart, A, Brown, B, Bandura, A, Ritter, P, Gonzalez, V, Laurent, D & Holman, H 1999, 'Evidence suggesting that a chronic disease self-management program can improve health status while reducing hospitalization: a randomized controlled trial', *Medical Care*, vol. 37, no. 1, pp. 5–14.

21. Lorig, K, Ritter, P, Stewart, A, Sobel, D, Brown, B, Bandura, A, Gonzalez, V, Laurent, D & Holman, H 2001, 'Chronic disease self-management program: 2 year health status and health care utilization outcomes', *Medical Care*, vol. 39, no. 11, pp. 1217–23.

22. Macdonald, W, Rogers, A, Blakeman, T & Bower, P 2008, 'Practice nurses and the facilitation of self-management in primary care', *Journal of Advanced Nursing*, vol. 62, no. 2, pp. 191–9.

23. Martin, C & Nisa, M 1996, 'Meeting the needs of children and families in chronic illness and disease: a greater role for the GP?', *Australian Family Physician*, vol. 25, no. 8, pp. 1273–5.

24. National Health Priority Action Council (NHPAC) 2006, *National Chronic Disease Strategy*, Department of Health & Ageing, Canberra.

25. Parliamentary Library of Australia 2007, *Practice nursing in Australia*, Parliamentary Library Research Paper no. 10 2007–08, Canberra Australia, viewed 1 June 2009, <http://www.aph.gov.au/library/pubs/rp/2007–08/08rp10.htm>.

26. Phillips, SM, Davies, JM & Tofler, GH 2004, 'NICS Heart Failure Forum: improving outcomes in chronic care', *Medical Journal of Australia*, vol. 181, no. 6, pp. 297–9, viewed 29 May 2009, <http://www.mja.com.au/>.

27. Piette, JD 2005, 'Helping chronically ill patients cope', *Medical care*, vol. 43, no. 10, pp. 947–50.

28. Prochaska, JO & DiClemente, CC 1986, 'The transtheoretical approach: towards a systematic eclectic framework', in JC Norcross (ed), *Handbook of Eclectic Psychotherapy*, pp. 163–200, Brunner/Mazel, New York.

29. Quit Victoria 2005, *The important role of health professionals in smoking cessation*, viewed 30 October 2009, <http://www.quit.org.au/browse.asp?ContainerID=health_profs>.

30. Redman, B 2004, *Patient self-management of chronic disease: the health care provider's challenge*, Jones and Bartlett Publishers, Sudbury MA.

31. Swerissen, H, Belfrage, J, Weeks, A, Jordan, L, Walker, C, Furler, J, McAvoy, B, Carter, M & Peterson, C 2006, 'A randomised control trial of a self-management program for people with a chronic illness from Vietnamese, Chinese, Italian and Greek backgrounds', *Patient Education and Counseling*, vol. 64, no. 1–3, pp. 360–8.

32. Vale, MJ, Jelinek, MV, Best, JD, Dart, AM, Grigg LE, Hare, D, Ho, BP, Newman, RW & McNeil, JJ 2003, 'Coaching patients on achieving cardiovascular health (COACH): a multicenter randomized trial in patients with coronary heart disease', *Archives of Internal Medicine*, vol. 163, no. 22, pp. 2775–83.

33. Wagner, EH, Austin, BT & Von Korff, M 1996, 'Organizing care for patients with chronic illness', *Millbank Quarterly*, vol. 74, no. 4, pp. 511–44.

34. Wagner, EH, Austin, BT, Davis, C, Hindmarsh, M, Schaefer, J & Bonomi, A 2001, 'Improving Chronic Illness Care: translating evidence into action', *Health Affairs*, vol. 20, no. 6, pp. 64–78.

35. Western Australian Department of Health 2009, *Chronic Disease Self Management Strategy*, Government of Western Australia, Perth, viewed 29 May 2009, <http://www.healthnetworks.health.wa.gov.au/abhi/project/self_management.cfm>.

36. Young, D, Furler, J, Vale, M, Walker, C, Segal, L, Dunning, P, Best, J, Blackberry, I, Audehm, R, Sulaiman, N, Dunbar, J & Chondros, P 2007, 'Patient Engagement and Coaching for Health: The PEACH study—a cluster randomised controlled trial using the telephone to coach people with type 2 diabetes to engage with their GPs to improve diabetes care: a study protocol', *BMC Family Practice 2007*, viewed 30 June 2008, <http://www.biomedcentral.com/1471-2296/8/20>.

37. Zwar, N, Harris, M, Griffiths, R, Roland, M, Dennis, S, Powell Davies, G & Hasan, I 2006, 'A systematic review of chronic disease management,' *Research Centre for Primary Health Care and Equity*, School of Public Health and Community Medicine, UNSW, viewed October 2009, <http://www.anu.edu.au/aphcri>.

Part four

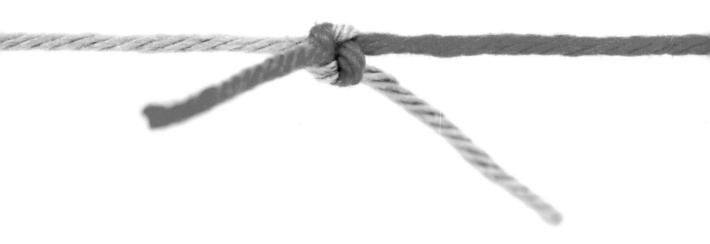

The way forward in practice nursing

Edited by Elizabeth Patterson

Chapter seventeen

Using evidence in general practice

by Donna Waters

Overview

This chapter introduces the concept of evidence-based practice and how it relates to research. It provides a brief explanation of the different research approaches to investigating a practice question or problem, and information about how to access and evaluate the evidence generated from research. The chapter then gives practical advice about how to implement this evidence in practice.

Objectives

At the completion of this chapter you should be able to:

- be more familiar with the language used in research and evidence-based practice;

- understand the differences between the skills and knowledge required for 'doing' research and 'using' evidence;

- have the skills to decide what is the best available evidence for the patient and practice context in which you work;

- better understand the relationship between evidence-based practice and quality care; and

- better appreciate the role of research in building the specialty of practice nursing.

Introduction

Nurses understand and welcome the concept of using research to improve their practice. Research utilisation literature has been around for a long time and, more recently, evidence-based practice (EBP) has placed the 'using' of research into a broader, and perhaps more realistic, framework. EBP is about using the findings from the best available evidence (preferably from good quality research) within the practice context. EBP recognises that the clinician and the patient or client are usually in the best position to judge the most appropriate use of evidence within the practice setting. Thus, EBP affirms the position of the patient or client or family at the centre of shared decisions about their health care. In acknowledging the complex nature of health care, EBP has contributed a range of useful resources that have attempted to address some of the obstacles nurses have previously encountered in research utilisation. These barriers are very familiar to nurses and include a lack of time to both use and conduct research, and a lack of knowledge and skill to interpret and implement research findings.

The origins of EBP are in evidence-based medicine (EBM), and although viewed by some as an extremely narrow approach (Miles, Loughlin & Polychronis 2008), the early definitions of EBP were clear (at least on paper) about placing the patient at the centre of health care decisions. The often quoted early definition of EBM is 'the conscientious, explicit and judicious use of current best evidence in making decisions about the healthcare of patients' (Sackett et al. 1997, p. 2). The essence of this definition has not really changed over the last ten years except to make the position of the patient more explicit, for example, 'the integration of the best research evidence with our clinical expertise and our patient's unique values and circumstances' (Straus et al. 2005, p. 1).

Reflections

What do you understand evidence-based practice to be about?
Is your understanding similar to the above definition of evidence-based medicine?
Do you think evidence-based medicine ultimately aims to improve health and health care?

Many nurses initially eschewed EBM because the type of research said to offer the 'strongest' kind of evidence (National Health and Medical Research Council 1995) was based on experiments or trials that used statistical methods (such as randomised controlled trials). This approach was difficult for some nurses to reconcile with nursing research models that had traditionally focused on care (rather than treatment) and which had tended to use more interpretive or qualitative methods. This initial judgment was probably overly simplistic, however, because it assumed that EBM was only about statistical (or quantitative) methods and that *only* research using these methods could offer the 'best' evidence for practice. As more health professionals focused on the overarching philosophy of EBM (to improve health and health care), the emphasis was able to move from who owned and defined the quality of evidence, to the more appropriate consideration of what is the most appropriate evidence to answer the kind of question the clinician or patient is asking.

It is only really during the last decade that the focus on the quality or strength of evidence has changed from being based on research method to one that considers the appropriateness of the evidence for the question, the clinician, the client and the context. The terms 'evidence-based practice' and 'evidence-based health care' reflect the development of this broader thinking and mirror changes in professional nursing from using research in practice (research utilisation) to making context-based, person-centred decisions based on appropriate evidence from research (EBP). The overarching principle of using the best available evidence to improve health care is one that appeals to all health professionals, and it is through their engagement and robust debate that EBP now presents as a broader genre. While different kinds of evidence are generally available; the most important goal of EBP is to use the best available evidence for the question or decision at hand, for the patient or client being cared for and for the context in which the care is provided.

Reflections

What kind of evidence do you think is the most appropriate to help you decide on treatment or therapy for wound care?

What advantages can you think of for using wound dressings that have been proven effective in controlled trials?

What kind of evidence do you think is appropriate to update your knowledge about caring for patients who have just been diagnosed with a life-threatening condition?

What is research and what is evidence?

The words 'research' and 'evidence' are often used interchangeably (Waters et al. 2009), but this usage is not always correct within the contemporary context of EBP. Research is a process. It is the thoughtful and systematic approach taken to investigating a question or conjecture and (while this may surprise you) it is probably something you have already done. Have you ever bought a car or a refrigerator? Think carefully about what you did—perhaps you measured the size of your garage or the space in your kitchen. Perhaps you compared fuel or energy efficiency, cost or colour? You might have studied a range of brochures to compare certain features. It is likely that you conducted a thoughtful and systematic approach to buying your car or fridge—you have done research!

A range of methods is used in research to permit a systematic approach to investigating a question or problem. Research methods are a lot like recipes—and there are particular methods for researching different kinds of problems or questions. In the broadest sense, the different approaches to research fall into two main categories; however, a third category is emerging and is described below.

1. **Quantitative research**   mainly collects data in numerical form (such as blood pressure readings, test results, height or weight) and uses statistical methods to group, analyse and describe the results.

2. **Qualitative research**   uses mainly textual or observational data from interviews, video, diaries or journals and analyses individual or group experiences and observations to develop theory or to elicit themes.

3. **Mixed methods**   research is emerging as a separate approach to research. As the name implies, mixed methods research uses either a combination of quantitative and qualitative methods or more than one quantitative or qualitative method sequentially or in combination.

There are many different research methods within each of the above categories and new methods are constantly being developed. But it is not the method that determines evidence. Research is a process or tool of discovery that uses different methods to investigate problems or questions—evidence is what is produced and used within the context of care.

When should evidence be implemented?

There are other distinctions that need to be made about when and how evidence is used. Once produced, new knowledge derived from research could simply be added to your existing knowledge base. This kind of professional practice knowledge is what might be put under the banner of continuing professional development. At other times, it may be that the research evidence produced is of good quality; that it is applicable to your general practice context and can be introduced relatively easily into current systems. At the other extreme, some research evidence may be so significant that it influences you, your practice team or state or federal health authorities to make a significant change to the way a current service or treatment is delivered. Sometimes, there is research evidence available but it is neither good quality nor applicable and, therefore, should not be regarded as evidence for practice (Fleming 2007). At other times, evidence may not be available or the research may not have yet been carried out. In this chapter, the term 'research evidence' is used to differentiate evidence that comes from good quality research, from evidence that is derived from other sources (such as expert opinion). It is an expectation of our national professional bodies that evidence-based practitioners will make an attempt to seek out and use the best evidence available, while acknowledging that this may not always be the best evidence possible (Gray 2001).

Example 17.1

When updating practice protocols for the management of newly diagnosed patients with diabetes the following questions should guide the process:

> Is there any new research available that helps in discussing options for managing and monitoring the ongoing care and treatment of newly diagnosed diabetic patients?

> If available, what is the quality of this research and is it applicable to the general practice context?

> If there is no good quality research evidence available, what would be another source of evidence practice nurses could use to help newly diagnosed clients adjust to their care and treatment program, such as information from the Australian Diabetes Foundation? How confident can practice nurses be in this source of evidence? Is this information based on research evidence? How would you know?

> If there is good quality research evidence available, will it be acceptable to patients and clients who attend this practice? Does it fit with my experience of managing diabetes and are the research recommendations practical and/or feasible within the context of primary health care?

What is evidence-based practice?

Although there may be many different individual views on what evidence actually is or what it means within a particular context, there is relatively little disagreement that basing practice on evidence from research is ultimately going to be a good thing for the patient or client. Definitions of EBP within nursing are typically broad, such as 'the systematic interconnecting of scientifically generated evidence with the tacit knowledge of the expert practitioner to achieve a change in a particular practice for the benefit of a well-defined client/patient group' (French 1999, p. 74). But it is a national competency requirement for nursing registration that practice is delivered within an evidence-based framework and that practice nurses 'provide evidence-based information, resources and education to assist individuals to make health care decisions' (Competency 2.4) and use the 'best available research to inform clinical care management' (Competency 3.1) (Australian Nursing Federation 2006, pp. 20–21). Identifying an evidence-based framework may not be as easy as it sounds because the answer to 'What is evidence?' is actually 'It depends!'

It is not new for nurses to want to use research to inform their practice, but previous approaches to research utilisation often failed to recognise the wider context in which the utilisation part was to occur. For example, how the research would be found; how its quality and applicability to context would be assessed; how it would actually be implemented; and what happened as a result. Further, research utilisation approaches rarely included the perspectives of the patient or client. These additional components are what define evidence-based practice and also serve to differentiate an evidence-based practitioner from a researcher.

Although the steps for doing research and using evidence parallel each other (see Table 17.1 below), the tasks, expectations and outputs are distinctly different. Both roles have similar motivations and both are demanding—but one has a finite end (doing the research and reporting the results) while the other is intended to be continually evolving (EBP).

Table 17.1 Contrasting the steps of research and evidence-based practice

A researcher	An evidence-based practitioner
– Asks a research question	– Asks a practice question
– Conducts a literature review	– Conducts a literature review or locates an evidence summary
– Determines the best method to use	– Determines the quality of the evidence
– Conducts the research	– Summarises the results
– Answers the question	– Answers the question
– Communicates/Publishes the results	– Applies the results in practice
	– Evaluates the outcome

Within the general practice context, an evidence-based practitioner uses the results of research to inform their diagnostic and treatment decisions, but also has an important role in translating evidence for clients. Patients and clients now have access to much the same information as clinicians (through the internet for example) but may need assistance with interpreting this evidence in order to meaningfully participate in their health care decisions. To this end, it is encouraging that a range of aids for evidence-based decision making are starting to become available for consumers.

The relationship between questions and evidence

Table 17.1 opposite shows that evidence-based practice and research both start (and sometimes end) with a question. This question arises out of a practice problem or issue—something that requires a search for new knowledge. Busy nurses do not generally spend time articulating the type of questions that go through their heads whenever they see a patient or client. But in general, there are two reasons why nurses might ask questions about practice. There are knowledge questions (to know more about a particular topic) and there are questions around clinical decisions or actions (practice questions).

Knowledge questions can draw on information from many places—including good quality research—but evidence-based practice generally refers to a specific kind of question that is based around a clinical encounter or decision occurring in practice.

If you think about how you actually apply your clinical knowledge, you can see how clinical practice questions fall into a range of different types, for example:

- How does this patient look to me?
- What have they told me?
- What are the possible causes of this complaint or illness?
- How should I diagnose or treat this problem?
- What are the benefits and harms of taking this action?
- Is this an appropriate course of action for this patient?
- What is the effectiveness of a treatment or therapy?
- What is the cost (to the practice and to the patient)?
- How will this decision affect the outcomes or quality of life for the patient?

- How do I assess the quality, safety and delivery of this care?
- What does the patient or client think or feel about this?
- What can I do to promote wellness?

Framing practice queries as answerable clinical questions is an important first step to EBP as the question describes what information is needed and where to look for it. For example, if the question is 'What is the best topical treatment for eczema?' some keywords to look for in the literature ('eczema' and 'topical treatments') are already defined and because we want to compare different treatments we should be thinking about the kind of study that would provide the best evidence for this treatment question (a randomised controlled trial would be best). It is possible to make clinical questions even easier to answer by breaking them up into chunks. Straus et al. (2005) propose using the PICO acronym to define the:

- P—**patient** or **problem**
- I—**intervention** or treatment
- C—what this is being **compared** to
- O—desirable **outcome**.

So our question above might become 'Is treatment A (the intervention) more effective than treatment B (the comparator) in healing eczema (the outcome) in otherwise healthy patients (patient group)?' In this example, healing might be defined by a range of outcomes including symptom reduction or healing times.

Reflections

It is helpful to spend some time thinking about the kind of questions you usually ask in your practice. This can save time in determining where you look for the answers, and eventually allows you to build a collection of good quality evidence resources for the practice.

Levels of evidence

The National Health and Medical Research Council (NHMRC) of Australia initially recommended an approach to judging the strength or quality of evidence in a series of texts supporting the development and use of clinical practice guidelines. The early 'quality of evidence' tables were based very much on defining the best evidence for treatment decisions (NHMRC 1995) and graded evidence according to 'levels'. Many health professionals refer to the

NHMRC Levels of Evidence, and these have recently been reviewed to include a broader range of 'quality of evidence' ratings for other types of clinical questions, such as those relating to screening or prognosis.

Locating evidence and deciding its quality

We have established that the quality of evidence should not be judged on the research method but on the basis of the question we are asking and the context in which it will be applied. In the real world, good quality evidence is not always available to answer every question. Availability can mean lots of things—we might not have time to search for the evidence or be able to find it. We might be working in a remote location and relying only on an outdated protocol because there is no access to the internet. On the other hand, there might be so much information available that our problem is more about having the time to decide on its quality. The kind (or strength) of research evidence that is available to us will determine the degree of confidence we have in applying it. But whatever way it is, our clinical experience will always be required in making that judgment.

The increasing availability of information via the internet (for example) has been one of the drivers behind the development of EBP. At one time finding evidence might have required visiting a library, conducting a search and waiting for a copy of a paper. Once you had the paper you may or may not have made an assessment of the quality of the research and you may or may not have judged its findings as important to your practice. Today, you can electronically search any of a number of databases to find online journals, books and other publications. But which of this now very large and accessible collection should you choose to inform your practice? In evidence-based practice this part of the process is called accessing and appraising (or critiquing) research literature. As shown in Table 17.1 on page 408, it involves conducting a search of research literature and determining the quality of the findings. Based on the premise that all clinicians are busy and not all will have the skills to search and appraise every piece of research related to an area of practice, a range of methods and resources have developed out of EBP to bring pre-appraised (quality checked) evidence to the point of care.

Reviews of evidence

The process of combining literature to produce a summarised collective result as the outcome is called a review. Different kinds of reviews produce different kinds of evidence for different kinds of questions. This is largely related to the kind of studies and the level of rigour applied to the selection and inclusion of literature within the review. The collection of systematic reviews of randomised controlled trials contained in the Cochrane Library (online) is a good example of reviews undertaken using highly structured and rigorous methods. However, the outcome of any review will be improved if systematic and transparent methods are followed (see List 17.1 below). The methods that are now applied to reviews of evidence (including clinical practice guidelines) have heralded a new era of transparency in determining the quality of research literature. It also means that someone else has done the hard work of collecting and appraising the research evidence contained in the review or guideline. But it is still up to the practice nurse—as the user of that evidence—to make a judgment on its overall quality, as would be required for a single research paper.

List 17.1 Evaluating a systematic review

- Who conducted the review? Are they well known in the field? Do they have credibility?
- Have they clearly outlined the question or aim of the review?
- Have they clearly outlined the inclusion and exclusion criteria for the literature that is to be included in the review?
- Where and how did they search for this literature?
- Did they search across a wide range of databases, and if not, was the place of searching appropriate?
- Did they go back far enough in the literature to capture any important changes?
- How was the information put together?
- What are their conclusions?
- Are these relevant and applicable to your practice?

Reflections

Find a systematic review of relevance to your practice. Try to evaluate this review using the questions listed in List 17.1 above.

Evidence summaries

Essentially shorter versions of the larger evidence review, evidence summaries are very useful for busy practitioners. They are intended to be short (one or two pages); easy to use (summarising a large amount of information in a user-friendly way); and accessible (easy and low cost to update). The first page of a Cochrane Review can be regarded as an evidence summary because it offers all the information needed to make a judgment on the conduct and quality of the whole review and its findings.

One of the most well-known types of evidence summaries used by nurses in Australia are the Joanna Briggs Institute Best Practice Information Sheets. These are generally a four-page booklet outlining the method of a review and a summary of the evidence relating to nursing practice questions. It is important to remember that evidence summaries should be subject to the same quality criteria as any other evidence review. Because it is hard to include a lot of information about searching, selecting and appraising a large amount of literature in a few pages, the authors of evidence summaries will often use figures, tables, keys, codes or icons to convey this information using a minimum number of words.

Evidence-based clinical practice guidelines

Clinical practice guidelines are a very common form of evidence summary used in the general practice context. What differentiates guidelines from reviews and other evidence summaries is that in addition to grading and summarising evidence, guidelines will usually include some form of instruction or advice to assist with their adaptation or implementation. There is a broad range of guidelines available from specialist foundations and national collaborations. But what constitutes a good guideline?

All EBP resources that aim to reduce the burden on clinicians by summarising and appraising evidence for use in practice are required to provide criteria on which their quality can be judged. List 17.2 below outlines some of the features of a good quality clinical practice guideline (NHMRC 1995).

List 17.2 Attributes of a good quality guideline
- The process of evidence selection is transparent.
- All relevant evidence is included.
- The evidence is the best available and is summarised.
- The trustworthiness and strength of the evidence is clear.
- There is a process for updating the evidence within the guideline.
- It describes the 'average' patient or client to whom recommendations apply.
- It outlines the clinical context in which the guideline can be used.
- It details the full range of possible client outcomes.

- It considers the expertise and resources (including cost) required to implement the guidelines.
- It grades recommendations based on the strength of the evidence.
- It provides detailed instructions, protocols, algorithms or flow charts for ease of use.
- It delivers options for flexibility, and adaptability to specific circumstances are suggested.
- It provides a profile of the development team.
- The details of the development process are accessible.
- It suggests a dissemination and evaluation plan.

There are many international organisations that develop and share evidence-based guidelines with evidence-based practitioners:

- New Zealand Guidelines Group (NZGG)
- National Institute of Clinical Studies (NICS) in Australia
- National Institute of Clinical Excellence (NICE) in the UK
- Scottish Intercollegiate Network (SIGN)
- Guidelines International Network (GIN) (refer to Useful resources on p. 420).

Similarly, there are internationally accepted standards of guideline quality such as those outlined in the AGREE (Appraisal of Guidelines Research and Evaluation) framework. All these organisations (except GIN) offer free online access to their guideline libraries, as well as resources for the development and appraisal of guidelines. It should rarely be necessary, therefore, for any health professional to write a new guideline from a blank slate. Searching for good quality guidelines is akin to searching for any other form of quality evidence. Start with a reputable international source, apply quality criteria to the selection and appraisal of the guideline and determine its applicability to your practice.

The increasing availability of good quality reviews, summaries and guidelines from reliable international sources means that nurses and other health professionals can save a lot of time by searching these in the first instance. Evidence resources are there to help but by necessity, reviews, summaries and guidelines will relate to a specific question or topic and to the average patient. Their quality is dependent upon how, where and why they have been prepared and it remains the responsibility of the clinician to use their expertise and judgment in applying the recommendations within the patient and practice context. Equally, evidence resources are aids to clinical decision making and, therefore, flexibility is in-built around patient, family and organisational values and goals. But you will not always find what you need. If you have not been able to find good quality summarised evidence for a particular kind of question that has arisen in practice, it remains your professional responsibility to ensure that any other evidence you use is appropriately critiqued for the validity of results and applicability to context. When applying this lesser quality evidence, it is important to remember that this was the best evidence available (not the best evidence possible) and the confidence and certainty with which the clinical team makes a decision based on this evidence should be moderated accordingly.

One of the most fundamental aspects of evidence-based practice is to actually use the evidence in practice. The two main ways in which this occurs are related to our previous discussion of the types of questions nurses ask. There is a continual stream of research evidence offering new knowledge for general practice. Keeping ourselves and our colleagues abreast of this new knowledge is a part of our legal and ethical responsibility. Other than restating the importance of using quality evidence to update professional knowledge, continuing professional education is not the focus of this chapter. The remainder of this discussion will focus on using evidence when the purpose of finding out new information has been driven by a need to improve quality or when new knowledge has such significant and important implications that a decision to change practice has resulted. This change may need to be made at the individual level (for example, the practice nurse) or at the organisational level (for example, the systems and processes used in the practice).

Implementing new knowledge in practice

Just because research is new or is of good quality doesn't necessarily mean it *must* be implemented. Similarly, performance and outcomes in certain areas of general practice may be travelling along very nicely and do not necessarily *need* to be changed. This brings us to the first stage in any evidence implementation process.

Stage 1: Determine whether there is need for change

Sometimes the need for change is obvious. Other than documenting what has occurred (if it is an isolated problem) or being alerted to quality issues through practice audits for example, the initial action is to identify exactly what the problem is. This is the same as asking a practice question and, as described above, is the most important first step to finding good quality evidence for ways of improving practice. A practice nurse should be familiar with audit and evaluation as tools for routine quality monitoring in general practice.

- **Audit** is a process of systematically collecting information on a specific outcome or process over a period of time. Continual tracking and review of audit data can alert health professionals to any changes in system or process and is integral to quality monitoring.

- **Needs analysis** is a more formal way of identifying what might need to change. Using a range of methods (for example, surveys) or tools (quality checklists), needs analysis aims to find gaps between what is happening now and what should be happening.

Stage 2: Make an implementation plan

A collaboratively developed implementation plan helps to keep everyone focused on the main aims and purpose, and implementing what was agreed. The plan is also a means of delegating roles and responsibilities to others and forms the basis for any business case or funding proposal that might be required to implement the change. For a researcher, the implementation plan is like the research method—it outlines who does what, when, how and why. The staging of implementation plans is also very important to their success. Sometimes it is important to pause in the change process to allow participants time to adjust to the change before moving onto the next stage.

Another important aspect of an implementation plan is the identification of barriers and enablers. Identifying all known barriers *before* making a change enables the practice nurse to prepare strategies to counter these should they occur (see List 17.3 below). This chapter began by placing EBP within the context of real life and the reality of life is that (a) people feel more comfortable working within a framework that they already know and (b) change is not always easy to achieve. In nursing, no more studies are needed on why nurses do not use research—what is needed are innovative and exciting models that assist nurses in achieving and sustaining practice change.

List 17.3 Elements of an implementation plan
- Clearly articulate what you are aiming to achieve.
- Identify all individuals who are likely to be involved in the change.

- Negotiate their role in planning and evaluating the implementation upfront—who will do what.
- Identify 'change champions'—these are people who can help make this change.
- If any supporting documents or resources are required, allow adequate time to develop or source these.
- Identify any possible financial implications—no one likes surprises!
- Allow a realistic time frame for the change process to occur.
- Determine how the success of an evidence-based individual or practice change will be evaluated.

An often neglected part of the implementation plan is planning for the outcome. Does the evidence-based intervention work? Has changing a practice solved the problem or improved the quality? It is important to decide what measures will be taken during and at completion of the implementation process as this will form part of the final decision about whether the time, effort and cost of implementing an EBP change has made a positive difference. It is also helpful to determine what level of outcome is important in determining success, for example, should the improvements be demonstrated at the individual, organisational, process or patient level. It is too late to think about this after the event!

Finally, the implementation plan should consider strategies for sustaining change if the outcome evaluation is positive. This might include incorporating a regular check of audit data on that particular practice initiative to see whether there is 'practice creep' (that very human trait of reverting back to old habits).

Stage 3: Implement the plan

This may sound silly but all the hard work and excitement of getting people together for a common goal around improving practice is wasted if the evidence doesn't actually get to the place it is supposed to go. A lot of work has already been done around how to implement evidence-based practice change and several models, frameworks and theories have been put forward (Grol & Wensing 2005; Grimshaw & Eccles 2008). Not surprisingly, none of this literature offers a simple solution or a guaranteed result, however, it does reveal key features of the most successful evidence implementation strategies (see List 17.4 overleaf).

List 17.4 Successful implementation strategies

- Focus on groups, not individuals.
- Implement good quality evidence that has been shown to improve practice in other contexts.
- Work best when the whole group recognises the need for change.
- The individual, organisation or patient (the context) is receptive to the change.
- The process of change is facilitated on a number of levels, such as addressing individual barriers, targeting different people at different times, providing education and staging practice change over time.

Stage 4: Evaluate the outcomes

Evaluation is a general term used to describe a structured approach to measuring professional, organisational or client-based outcomes. In this context any one of a range of evaluation methods could be used (perhaps client surveys or the analysis of audit data before and after the practice change) to determine the success of evidence implementation.

The successful implementation of evidence is not something that can be done by one person, and it requires a great deal more effort than simply bringing the new knowledge to others and expecting them to use it. Hopefully, the importance of making an evidence implementation plan to guide the very active process of engagement and implementation, followed by the need to demonstrate that change has occurred and has achieved the desired outcome, is apparent. It may also be a requirement of those who are funding your practice change. Further, it is implied that practice improvement will continue to occur with the generation of new knowledge. So, evidence-based practice has no end because once the evidence is implemented, the question arises again—has the implementation been successful?

The evaluation of evidence implementation can take many forms—and it is here that the evidence-based practitioner might take on the role of researcher. Structured evaluation with clear goals and outcomes is a research method. In a recent study to ascertain the place of knowledge and evidence in Australian general practice nursing, Mills, Field and Cant (2009) recommend drawing on the predominantly oral culture of Australian nurses and more formally recognising a role for knowledge transfer agents in the career structure of practice nurses to champion evidence implementation in general practice. There are many excellent resources that assist in the search for and use of evidence in general practice. Knowledge about EBP is growing and changing all the time so the best way to keep up to date is to regularly check international organisations that maintain online resources for EBP.

Reflections

Identify a change in practice that you would like to implement in your workplace and work through Stages 1 to 4 as outlined above.

Conclusion

More than a decade ago a Canadian nurse, Carole Estabrooks (1998, p. 30) wrote:

> *The practice context is complex, people are complex, and clinicians are complex. The best evidence will most probably come in different forms, in different situations and contexts—and knowing how to decipher this complexity, how to match situation and context with appropriate evidence requirements will perhaps be the most important requirement of the 21st-century practising nurse.*

The poignancy of these words resonates today and will probably continue to do so into the future. Aside from a mostly welcoming attitude to EBP and a desire to provide the best care and service to patients or clients, it is also a competency requirement in Australia that nurses and midwives use research and other forms of evidence to continuously improve their knowledge and practice. This sits within a context where patients and clients have access to the same health information as clinicians and are finally gaining a voice in decisions about their care. Evidence-based practice encourages thinking about practice. It is not judged by whether a randomised controlled trial or other research method is used, but by the appropriateness of evidence to certain kinds of questions, its acceptability to patients or clients and its applicability to context.

Key messages

Research is a process or tool of discovery that uses different methods to investigate problems or questions—*evidence* is what is produced and used within the context of care.

EBP recognises that the clinician and the patient or client are usually in the best position to judge the most appropriate use of evidence within the practice setting.

While different kinds of evidence are generally available, the most important goal of EBP is to use the best available evidence for the question or decision at hand for the patient or client being cared for and for the context in which the care is provided.

It is an expectation of national nursing professional bodies that evidence-based practitioners will make an attempt to seek out and use the best evidence *available*, while acknowledging that this may not always be the best evidence *possible*.

Useful resources

Joanna Briggs Institute
http://www.joannabriggs.edu.au/

Cochrane Collaboration
http://www.cochrane.org/

The New Zealand Guidelines Group
http://www.nzgg.org.nz/

National Institute of Clinical Studies
http://www.nhmrc.gov.au/nics/

National Institute of Clinical Excellence
http://www.nice.org.uk/

Scottish Intercollegiate Network
http://www.sign.ac.uk/

Guidelines International Network
http://www.g-i-n.net/

Appraisal of Guidelines Research and Evaluation
http://www.agreetrust.org/

A useful text for patient-based decision making:
Irwig, L, Irwig, J, Travena, L & Sweet, M 2008, *Smart Health Choices: Making sense of health advice*, Hammersmith Press, London.

References

1. Australian Nursing Federation 2006, 'Competency Standards for nurses in general practice', viewed 23 January 2010, <http://www.anf.org.au/nurses_gp/toolkit_complete.pdf>.

2. Estabrooks, C 1998, 'Will evidence-based nursing practice make practice perfect?', *Canadian Journal of Nursing Research*, vol. 30, no. 1, pp. 5–36.

3. Fleming, K 2007, 'The knowledge base for evidence-based nursing: a role for mixed methods research?', *Advances in Nursing Science*, vol. 30, no. 1, pp. 41–51.

4. French, P 1999, 'The development of evidence-based nursing', *Journal of Advanced Nursing*, vol. 29, issue 1, pp. 72–8.

5. Gray, JAM 2001, *Evidence-based healthcare: how to make health policy and management decisions*, 2nd edn, Churchill Livingstone, Edinburgh, UK.

6. Grimshaw, J & Eccles, MP 2008, 'Knowledge translation of research findings', in *Effective dissemination of findings from research: a compilation of essays*, Institute of Health Economics, Alberta, Canada, pp. 8–24, viewed 23 January 2010, <http://www.ihe.ca/>.

7. Grol, R & Wensing, M 2005, 'Characteristics of successful innovations', in R Grol, M Wensing & M Eccles (eds), *Improving patient care: the implementation of change in clinical practice*, Elsevier, Oxford, pp. 41–58.

8. Miles, A, Loughlin, M & Polychronis, A 2008, 'Evidence-based healthcare, clinical knowledge and the rise of personalised medicine', *Journal of Evaluation in Clinical Practice*, vol. 14, pp. 621–49.

9. Mills, J, Field, J & Cant, R 2009, 'The place of knowledge and evidence in the context of Australian general practice nursing', *Worldviews on Evidence-based Nursing*, vol. 6, no. 4, pp. 219–28.

10. National Health and Medical Research Council (NHMRC) 1995, *A guide to the development, implementation and evaluation of clinical practice guidelines*, Australian Government Publishing Service, Canberra.

11. Sackett, DL, Straus, SE, Richardson, WS, Rosenberg, W & Haynes, RB 1997, *Evidence-based medicine: how to practice and teach EBM*, Churchill Livingstone, Edinburgh.

12. Straus, SE, Richardson, WS, Glasziou, P & Haynes, RB 2005, *Evidence-based medicine: how to practice and teach EBM*, 3rd edn, Churchill Livingstone, London.

13. Waters, DL, Rychetnik, L, Crisp, J & Barrett, A 2009, 'Views on evidence from nursing and midwifery opinion leaders', *Nurse Education Today*, vol. 29, no. 8, pp. 829–34.

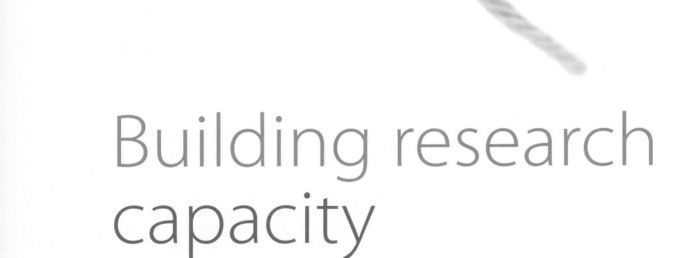

Chapter eighteen

Building research capacity

by Elizabeth Patterson, Elizabeth Halcomb, Rosemary Mahomed, Judy Evans and Katrina McNalty

Overview

This chapter provides five stories from academic and practising nurses about their journeys along research pathways that have built personal research capacity and contributed to current knowledge about practice nursing in Australia. These stories have been presented because they illustrate how research activities facilitate networks and collaborations between researchers, educators and clinicians, and hence, develop the discipline. The stories describe various levels of expertise and commitment to nursing research by five nurses, all with a strong desire to progress the body of knowledge supporting nurses working in general practice. Their experiences range from academic, professional, skilled researcher and mentor to novice nurse researcher gaining the skills to participate, manage and implement research into their working environment to influence patient outcomes at a practice level.

Objectives

At the completion of this chapter you should be able to:

- understand how research has contributed to the development of an evidence base for general practice nursing in Australia;

- explore ways in which you could contribute to the development of practice nursing knowledge through research activities;

- identify how research capacity has been, or could be, built in your practice; and

- discover a variety of resources to support your research development.

Introduction

In general practice there is a variety of opportunities for nurses to undertake research and research training. Practice nursing has been described in the National Nursing and Midwifery Specialisation Framework as an area that meets some, but not all, criteria necessary to be described as a nursing specialty (National Nursing and Nursing Education Taskforce 2006). The criteria dictate that specialty practice is based on a core body of nursing knowledge, which is being continually expanded and refined. Hence, mechanisms are required to support, review and disseminate research. The contribution of nurses to knowledge development and evidence-based practice is important for the development of practice nursing as a specialty and the development of skilled nurse researchers.

C A S E   S T U D Y

ELIZABETH PATTERSON

I first became interested in primary health care while undertaking a Masters of Health Science in the early 1990s. Prior to this my experience was limited to acute care and I had little experience of nursing outside of the hospital. This degree opened a whole new sphere of knowledge and skills about both primary health care nursing and research methodologies, and facilitated my first venture into research.

On completion of that degree I was keen to continue with research training and was particularly interested in further exploring primary health care in Australia. To achieve this I sought the advice of Professor Chris Del Mar who, at that time, led a university-based primary health care centre. As Chris had come from the United Kingdom where nursing roles in primary care were more established, he stimulated my interest in the roles of nurses in Australian general practice settings.

Under the initial guidance of Professors Chris Del Mar and Jake Najman, and later Professors Anne McMurray and Carol McVeigh, I undertook a PhD study, 'Primary health care nursing: A case study of practice nurses'. This research explored the role of Australian practice nurses and the factors that could facilitate or hinder their development and contribution to primary health care. This study resulted in four publications (Patterson, Del Mar & Najman 1999a, 1999b, 2000; Patterson & McMurray 2003) which complemented and added to knowledge generated from previous studies about a variety of community-based nursing roles. Undertaking this research project introduced me to the complexities of gaining entrance to general practice settings for research purposes, recruiting participants, receiving a good response rate from posted questionnaires and finding mutually convenient times and places to interview very busy general practitioners and practice nurses. Learning how to navigate the journey of study design, data collection and data analyses added to my early expertise in research.

My PhD set me on a journey which led to meeting other researchers interested in the rapidly developing field of practice nursing and in being part of networks and collaborations to advance the knowledge in this area. Shortly after completing my PhD I developed and convened university-based postgraduate education programs for practice nurses with some of the graduates progressing to become involved in research training. You will read stories from two of these graduates—Rosemary Mahomed and Judy Evans—later in this chapter.

In 2003, I was very privileged to be invited to be one of the keynote speakers at the inaugural Royal College of Nursing, Australia (RCNA) National Practice Nurse conference in Bunbury, Western Australia. At that conference I met Elizabeth Halcomb, who was embarking on her PhD studies, and her principal supervisor Professor Patricia Davidson. Since that time we have consolidated our research partnership and jointly contributed to synthesising and analysing general practice nursing knowledge development (Davidson, Halcomb & Patterson 2007; Halcomb, Patterson & Davidson 2006; Halcomb, Davidson & Patterson 2007). One of my PhD examiners was Professor Desley Hegney and as a result of that initial relationship I have journeyed further down the research pathway with her and others exploring consumers' perceptions of potential expanded roles for practice nurses and, more recently, trialling a nurse-led model of chronic disease management in general practice. At one of the national practice nurse conferences, Desley and I met Dr Kay Price, who had also researched consumers' perceptions of practice nurses. We agreed to aggregate our findings and publish these results together (Hegney et al. 2004; Patterson et al. 2005; Patterson, Price & Hegney 2005; Price, Patterson & Hegney 2006).

In 2006 a research team led by Professor Hegney, and of which I am a principal investigator, was awarded an Australian Research Council (ARC) Discovery grant to trial the feasibility, acceptability and cost effectiveness of nurse-led models of chronic disease management in general practice. This study involves three general practices across two states, and three universities in Queensland, and includes academic and practising nurses and general practitioners. The funding for this study has allowed the inclusion of two PhD students and later in this chapter you will read the story of one—Rosemary Mahomed. One of the practice nurses, Katrina McNalty, who is trialling this expanded role in her practice also shares her story of what it is like to take part in a multidisciplinary, multisite study and what it has taught her about the research process. Rosemary and Katrina have respectively presented their experiences at the 2007 and 2008 National General Practice Nurse Conferences. Currently data analysis is still in progress but an account of a pilot study to test the patient recruitment process for this study (Eley, Hegney & Patterson 2005) and an interim report (Eley et al. 2008) have been published.

My publications and conference presentations about practice nursing led to an invitation to join another team of researchers in Melbourne. Dr Lena Sanci has been successful in securing Australian Primary Health Care Research Institute (APHCRI) and National Health and Medical Research Council (NHMRC) funding to conduct studies related to risk taking and counselling of adolescents in primary care. Both of these studies involve the contribution of practice nurses and have provided opportunities for research training to practice nurses. Judy Evan's story provides more information about these projects.

Becoming involved in research has opened doors I might never have ventured through and linked me to other clinicians and academics who, together, have achieved outcomes not probable by any one individual. My own research capacity has been developed through the mentorship and leadership of others and I, in turn, am now mentoring others and contributing to building research capacity through PhD supervision and membership of the Australian Practice Nurse Association (APNA) Research and Policy Committee.

ELIZABETH HALCOMB

My clinical nursing background is primarily in acute care, with the majority of my nursing experience being in the intensive care unit and trauma department of a major metropolitan hospital. In 2001 I embarked on a PhD within the School of Nursing at the University of Western Sydney. My supervisor, Professor Patricia Davidson, was an investigator on the National Health and Medical Research Council funded *Chronic Heart Failure Assistance via Telephone (CHAT) Study* (Yallop et al. 2006). The researchers working on this project had identified the emerging role of practice nurses and, in light of the lack of attention being paid to these nurses, were keen to further investigate this specialty group. This led to the development of my PhD project 'Carving a niche for Australian Practice Nurses', which was comprised of three discrete yet interrelated investigations that explored the role of practice nurses in the management of chronic heart failure (Halcomb 2005).

The *Australian Practice Nurse and Chronic Heart Failure (APACHE) Study* was the first national survey that sought to explore the demographics of the practice nurse workforce and understand the current role of nurses in general practice (Halcomb et al. 2008).The next phase was the *Western Sydney Cardiac Awareness Survey and Evaluation (WESTCASE)*, which explored the epidemiology of heart failure in Australia and the current general practice management of heart failure in Western Sydney (Halcomb et al. 2004). Finally, a consensus development conference was held to synthesise the research evidence and expert opinion and develop a model of chronic disease management for Australian general practice (Halcomb & Davidson 2006; Halcomb et al. 2007).

Undertaking this project allowed me to develop an insight into some of the challenges faced by practice nurses, both in terms of clinical practice issues and the rapidly evolving nature of the specialty. Since these early days I have been privileged to have been involved with and witnessed a number of significant developments. Perhaps the most obvious of these is the growth in practice nurse numbers and the improved organisation of state-based and local practice nurse groups. In addition to the obvious networking benefits of practice nurse groups, their development is significant to me as a researcher as I am now better able to identify practice nurses who may be willing to participate in various projects.

Since 2003, the Royal College of Nursing Australia (RCNA) has held annual general practice nurse conferences. The content of the presentations delivered at these conferences shows the evolution of the specialty of practice nursing and the emergence of skills in research and evaluation among clinical nurses (Halcomb et al. 2006; Halcomb et al. 2007). However, these presentations have also highlighted the potential for nurses to enhance the evaluation of their practice through further development of research skills. These conferences have also provided excellent networking opportunities for clinicians, divisional staff and academics, as Elizabeth Patterson has alluded to previously.

I am privileged to be an active member on a number of committees for APNA. In particular, the development of a research and policy committee has demonstrated the organisation's commitment to taking a proactive role in research and policy development in primary care. With the rapid changes currently occurring in Australian primary care it is vital that nurses contribute to the debate and actively participate in decision making and policy development. It is to this end that research evidence can support nurses in advocating for best practice and evidence-based models of care.

APNA has also taken a proactive role in endorsing, commissioning and undertaking research. A number of researchers working in the area of practice nursing have sought APNA endorsement of their projects. Before being endorsed, such projects are reviewed by members of the research and policy committee to ensure that they are consistent with APNA's strategic goals. This process allows APNA to constructively contribute to the development of projects and ensure that projects recruiting its members are relevant and meaningful. In terms of its own contribution to the research landscape, APNA has recently completed a number of projects focused on gauging the perceptions of nurses about the association, evaluating the Australian Government's continuing professional development program and the development of a tool to measure consumer satisfaction with nursing in general practice. Each of these projects will contribute to the body of knowledge around practice nursing in Australia.

As a result of my publications, presentations and networking at practice nurse events I have developed collaborations with several industry groups and individual practice nurses. In such collaborations I have been able to provide academic mentorship and support to facilitate the conduct and evaluation of small-scale research projects that have been identified by the partner. By working together we have been able to learn from each other and complete projects that neither of us would have been able to achieve so easily on our own. Some of these projects include evaluation of continuing education for practice nurses (Halcomb, Meadley & Streeter 2009), evaluation of an immunisation training program and the impact of the Healthy Kids checks.

Given the relative infancy of practice nursing in Australia it is vital that we all contribute to the evaluation of our current practice and trial new interventions and models of care that contribute to the evidence base for our practice. Such research needs to be based on established research principles and published in the peer-reviewed literature to maximise its contribution to the discipline and disseminate the findings. I am not suggesting that all nurses need to conduct their own research, but rather that all nurses need to seek opportunities to contribute to the development of the body of knowledge around practice nursing. This contribution may be by participating in research, acting as a consultant to a project, providing feedback to researchers about study findings, implementing research in the workplace, or by conducting their own research.

In 2008 I led a team including Professors Patricia Davidson and Nicholas Zwar which was successful in gaining a grant from the University of Western Sydney to explore the use of chronic disease item numbers by general practice nurses. This evaluation considers not only the tasks that practice nurses are undertaking related to chronic disease management, but also the consumer and GP perceptions of the practice nurse role. While the practice nurse workforce has been identified as a strategy to improve chronic disease management in general practice, there has been no formal evaluation of these services within the context of the Australian health system. Undertaking a baseline evaluation of current practice, practice nurses' education and training needs, the barriers and facilitators to service provision and the acceptability of interventions to both consumers and GPs will both inform clinical practice and provide important preliminary data to support subsequent larger investigations in the future.

Also in 2008 a research team, of which I am a member, led by Professor Nicholas Zwar was awarded a project grant by the National Health and Medical Research Council to test the uptake and effectiveness of practice nurse assisted support for smoking cessation. This cluster randomised control trial compares the relative effectiveness of (1) Quit in general practice intervention, involving the GP, Quitline and practice nurse support; (2) brief intervention by general practitioner and Quitline referral; and (3) usual care. In addition to the information that this study will provide about smoking cessation, the findings of this study will be significant for practice nurses. Study findings will provide evidence to guide the development of the role of the practice nurse in smoking cessation. Such evidence will allow policy making to be guided by best practice rather than simply being reactive to address perceived deficiencies in the current health system.

In my role as a peer reviewer of manuscripts and grants it is apparent that there is a growing interest in research that evaluates various interventions involving the practice nurse. Such work is important in providing an evidence base for current clinical practice and strategic directions for practice change. However, it is vital that clinical practice nurses and practice nurse researchers actively participate in the design, implementation and conduct of such projects to ensure that they are relevant to the nursing profession and consider the specific needs of nurses as well as other disciplines within general practice.

From this story I hope that you take two messages. First, that research is an important component of evidence-based practice. Together with clinician judgment and individual and community preference, well-designed research provides an important tool to inform best practice (Sackett et al. 1996). By striving for evidence-based practice we can ensure that we implement the most effective interventions for our clients within the most effective use of our resources. Second, it must be recognised that research is not a solo pursuit. The conduct of high-quality research relies on well-designed studies supported by enthusiastic participants who are committed to the conduct of the study. A well-designed study is often the result of the collaboration of a number of people with a range of different skills, from research design to clinical expertise and data analysis techniques. While not all nurses necessarily need to conduct their own research, all nurses need to be informed consumers of research and active participants in the development of the knowledge base that will inform their clinical practice.

ROSEMARY MAHOMED

I have been a practice nurse working part-time in a solo general practice since 2000. After a 20-year break from study I began a post-registration nursing degree in 2001. My research journey started in 2006 when, as part of a Master of Community Health Practice, I was required to undertake a research project. While researching for assignments during course work for the degree I became aware that, although chronic disease self-management courses were available and seemed to offer benefits to patients, participation rates for the courses were low. As this was an area very relevant to general practice I based my research on this area of interest. I think it is very important to choose an area of inquiry that really interests you or will be useful to your practice as it helps maintain your enthusiasm for the research which can become a very large part of your life. Ethical considerations meant that I was unable to approach patients from my practice for participation in the research and so I drew on friendships and connections to gain access to patients of other general practices. The GPs and staff at these practices were very helpful in identifying possible participants and sending out the letters of invitation for me. Divisions of General Practice network meetings, workshops and nursing conferences give practice nurses opportunities to build networks with staff from other practices which can be drawn on when you need help with recruiting participants, either patients or other health professionals. I have also found that the patients have been incredibly generous in giving their time and sharing their thoughts in order to help me in my research.

I presented the findings of my master's research at the 2006 RCNA National General Practice Nurse Conference which was a new and challenging experience. At the conference I was encouraged to apply for a PHCRED (Primary Health Care Research and Evaluation Development) bursary to write up my research for publication. I was successful in obtaining this and it helped give me the impetus to keep writing when I found it difficult and might have given up. This was my first attempt at writing for publication and although it was very challenging and took longer than I had anticipated it was another new skill that I learnt. With the invaluable help of my supervisors, Professor Elizabeth Patterson and Associate Professor Winsome St. John, I produced an article which was accepted by the *Australian Journal of Primary Health* (Mahomed, Patterson & St. John 2008).

After completing the master's degree I was offered the opportunity to undertake a PhD as part of an ARC funded project trialling practice nurse-led chronic disease management. Although I did not have any specific plans to undertake further study at the time, this is a subject of particular interest to me as chronic disease management constitutes a large part of my job as a practice nurse and so I was interested in pursuing the research. My part in this project has been to develop a grounded theory of patient satisfaction with practice nurse-led chronic disease management and assess the acceptability to patients of the model of care being trialled. The 2007 RCNA National General Practice Nurse Conference in Hobart and the 2009 General Practice and Primary Health Care Conference in Melbourne provided opportunities for me to present my research to a wide audience of health professionals and academics. Being part of a research team has had many advantages, including providing support and offering many opportunities to learn and network with other researchers. Undertaking a PhD can be a rather solitary experience but being part of a research team and having supportive supervisors helps overcome this.

I am a person who likes to find out the answers to the 'why' and the 'how' questions behind statistics and so am drawn to qualitative research which gives researchers a framework to explore issues of interest in depth from the participants' perspective. I think that qualitative research is particularly suited to nursing research as it shares a people-centred approach with nursing. I chose grounded theory as the methodology for my PhD. It has been said that the best way to understand grounded theory is to do it and I have certainly found that to be true. It has been fascinating and exciting to see how it works in practice and how it makes sense as you use the techniques specific to this methodology. Undertaking a PhD has been a huge learning experience in all sorts of different areas from the theoretical, such as understanding the philosophies of different research methodologies to the practical, for example, mastering qualitative interviewing techniques. It has also enabled me to develop skills, such as making formal presentations, writing for publication and qualitative analysis, as well as learning more about the process and practicalities of research in the real world of general practice. Skills I have developed as a practice nurse have also been useful when undertaking research. Practice nurses are already adept at working as part of a team with other disciplines and this experience helps when negotiating the practicalities of research.

JUDY EVANS

When I was approached to apply for a PHCRED research fellowship my first thought was: why would I want to do research? As I considered the idea and I started to look at how I used research in my daily work, I was shocked at my own ignorance. In daily practice I felt that I worked in a vacuum of evidence and was often reliant on a history of 'we have always done it this way' or I remember 'reading it somewhere'. So, I completed my curriculum vitae, lodged my application and waited to hear if I was successful in obtaining an interview. As I waited I pondered what qualities a suitable candidate would need to undertake the fellowship. I also thought that this could possibly be an opportunity in disguise. I did an internet search using the words 'practice nurse', 'chronic disease management' and 'Australian Government health policy' and saw that there was a body of work that had been undertaken by Australian nursing academics but the bulk of the work had been informed by United Kingdom academic studies. I considered who was conducting this research and if they were representative of nurses who work in general practice.

This position was made available through funding from the PHCRED program. The offer was a part-time position with remuneration similar to my clinical role. At the time I was working as a practice nurse full-time and negotiation with my employer allowed me to successfully combine both roles. My employer fully supported my application as she saw the value of this education for me personally, but also the skills that I would bring back to the practice.

Despite my anxiety, I presented for the interview. I answered the questions honestly but with an obvious change in my focus, and I started looking forward to what I thought would add to my future nursing experience. The questions were around my vision which I realised, at the time, was one that I could not articulate well. I had many years of practice nursing experience but little knowledge of the large scope of work that was informing the government policy that eventually would impact on my nursing role.

I was awarded the fellowship: now the journey would start. What I did not fully recognise at the time was that this was an amazing opportunity. Developing a research question seemed initially to be easy, however, this was to be my first lesson in the many challenges of research. It seemed I had a lot to learn. The first hurdle was that I had too many questions to ask and it was a difficult process to choose and refine just one. I also learnt the golden rule that a research question had to be 'answerable and researchable'.

While working on my own research question I was asked to be a part of the research team for two APHCRI-funded projects—the PANACHE and the PARTY projects. The PANACHE project (Practice Nurse Adolescent Clinics for Health Evaluation) evaluated the acceptability, economic and organisational impacts of nurse-led clinics in the area of adolescent health. The PARTY project (Prevention, Access and Risk Taking in Young People) assessed the effectiveness and acceptability of a screening, counselling and systems change intervention to address the problem of adolescent health-risk behaviours presenting in general practice. An integral aspect of this research was a feasibility study of the role of the practice nurse in preventive health for young people. The PANACHE project was linked to the larger PARTY project in that both studies evaluated the impact of practice nurse-led health care clinics.

Through these two projects I learned many of the fundamentals of research; how to run focus groups, apply for ethics approval, write plain-language statements, recruit participants and work within a team of researchers while discovering the true meaning of the words 'barriers' and 'facilitators'. These two projects, plus my own research project, were core to what I believed was preventing advancement of nursing in general practice. What was not known was the evidence of the acceptability of an expanded role for practice nurses to nurses themselves, general practitioners, patients and their families. By answering these questions, what would potentially follow would be the evidence and practical information (economic and organisational) about setting up and running nurse-led health clinics. These projects will also inform policy development for practice nursing in primary health care.

So, as I worked within these two projects I refined my research question. I wanted my research question to examine the collaborative frameworks and professional recognition between members of the clinical team, which are essential to further develop the role of the practice nurse in being an active partner in clinical decision making and health management. What I knew was that the emerging role of the practice nurse had occurred over a short period of time and the necessary frameworks of communication, collaboration and teamwork needed to be explored and questioned. I started reading the literature and became engrossed in the amazing work that was being done around the world in primary health care. In Australia general practice was looking at the role of the practice nurse to provide solutions to the diverse problems in delivering high-quality and reduced-cost health care to patients. What became evident was that the most effective nursing model of care in general practice was not well defined.

My research question took time to develop and the focus shifted over a 12-month period. At times this was very frustrating and required many meetings that pulled the minutia of the wording apart and tried to reassemble them into a sentence of clarity and focus that also was researchable. I finally designed my research question around how the practice nurse is recognised, within the clinical team, as a professional who contributes to patient health outcomes.

During this journey there were times that I felt like an imposter. What was I doing in an environment of highly skilled researchers? What could I contribute? However, I was supported and encouraged by a team of primary care researchers who really wanted the contribution of nurses. I also learned that even a small study has impact. Although my project was small the question evoked great interest from other Australian researchers and had the potential to grow into a bigger study.

At the conclusion of my 12-month fellowship I reviewed what I had learned and what had changed in my approach to research. This opportunity had provided an insight into the complexity in developing research questions, and it also highlighted to me that nurses need not only to be involved in the development of our profession, but also in the research that will provide the evidence that general practice will benefit from additional nursing services. Nurses need to contribute to the debate and the evidence that comes from appropriate and well-designed research. When I now look at a research article I look first at who wrote it, what institution they are from, and what is the date of publication (currency). I then look at the reference list to see what articles I recognise and what articles I need to source.

I presented my findings at two Primary Health Care Research and Information Service (PHCRIS) conferences and received positive feedback from a range of highly respected researchers. This experience reaffirmed my desire to continue to study and I encourage nurses to take opportunities when they present. In spite of my fears and feelings of being inadequate I was encouraged and supported to continue on this learning pathway. Although there were times I suffered from the 'imposter syndrome' I have gained insight and skills that have contributed to my professional development and my interest and passion for ensuring that nurses lead the development of the nursing profession.

KATRINA McNALTY

Of my five years working as a practice nurse, the last two have been involved in an ARC-funded research project trialling practice nurse led management of chronic disease. It is a model of care being trialled for patients with the long-term conditions of hypertension, diabetes or ischaemic heart disease. The study is investigating how practice nurse-led management of long-term illness compares with the way long-term illnesses are usually managed in general practice, that is, by a general practitioner. Initially when asked to be the practice nurse to lead this new initiative, there was a feeling of nervousness, self-doubt and thinking 'why do I need to take part in research'? It was then that I thought none of these feelings would be present if I didn't care and I then realised that obviously this was important and taking part would be an enriching experience. The last two years for me have been extremely rewarding as I have discovered what research means to me. The term 'research' encompasses many different meanings, terms and phrases, but a few words that I like to carry with me are: human activity, discovering, interpreting, developing and advancement of human knowledge. I have discovered a whole new aspect to nursing, have interpreted many different results, developed my teaching and communicating skills and advanced my level of knowledge, not just about nursing practice but also about the research process.

Until given the opportunity to join a research team and take part in a research project, I had never given much time to appreciating or understanding the importance research has in our professional lives. I had never really appreciated that research is used to support nursing practices as it places emphasis on the use of evidence to support and improve our role in ensuring high-quality care and outcomes for our clients. This evidence can be used not only to support why we are in general practice but also to expand our roles and gain the respect and trust that, as professionals, we deserve.

This is not only from our colleagues in the health care team but also from the general public. For example, participants in the project came with mixed feelings so we spent time educating them that practice nurses are skilled professionals who are competent to see patients independently. Once this hurdle was overcome, reassurance was provided that the nurse would always be in regular contact with the doctor. It was interesting to note the difference in reactions, with some patients jumping at the chance to see the nurse, while some took the definite 'no' stance and others wanted permission from their GP to join.

The initial patient education about the project, including the guidelines under which the nurse consultations would run, was delivered by the GP. It was explained that the nurse consultations would be guided by the GP management plan, where the areas of responsibility are clearly defined, patient targets set, and reviews conducted at six monthly intervals by the GP and the practice nurse. The GP management plan was essential in providing safety and security in defining the nurse's boundaries. The initial consultation between GP, nurse and patient was very important as it formed the opportunity for the doctor to hand over the care to the nurse, which seemed very significant for the patients.

Conducting one-on-one consultations brought a whole new aspect into my everyday life. Earning the trust and respect from the patients was the initial hurdle, but as the patients became accustomed to the new process it was easy to see the relationship grow and the trust and respect along with it. For older, long-term patients who have only seen the one doctor it was a challenge for them to accept the new nurse consultations. The relationships grew to a point where the patients were sad and disappointed when the 12-month project finished and they returned to 'usual care'.

Implementing the research project into the practice brought about many changes which were difficult and time consuming. Ultimately the changes were positive and forced us to review procedures and policies, with the outcome being improved quality of care. For example, the practice had to take into account the extra activity, particularly in the waiting room, with the extra person conducting consultations, making sure it remained a friendly environment for the patients. As with most general practices, finding an appropriate space for the nurse to conduct the consultations proved trying at times so new rosters for sharing the treatment rooms and resources were drawn up. Without being involved in the research project our practice, particularly the nursing services, might never have grown to its full potential.

Being involved in the project has also led to opportunities to increase my knowledge base. Being involved with the investigators, and with the support and education we received through the university, has allowed me to expand my role as a practice nurse and open up a whole new field of nursing and understanding about research. Chronic disease management is often considered difficult and time consuming. However, through the research project I have realised what a difference practice nurses can make through prevention, support and monitoring patients' conditions, all of which can have a huge impact on their lives.

Undertaking this research in our practice also affected the reception staff who arrange appointments for the nurse consultations. Education also had to be given on the relevant item numbers, when to bill, and the requirements for billing the items involved. The receptionists also had to adjust to the fact that patients could ring and request an appointment to see the nurse only. A system was devised to note those patients being cared for by the nurse, not only for the reception staff when booking patients in, but for the doctors as well when they conducted their consultations with the patients.

Participation of our practice in the research project was undertaken with full staff support, which led to improved teamwork and cooperation. Our practice had been involved with this research project from the early days. Many staff meetings were held to discuss the various situations and the impact the project would have on the staff and the practice as a whole to prepare us for the adventurous road ahead. Our practice is always open and prepared for new initiatives; the research project has encouraged us to constantly review our practices to ensure we are delivering the best quality of care and to keep developing as a patient-centred team.

Being at the frontline of data collection was sometimes daunting; however it reminded me that every one has an important role within the research team regardless of how minor or major the input. It is a collaborative effort that no one effort alone can produce—we are all responsible for the development and collection of data to gather evidence to improve our profession. Without research our profession will not grow to its full capacity. I believe that everyone should take on this challenge as this could build a new career, a new you, a new practice and even a new world.

Discussion

These stories illustrate that developing personal, organisational or professional research capacity is often the result of intrinsic drives to improve knowledge and practice combined with extrinsic motivators such as the introduction of new national policies, the availability of a research funding steam or the establishment of an informal professional networking/mentoring research group or formal body (like APNA's Research and Policy Development Committee). Macfarlane et al. (2005) have suggested that general practices, in developing research capacity, can be mapped to a model of organisational development that has distinct but overlapping phases that are not necessarily linear—creative energy, concrete planning, transformation, consolidation and collaboration. Movement between these phases can be triggered by both internal and external influences.

Phase 1—'creative energy' can be triggered by just one practitioner's interest or concern about a practice issue or an invitation to participate in a trial. Macfarlane et al. (2005) contend that strong motivation and interest is present from the outset with a planned approach to training and personal development following. This is evident in most of the stories you have just read. Moving to the next phase of 'concrete planning' is often stimulated by a particular 'champion' with the skill, interest, leadership abilities and influence to plan strategically for the practice's future involvement in research. Training opportunities, local networks of researchers or perhaps a grant may also emerge in this phase. The third phase of 'transformation' is realised by a practice following through their plans and becoming an organisation with a new culture and infrastructure to support research activities. This phase is associated with major changes in systems, roles, knowledge and skills—all alluded to in Katrina's story. Phase 4—'consolidation' is often marked by a formal milestone such an award or achieving a particular research practice status and where research is integral to the practice's identity. Moving to the final phase of 'collaboration and linkage' involves actively linking to the wider research community and contributing to the strategic development of research both locally and nationally (Macfarlane et al. 2005).

Although this model of research development presented by Macfarlane et al. (2005) refers to organisations (general practices) it can probably be adapted to individual research development. For example, they identify triggers for development as enthusiasts and innovators, the diffusion of ideas, seed funding, vision, leadership, infrastructure, skills training, incentives and opportunities to collaborate—all equally applicable to an individual as to an organisation. Similarly, barriers such as conflicting priorities, lack of time, unsuccessful grant applications and breakdowns in collaboration can be cited as setbacks to research development by individuals as well as organisations.

Conclusion

Each of the five stories provides evidence of how particular individuals have developed their capacity to engage in research activities and all illustrate the importance of networking and mentorship in building and sustaining research knowledge and skills. When clinicians, researchers and educators come together to develop, test and disseminate new knowledge, development of the discipline gains momentum and credibility is enhanced. Engagement with research is essential in improving health outcomes and influencing policy. The reform agenda identified in the final report of the National Health and Hospitals Reform Commission (NHHRC), *A healthier future for all Australians* (NHHRC 2009) provides fertile research ground for practice nurses to explore expanded roles and provide evidence of their vital contribution to primary health care.

Reflections

How can I relate to these stories?

How have research findings contributed to my practice development?

What resources can I use to access research related to my practice?

What opportunities are available to me to develop my research skills and ability to use research in my practice?

Am I aware of what research is, or has been, undertaken in my practice or division?

Key messages

Research is an important component of evidence-based practice.

Practice nurses need to be active participants in the development of the knowledge base that will inform their clinical practice.

Developing research skills benefits the practice nurse, the general practice and the nursing profession.

Useful resources

PHCRED Strategy
http://www.phcris/phcred/

ROAR: Roadmap of Australian Primary Health Care Research
http://www.phcris.org.au/ROAR/

Australian Primary Health Care Research Institute
http://www.anu.edu.au/aphcri/

National Institute of Clinical Studies (NICS)
http://www.nhmrc.gov.au/nics/asp/index.asp

Joanna Briggs Institute
http://www.joannabriggs.edu.au/about/home.php

Cochrane Collaboration
http://www.cochrane.org/

Evidence-Based Practice Tutorial (University of Minnesota)
http://www.biomed.lib.umn.edu/learn/ebp/

Evidence-Based Nursing (University of North Carolina)
http://www.biomed.lib.umn.edu/learn/ebp/

Nursing research related sites
http://medi-smart.com/research-orgs.htm

WEB Centre for Social research methods
http://www.socialresearchmethods.net/

References

1. Davidson, P, Halcomb, E & Patterson, E (eds) 2007, *Contemporary Nurse: Advances in General Practice Nursing*—special issue, vol. 26, no. 1. e-Content Management Pty Ltd.

2. Eley, DS, Del Mar, CB, Patterson, E, Synnott, RL, Baker, PG & Hegney, D 2008, 'A nurse led model of chronic disease care—an interim report', *Australian Family Physician*, vol. 37, no. 12, pp. 1030–2.

3. Eley, D, Hegney, D & Patterson, E 2005, 'Patient recruitment for a practice nurse study', *Australian Family Physician*, vol. 34, no. 11, pp. 991–2.

4. Halcomb, EJ 2005, *Carving a niche for Australian practice nurses in chronic heart failure management*, unpublished PhD thesis, University of Western Sydney, Australia.

5. Halcomb, EJ & Davidson, PM 2006, 'The role of practice nurses in an integrated model of cardiovascular disease management in Australian general practice', *Australian Journal of Primary Health,* vol. 12, no. 2, pp. 44–54.

6.   Halcomb, EJ, Davidson, PM & Patterson, E 2007, 'Exploring the development of Australian general practice nursing: where we have come from and where to from here?', *Contemporary Nurse*, vol. 26, no. 1, pp. 145–53.

7.   Halcomb, EJ, Davidson, PM, Salamonson, Y & Ollerton, R 2008, 'Nurses in Australian general practice: Implications for chronic disease management', *Journal of Nursing and Healthcare of Chronic Illness,* in association with *Journal of Clinical Nursing*, vol. 17, no. 5A, pp. 6–15.

8.   Halcomb, EJ, Davidson, PM, Yallop, J, Griffiths, R & Daly, J 2007, 'Strategic directions for developing the Australian general practice nurse role in cardiovascular disease management', *Advances in Contemporary Nursing*, vol. 25, no. 2, pp. 125–135.

9.   Halcomb, EJ, Edwards, P, Davidson, PM, Daly, J, Griffiths, R & Tofler, G 2004, *Audit of heart failure management in general practice: Highlighting a potential role for the practice nurse (Free paper)*, paper presented at the Royal College of Nursing, Australia 2nd National General Practice Nurse Conference: Working together—Improving Primary Care through Teamwork, Wollongong, New South Wales.

10.   Halcomb, EJ, Meadley, E & Streeter, S 2009, 'Professional development needs of general practice nurses', *Advances in Contemporary Nurse Education*, vol. 32, no. 1–2, pp. 201–210.

11.   Halcomb, EJ, Patterson, E, & Davidson, PM 2006, 'Evolution of practice nursing in Australia', *Journal of Advanced Nursing*, vol. 55, no. 3, pp. 376–88.

12.   Hegney, D, Eley, R. Buikstra, E, Rees, S & Patterson, E 2006, 'Consumers' level of comfort with an advanced practice role for registered nurses in general practice: A Queensland, Australia study', *Australian Journal of Primary Health*, vol. 12, no. 3, pp. 55–62.

13.   Hegney, D, Price, K, Patterson, E, Martin-McDonald, K & Rees, S 2004, 'Australian consumers' expectations for expanded nursing roles in general practice—choice not gatekeeping', *Australian Family Physician*, vol. 33, no. 10, pp. 845–9.

14.   Macfarlane, F, Shaw, S, Greenhalgh, T & Carter Y 2005, 'General practices as emergent research organizations: a qualitative study into organizational development', *Family Practice*, vol. 22, pp. 298–304.

15.   Mahomed, R, Patterson, E & St John, W 2008, 'Factors influencing possible participation in chronic disease self-management courses', *Australian Journal of Primary Health*, vol. 14, no. 3, pp. 19–26.

16.   National Health and Hospitals Reform Commission (NHHRC) 2009, *A healthier future for all Australians*, viewed 7 January 2010, <http://www.health. gov.au>.

17.   National Nursing and Nursing Education Taskforce 2006, 'A National Specialisation Framework for Nursing and Midwifery: defining and identifying specialty area of practice in Australia', viewed 21 January 2010, <http://www. nnnet.gov.au/>

18. Patterson, E & McMurray, A 2003, 'Collaborative practice between nurses and medical practitioners in Australian general practice: Moving from rhetoric to reality', *Australian Journal of Advanced Nursing*, vol. 20, no. 4, pp. 43–8.

19. Patterson, E, Del Mar, C & Najman, J 1999a, 'A descriptive study of nurses employed by general practitioners in south-east Queensland', *Australian Journal of Advanced Nursing*, vol. 17, no. 2, pp. 13–20.

20. Patterson, E, Del Mar, C & Najman, J 1999b, 'Nursing's contribution to general practice: general practitioners' and practice nurses' views', *Collegian*, vol. 6, no. 4, pp. 33–9.

21. Patterson, E, Del Mar, C & Najman, J 2000, 'Medical receptionists in general practice: who needs a nurse?', *International Journal of Nursing Practice*, vol. 6, no. 5, pp. 229–36.

22. Patterson, E, Forrester, K, Price, K & Hegney, D 2005, 'Risk reduction in general practice and the role of the receptionist', *Journal of Law Medicine*, vol. 12, no. 3, pp. 340–47.

23. Patterson, E, Price, K, & Hegney, D 2005, 'Primary health care and general practice nurses: What is the nexus?', *Australian Journal of Primary Health*, vol. 11, no. 1, pp. 47–54.

24. Price, K, Patterson, E & Hegney, D 2006, 'Being strategic: utilising consumer views to better promote an expanded role for nurses in Australian general practice', *Collegian*, vol. 13, no. 4, pp. 16–21.

25. Sackett, D, Rosenberg, W, Muir Gray, J, Haynes, R & Richardson, W 1996, Evidence-based medicine: what it is and what it isn't', *British Medical Journal*, vol. 312, no. 7023, p. 71.

26. Yallop, J, Chan, B, Piterman, L, Tonkin, A, Forbes, A, Davidson, PM, Clark, R, Halcomb, EJ, Nagle, A, Stewart, S, Croucher, J, Krum, H & on behalf of the CHAT Study Group 2006, 'The chronic heart-failure assistance by telephone (CHAT) study: Assessment of telephone support for vulnerable patients with chronic disease', *Asia Pacific Journal of Family Medicine*, vol. 5, no. 2, viewed 21 January 2010, <http://www.apfmj-archive.com/afm5_2/afm38.htm>.

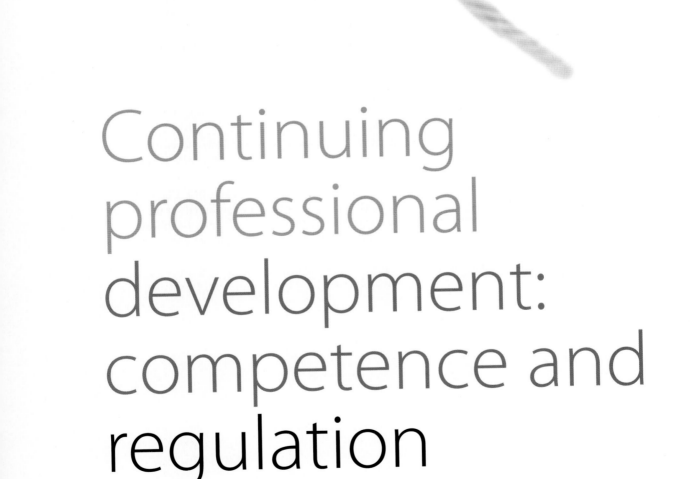

Chapter nineteen

Continuing professional development: competence and regulation

by Stephanie Fox-Young

Overview

In this chapter, continuing professional development (CPD) requirements from four professions (nurses, teachers, general practitioners and engineers) are examined to identify key components of CPD and competence. The regulation of CPD as an indicator of the maintenance of competence are considered as well as alternative models of regulation of CPD. Current knowledge of the costs of, benefits from, barriers to and effectiveness of CPD are also explored.

Objectives

At the completion of this chapter you should be able to:

- have enhanced understanding of the origins and scope of continuing competence/professional development requirements;

- have increased knowledge of the varieties of continuing professional development practices and strategies available for maintaining competence; and

- better appreciate the regulatory frameworks surrounding continuing competence.

Introduction

The focus on CPD, also known as continuing professional education, is a recent stage in the regulation of professions. An assumption that professionals will engage in lifelong (or at least career-long) learning has existed for a long time, but this has not always been accompanied by an expectation that professionals will be able to produce evidence of a range of professional activities to demonstrate that they meet their profession's standards. Rather, most people have assumed that an ethical professional would ensure that their knowledge and skills remained up to date, and that a well-educated person (as professionals were understood to be) would be likely to engage in ongoing education.

Definitions

Competence is defined by the Australian Nursing and Midwifery Council (ANMC 2009) as the combination of skills, knowledge, attitudes, values and abilities that underpin effective and/or superior performance in a profession/ occupational area and context of practice.

Continuing competence is defined by the International Council of Nurses (2005) as the ongoing ability to integrate and apply the knowledge, skills, judgment and personal attributes required to practice safely, competently and ethically in a designated role and setting. ANMC (2009) extends this definition to include the ability of nurses and midwives to demonstrate that they have maintained their competence to practise in relation to their context of practice, and the relevant ANMC competency standards under which they gain and retain their licence to practise.

Continuing professional development (CPD) involves the active learning of new skills or knowledge. It is the ongoing, systematic learning process that nurses and midwives undertake to maintain their competence to practise and enhance their professional and personal skills and knowledge. The CPD cycle involves reviewing practice, identifying learning needs, planning and participating in relevant learning activities, and reflecting on the value of those activities (ANMC 2009).

Regulation is all of those legitimate and appropriate means—governmental, professional, private and individual—whereby order, identity, consistency and control are brought to the profession. The profession and its members are defined; the scope of practice is determined; standards of education and of ethical and competent practice are set; and systems of accountability are established through these means (International Council of Nurses 2005).

Background to regulation of continuing professional development

For as long as there have been professions, there have been social expectations about the standards of practice and conduct of professionals. However, it has only been a recent development, that is, in the last 20 to 30 years, that there has been an expectation that professionals will not only be professional by maintaining standards, they will also need to be monitored on a regular basis to ensure that those standards of professionalism are being adhered to, and that they can provide evidence to prove their professionalism on a regular basis. Until relatively recently in many places including Australia, registration was a lifelong 'award' bestowed on a person who had undergone a particular educational preparation. A person with a recognised qualification was assumed to be a professional who would therefore conduct themselves in accordance with expected standards of practice.

Until the 1990s, in many pieces of legislation governing professions, there were clear expectations that certain conduct would be avoided (misconduct, malpractice, and conduct likely to cause harm to the image of the profession or to bring the profession into disrepute). However, the expectation that a professional would remain competent may have been assumed but was not always openly stated.

Even in the early 1990s, the *Nursing Act* in Queensland, for example, required evidence of recent practice for re-registration after a period of absence from practice, but did not specifically identify continuing competence as a requirement for registration (*Nursing Act 1992 (Qld)*). Certainly for initial registration, nurses were expected to be competent, and by implication this could be extended to current practitioners, but competence was not specifically part of any requirement for renewal of registration on an annual basis. Essentially this meant that registrants who renewed their licences on time every year were not ever required to demonstrate that they had practised nursing at any time since they were initially registered.

It was not until some years after the *Nursing Act 1992 (Qld)* was introduced that recent practice requirements for continuing registration were implemented, following consultation with key stakeholders. Additionally, by then, the concept of recent practice had been interpreted as an indicator of continued competence (Queensland Nursing Forum 1998). The argument for this change was that the public would be more concerned about the competence of the professional's practice than about whether the professional had recently engaged in professional practice. Additionally, there was a change regarding monitoring of standards. Instead of simply waiting for exceptions to be reported to the appropriate authorities for action, there was a positive expectation that any professional would be able to provide evidence, if asked, not only of recent practice, but also of their ongoing adherence to standards of practice and competence, including participation in CPD.

Some of the reasons for this shift in expectations can be found in the consumer movement, in the publicity associated with cases of professionals behaving unprofessionally or incompetently, and in the increased interest in professional accountability. Consumers were wary of trusting professionals to regulate themselves, seeing evidence in the media in a variety of professions of people who were, if not actively protecting their colleagues, then at least not reporting them to appropriate authorities either. A doctor in New Zealand in the 1970s was a case in point. The doctor believed that carcinoma in situ did not lead to cancer of the cervix and was therefore, as part of a research project, not treating women with abnormal Pap smears (Paul 1988). Many health professionals were aware of this doctor's practice, and some tried to have action taken, without success. It took the concerted efforts of professionals and journalists to bring the matter to the attention of authorities who then established a judicial inquiry into the matter in the public interest.

So, self-regulation became suspect. And, with greater consumer awareness, particularly as information became more accessible through technology, it became evident that some professionals had not engaged in any, or sufficient, continuing education. This was even more concerning because it was also obvious that the ability of professionals to maintain competence in a rapidly changing environment would be compromised if they did not take active steps to keep their knowledge and skill current.

While some employers had certain expectations regarding annual competence, for example, for nurses in basic life support, medication calculations, manual handling and fire safety, not all professionals were employees, and not all employers were necessarily putting systems in place to monitor competence. Some employers may also have undertaken annual performance appraisal with their staff, and many professionals would have engaged voluntarily in peer review. But the public wanted to have some means of assurance that all the professionals they consulted were competent to provide the services they were seeking. The expectation therefore moved from exception reporting of incompetence to proactive provision of evidence of competence. As most professions already had regulatory systems in place, it was reasonably simple for those regulators to take on the additional roles required to implement this change. However, the links between continuing competence and continuing professional development, while sensible on the surface, had not necessarily been demonstrated by research.

What CPD is required for professionals?

Table 19.1 below summarises the CPD requirements published by the Australian Nursing and Midwifery Council in its Continuing Competence Framework (2009); the Queensland College of Teachers' Continuing Professional

Table 19.1 Requirements for CPD and recent practice across four professions

Nursing (Australian Nursing and Midwifery Council, 2009)	Teaching (Queensland College of Teachers, 2008)
20 hours CPD in 1 year, 60 hours over 3 years (Participation in mandatory continuing education, such as basic life support training or manual handling, should not be counted as CPD **unless** active learning of new knowledge or skills has taken place)	30 hours CPD per year (reduced requirements for teachers not working full-time—may be employer directed and supported, school supported, or individually identified)
Practice within the last 5 years, quantity not specified	200 hours practice in last 5 years
Examples of appropriate CPD activities	
– Reflecting on feedback, keeping a practice journal – Acting as a preceptor/mentor/tutor – Participating on accreditation, audit or quality improvement committees – Undertaking supervised practice for skills development – Participating in clinical audits, critical incident monitoring, case reviews and clinical meetings – Participating in a professional reading and discussion group – Developing skills in IT, numeracy, communications, improving own performance, problem solving and working with others – Writing or reviewing educational materials, journal articles, books – Active membership of professional groups and committees – Reading professional journals or books – Writing for publication – Developing policy, protocols or guidelines – Working with a mentor to improve practice	– Active contribution to education system initiatives, pilots, trials and projects – Courses, workshops (including school-based), conferences, vacation schools or online courses relevant to teaching context – Syllabus, curriculum and assessment professional development conducted by state studies authority or employer – Training for and development from participation in national and state test marking, studies authority and school-based teacher consistency of judgment procedures – Formal presentations to colleagues on classroom practices, research findings or contemporary issues in education – Leading school-based curriculum and/or policy development – Preparation for and development through providing collegial professional support for pre-service or beginning teachers as part of supervising/mentoring role – Educational research/action research projects

Continued >

Table 19.1 *continued*

Examples of appropriate CPD activities	
– Presenting at or attending workplace education, in-service sessions or skills workshops – Undertaking undergraduate or postgraduate studies which are of relevance to the context of practice – Presenting at or attending conferences, lectures, seminars or professional meetings – Conducting or contributing to research – Undertaking relevant online or distance education	– Active involvement in approved overseas teacher exchange, encompassing pre-preparation, on-site professional development and subsequent reporting – Professional reading linked to activities, such as research, preparation of articles, presentations to colleagues and professional practice – Formal study leading to a qualification in education or field related to teaching area.
General practitioners (RACGP)	*Engineers* (*Engineers Australia*, 2009)
To maintain certification with RACGP Minimum of 130 points for the triennium which must include: – Two category 1 activities and – Completion of basic cardiopulmonary resuscitation course	150 hours of structured CPD in the last three years. Of the 150 hours, – at least 50 hours must relate to the individual's area of practice – at least 10 hours must cover risk management – at least 15 hours must address business and management skills – the remainder must cover a range of activities relevant to the individual's career.
Practice requirements not specified.	For academics/educators, 40 hours industry involvement in past 3 years required
Examples of CPD activities	
Category 1 options 1. Active learning module (40 points) 2. Clinical audit (40 points) 3. Evidence Based Medicine Journal Club (40 points) 4. GP research (40 points) – Principal investigator – GP research participant 5. Learning plan (one per triennium capped at 40 points) 6. Rapid Plan, Do, Study, Act (PDSA) cycle (40 points) 7. Small group learning (40 points) 8. Supervised clinical attachment (40 Points)	1. Formal postgraduate study or individual tertiary course units not undertaken for award purposes (no limit to hours that can be claimed, must include assessment) 2. Short courses, workshops, seminars and discussion groups, conferences, technical inspections and technical meetings (no limit to hours that can be claimed) 3. Learning activities in the workplace that extend competence in the area of practice (maximum of 75 hours can be claimed, and normal work activities applying current knowledge cannot be claimed) 4. Private study which extends your knowledge and skills (maximum 18 hours claimable, records must be kept)

Examples of CPD activities	
9. Higher education relevant to general practice (Australian Qualifications Framework accredited) – Graduate certificate (60 points) – Graduate diploma (90 points) – Master's degree (120 points) – Doctor of Philosophy (PhD) (150 points) 10. RACGP assessment activities (150 points) – FRACGP by examination – FRACGP by practice based assessment – FARGP **Category 2 options** Endorsed or accredited provider of Category 2 activities (each activity capped at 30 points) Unaccredited activities Self-recorded activities (minimum of 10 hours education for 20 points for the triennium)	5. Service to the engineering profession (maximum 50 hours, can include serving on boards, committees, accreditation panels, reviewing publications, mentoring colleagues, preparing submissions) 6. The preparation and presentation of material for courses, conferences, seminars and symposia (up to 45 hours per paper/presentation can be claimed, up to 75 if peer reviewed. Must be outside normal work requirements) 7. Practitioners employed in tertiary teaching or academic research (must be able to demonstrate 40 hours of industry involvement in the 3-year period, through, for example, consultancy services, joint industry–university research collaboration, supervision of students' industry based design projects/field trips, secondment) 8. Any other structured activities not covered by 1–6 above that meet the objectives of the CPD policy (must be supported by documentary evidence with clear justification)

Development Framework policy (2008); The Royal Australian College of General Practitioners' QA&CPD Program, 2008–2010; and *Engineers Australia* in its 'Continuing professional development policy' (2009).

However, as can be seen from a superficial examination of the table, while there are similarities across these four professions, there are significant differences as well. The most obvious is the expectation of hours (or points) of CPD—ranging from 60 to 150 hours in a three-year period. All four professions are expecting continuing professional development activities to be undertaken. However, they are not overly restrictive or prescriptive about what are acceptable types of CPD, nor do they define what mixture of activities is best, although the engineers and general practitioners have made more of an attempt to identify that optimal mix.

Competence and CPD

Four examples are presented below to shed light on the subjectivity involved in judging whether what an individual has done is sufficient to maintain their competence. None of the examples are profession specific, although obviously some are health related.

Example 19.1 Lesley

> Completed initial professional qualification 10 years ago.

> Always displayed an enquiring, open mind and a willingness to ask questions about things not understood or known.

> Practice is informed by knowledge gained from expert colleagues and from reading in order to satisfy curiosity or to answer specific questions.

> Actively participates in the state branch of the relevant professional association and attends meetings but has not stood for office.

> Has not undertaken any formal extended study, nor been to any conferences, nor kept records/a reflective journal regarding questions raised or reading engaged in.

> Works 24 hours per week, and colleagues, if asked, would report that Lesley is definitely competent.

Example 19.2 Kim

> Works between 32 and 48 hours per week as a casual reliever/locum through an agency.

> Has attended all required annual 'competence credentialing' sessions, but has not undertaken any formal study since graduating with a degree eight years ago.

> Attends in-service sessions whenever they are offered, but on an ad hoc, unplanned basis.

> Does not read professional journals because there is 'no time', and does not attend conferences because they are 'too expensive'.

> It would be difficult to find a colleague who could report on Kim's competence, because of the nature of casual relieving employment, but facilities continue to request Kim as a reliever.

> Clients have written letters praising Kim's commitment.

Example 19.3 Alex

> Graduated six years ago, and has changed employer every two years since then.

> Has maintained a reflective journal which was started during full-time pre-registration study, but has not read any journal articles for at least three years.

> Intends to undertake further study, but is still looking for the 'right' program.

> Mentored a student last semester and really enjoyed the experience. The student reported that Alex was the best mentor thus far allocated in the course of the degree.

> Went to several conferences during the first year of practice, but found they were 'boring' and 'not relevant', and so has not attended any others.

Example 19.4 Lee

> Graduated 20 years ago and worked full-time for 17 years.

> Stopped working three years ago to care for parent suffering senile dementia.

> Has maintained professional contact through reading journals, especially in the areas of gerontology and palliative care.

> Maintains contact with professional colleagues via email and phone, often seeking advice in relation to role as carer.

> Intends to return to work, but unable to predict when that may happen.

> Would like to undertake further study in the area of palliative care, but is concerned about the length of time absent from professional practice, and the difficulty of regaining 'lost' skills.

Two questions may help to clarify the difference between competence and evidence of competence:

1. Could you say, with any certainty, whether Lesley, Alex, Kim or Lee is competent or not, on the basis of the information available?

2. Do you think the evidence in any of the four cases actually reflects their actual level of competence?

Each is undertaking activities that would 'fit' for at least one of the professions listed in Table 19.1 on page 445, although in some cases, just barely. It is clear, however, that each would have difficulty providing evidence of their competence. Lesley may be able to ask a colleague to provide a report, and this may include reference to seeking knowledge from expert colleagues, but may not capture the other informal education activities completed. Kim could supply the letters from clients, but would also be wise to seek certificates of attendance at the in-service sessions if not already obtained. Alex could provide the student's comment and the reflective journal but would be more certain of this being accepted if there was reference to reading or conference attendance in the journal. Providing a professional service for a family member is often difficult to use as evidence of professional practice, which is more usually undertaken in paid employment or on a fee-for-service basis. Although Lee is using newly learned skills and knowledge related to professional practice, written references from the colleagues consulted in the last three years would be necessary in order to supply the evidence of continued competence, and a reflective journal demonstrating how the new knowledge is relevant to future professional practice would also be useful.

Does CPD improve practice?

The evidence of the effectiveness of CPD in improving patient outcomes is, at best, mixed. Most studies report student satisfaction, many report changes in knowledge, but very few have reported improvements in patient outcomes, possibly because of the difficulties of attributing changes in patient outcomes to an educational program or experience undertaken by the practitioner.

According to Barriball, While and Norman (1992) there is a strongly held assumption that continuing professional education in nursing has benefits for nurses, clients and the health care service. However, they concluded that there was a lack of research evidence about nurses' perceptions of their continuing professional education needs and the perceived outcomes of continuing professional education in terms of changes in knowledge, attitudes, skills, job satisfaction, staff retention and career development (Barriball, While & Norman 1992). Barriball, While and Norman (1992) also noted that the impact of CPD on patient care had rarely been measured. Similarly, only one of the 18 studies included in a Cochrane review of the effect of educational outreach measured a patient outcome (Thompson O'Brien et al. 2001).

More recent studies have also reported difficulties with making the link between CPD and competence and improved patient outcomes. In a study of 43 graduates of a post-registration nursing degree, 77% reported that they had used new skills in practice, and that their practice had changed (Hardwick & Jordan 2002). However, when questioned, the graduates identified research skills rather than practical or clinical skills as examples; that is, their academic knowledge had increased, but not necessarily their clinical competence.

In one of the few studies that have evaluated patient outcomes, Cleland et al. (2009) reported a randomised clinical trial into whether continuing education improved physical therapists' effectiveness in treating neck pain. Only 19 therapists participated in the study involving a two-day course, with or without follow-up sessions. The outcome measures included patient-reported reduction in disability, pain and number of visits, all taken from 511 patient records, 283 being treated by therapists who received the follow-up sessions and 228 in the control group. Patients treated by the therapists who received the additional follow-up sessions reported greater reduction in disability and had fewer post-treatment visits, although there was no significant difference in reported pain between the two patient groups (Cleland et al. 2009).

Similar issues were identified in a meta-analysis of 31 studies involving 61 educational interventions undertaken by Mansouri and Lockyer (2007). The effect size of continuing medical education on physician knowledge was found to be a medium one; however, the effect size for physician performance and patient outcome was reported to be small. There was a larger effect size reported when the interventions were interactive, used multiple methods, and were designed for a small group of physicians from a single discipline (Mansouri & Lockyer 2007); however, as the authors noted, this would increase the cost of the educational interventions significantly.

Is there evidence that professionals are engaging in CPD?

One of the arguments against regulation is that a burden is imposed on the whole of a group in order to manage the few who do not comply with the accepted standards of a profession. The issue is one of trust—whether the public trusts the profession, as well as whether members of the profession trust each other to be undertaking sufficient CPD (however much or little that may be) to maintain their competence.

There are few reports of the level of CPD participation. Those that exist raise more questions than they answer. Following interviews with 289 nurses in the United Kingdom, Barriball and While (1996) reported that the evidence suggested that enrolled nurses and those working part-time and on night duty consistently attend less continuing professional education than their more senior, full-time and day-duty colleagues. However, this study used five days in a year as the benchmark for CPD participation, and reported only those who had completed less than that (11% of registered nurses) rather than reporting those who had not done any at all. It is possible, but not reported, that there were no participants who had omitted CPD entirely.

In 2005, in a voluntary scheme, 17 983 of 22 479 Canadian registered nurses (more than 80%) identified one or more indicators of the Canadian Registered Nurses Association Nursing Practice Standards for which they would develop and implement a learning plan. Over 16 000 (89% of the 17 983) reported in 2006 that they had implemented learning plans in that year (*Alberta RN* 2007). The main question this raises is whether the 20% who did not participate initially and the 11% of participants who did not report implementing a plan had undertaken any CPD in that year, or not.

What are the barriers to the uptake of CPD?

There do not appear to be any studies linking intention to change practice with educational interventions. There are also few studies that consider opportunity and accessibility as factors, and most of these were published in the early to mid 1990s.

Yuen (1991) compiled a list of the common obstacles for CPD:

1. inability to convince nurse managers that staff development is of vital importance for the service
2. failure to encourage qualified nurses to value their own continuing personal and professional development

3. failure to recognise that the training personnel also need help
4. lack of appropriate criteria for nurse managers to select staff for continuing nursing education programs
5. ineffective methods for publicising programs
6. little systematic attention to identifying educational and training needs
7. inadequate evaluation of effectiveness of staff development programs
8. lack of coherent staff development programs
9. inadequate funding for staff development.

Reflections

What are the barriers to your own professional development?

Hogston (1995) interviewed 18 participants and reported that these nurses readily identified the factors which may hinder them from reaching their full potential. These included financial restrictions and a reluctance by managers to fund courses they perceived to be irrelevant. Hogston (1995) suggested that CPD, therefore, risked being dictated by the needs of others rather than being used as a process of professional development, because professional development depended on an individual's ability to gain financial support to attend courses rather than on their need for learning.

Barriball and While (1996) noted that difficulty in obtaining study leave, low staffing levels, lack of support from managers, the late advertisement of CPD events, the poor availability of funds, as well as personal circumstances and domestic responsibilities of practitioners were all obstacles to accessing continuing professional education.

Fear of appearing incompetent was identified as another barrier that should not be underestimated (Perry 1995). Perry concluded that a positive impact of CPD on practice was dependent on:

*   sensitive and accurate needs assessment in the first instance;
*   innovative and effective implementation, both in terms of teaching process and content;
*   adequate funding and a supportive environment; and
*   evaluation procedures which address actual intended outcomes.

Taking a longer view of CPD and its effects on patient outcomes, barriers to the uptake of continuing professional education were noted by Nolan, Owens and Nolan (1995) to be made worse by the complexity of introducing change into practice. Dissatisfaction and scepticism can occur if staff are prevented from applying what they have learned. This not only negates the benefits of attending CPD but, according to Nolan, Owens and Nolan (1995), actually results in counterproductive effects, including frustration and disillusionment. An educated, motivated practitioner operating in an organisational culture that values and supports change is, for Nolan, Owens and Nolan (1995), the recipe for successfully changing practice.

Reflections

What strategies have you used to introduce changes into your practice and what was the outcome?

Is CPD cost-effective?

Cost is often identified by professionals as a barrier to participation in CPD, although it is not an excuse readily accepted by regulatory authorities. Cost-effectiveness is an equally significant issue.

Just in terms of study leave, if each professional required three days of study leave per year to undertake CPD, Australia could be looking at funding more than 600 000 days of study leave for nurses alone, not including funding other support for study, such as fees, travel and learning materials. Moreover, there are the costs of accrediting providers of CPD, and possibly of accrediting CPD programs or packages as well. While these costs are spread across the individual, the employer and the taxation system (where self-education may be a claimable expenditure), the cost is significant for an activity that is not yet proven to have benefits in terms of patient outcomes.

Prystowsky and Bordage (2001) found that leading journals in medical education contain little information concerning the cost and products of medical education; that is, provider performance and patient outcomes. Similarly, Cleland et al. (2009) reported that they had not examined the cost-effectiveness of their educational interventions for physical therapists, nor had they tried to separate whether all interventions were necessary for success, which would be a necessary step to be able to calculate cost-effectiveness. Thompson O'Brien et al. (2001) concluded in their Cochrane review that as cost-effectiveness had not been well evaluated, further research was necessary. Nevertheless, CPD requirements are in place and are not likely to disappear in the future.

Reflections

To what extent do you access education resources in the published literature or online?

Regulating CPD in nursing in Australia

Hogston (1995) argued that CPD would only improve quality of care if nurses used it as a learning process and not as a function that is demanded because of regulatory legislation. According to Pearson et al. (2002, p. 363) 'besides anecdote and local evaluation' there is little evidence to suggest that one method of monitoring continuing competence is better than another, and there is no profession that has found a reliable, easy to administer and acceptable (to the profession and the public) way of doing so.

In the statutory model, which is the current model for nursing and midwifery in Australian jurisdictions and the model to be implemented nationally 2010, a nursing and midwifery regulatory authority, functioning under legislation, regulates practice based on standards developed through consultation. Currently it monitors by self-report and auditing, plus active reporting of incompetence, the latter being likely to become mandatory with national registration. The regulator may revoke a professional's licence or impose conditions on practice if they are found through either audit or active reporting not to be meeting expected standards.

Reflections

What method do you use to record your CPD activities?

Portfolios

Keeping a professional portfolio has been recommended as a means of recording and providing evidence for engagement in CPD (Andre & Heartfield 2007; ANMC 2009). The ANMC suggest a portfolio should contain the following elements:

- professional history, such as curriculum vitae, job descriptions, registration certificates, educational transcripts and awards, employment records;
- professional activities, such as presentations and publications, membership and roles in professional organisations, awards and commendations, research

activities, and any other documents demonstrating relevant professional achievements; and

• evidence of participation in a professional review process, practice undertaken and CPD.

Examples of portfolios can be found on the Nurses Board of Victoria website (refer to Useful resources on p. 458).

Conclusion

Either through personal experience of incompetence in health practitioners or through media reports of incompetence, no matter how small the percentage of professionals who are not competent, consumers have come to expect that monitoring of professionals' continued competence should occur.

Although CPD is widely used as an indicator of continued competence and, on the surface, should have a positive impact on health outcomes, the evidence is not compelling. CPD will, however, continue to be a requirement for maintaining a licence.

What this suggests is that there is a need for CPD providers to evaluate not only their participants' satisfaction, but also the longer term effects of CPD on the professionals' practice and health outcomes of the professionals' clients. There is also an argument for the cost-effectiveness of CPD and of regulating continuing competence through CPD to be thoroughly evaluated in the future. In the meantime, nurses in every practice setting will need to ensure that they collect, collate and can produce evidence of their own CPD activities.

Reflections

Table 19.1 on page 445 lists the activities that are considered effective CPD activities. Which of these would be most relevant for your practice setting? Are there activities that you currently do (for example, practice audits) that would meet the standards?

CASE STUDY

Name of nurse
Ellen Rowatt

Practice
Woori Yallock Medical Centre, Woori Yallock, Vic.

CPD ACTIVITIES

Pap smear course
Immunisation course
Wound management course
Domestic violence counselling
Certificate IV in Workplace Training and Assessment
Post Graduate Certificate of Women's Health
Post Graduate Diploma of Primary Health Care
Master of Primary Health Care

IMPETUS FOR CPD

I was aware that when I commenced practice nursing I would need to develop and maintain skills in many diverse areas. Initially, the education was acknowledgment of my professional responsibility to ensure competence, but the course that I am presently completing (Master of Primary Health Care) has provided a comprehensive base that can be applied to many areas of my work. It has also increased my overall understanding of nursing as a profession and the often complex care needs required by patients which has, in turn, greatly increased the confidence of patients.

Nurses in general practice are often isolated from colleagues and there is limited opportunity for information exchange, therefore, continuing education also offers peer support and feedback which is invaluable. Practice nursing continues to evolve as a profession with a community and professional expectation of advanced competence and regulation.

BENEFITS OF CPD

Continuing professional development has increased the depth and confidence of my nursing practice that has had multiple benefits for me personally, the people I care for and the practice. I do not perceive practice nursing as 'task orientated', but as integrated and holistic care of the whole person and their family, which includes education, support, networking and physical care. The depth of knowledge required when approaching nursing from this viewpoint can only be genuinely acquired by gradually developing layers of knowledge, each built on the previous one. I am always surprised by the development of my practice after further education, even if it has been in an area that I have felt confident about. The authority gained by further study has given me greater scope when discussing health issues with patients, which has translated into a high degree of integrity for myself and the practice. I personally feel that continuing education is a professional responsibility that cannot be emphasised too much, and should be acknowledged as an ongoing need during undergraduate years.

Key messages

CPD requirements are in place and are not likely to disappear in the future.

Nurses in every practice setting will need to ensure that they collect, collate and can produce evidence of their own CPD activities.

A variety of options is available for practice nurses to undertake CPD activities.

Useful resources

Australian Nursing and Midwifery Council Continuing Competence Framework
http://www.anmc.org.au

Royal College of Nursing Australia
http://www.rcna.org.au> (3LP site)

Australian College of Midwives
http://www.midwives.org.au

Nurses Board of Victoria (proformas)
http://www.nbv.org.au

References

1. *Alberta RN* 2007, 10 000 members report on impact of continuing competence program on practice, results of survey, vol. 63, no. 1, p. 6.

2. Andre, K & Heartfield, M 2007, *Professional portfolios: evidence of competency for nurses and midwives*, Churchill Livingstone, Elsevier, Sydney.

3. Australian Nursing and Midwifery Council 2009, 'Continuing Competence Framework', *Australian Nursing and Midwifery Council*, viewed 8 August 2009, <http://www.anmc.org.au/>.

4. Barriball, KL & While, AE 1996, 'Participation in CPE in nursing: findings of an interview study', *Journal of Advanced Nursing*, vol. 23, pp. 999–1007.

5. Barriball, KL, While, AE & Norman, IJ 1992, 'Continuing professional education for qualified nurses: a review of the literature', *Journal of Advanced Nursing*, vol. 17, pp. 1129–40.

6. Cleland, JA, Fritz, JM, Brennan, GP & Magel, J 2009, 'Does continuing education improve physical therapists' effectiveness in treating neck pain: a randomised clinical trial', *Physical Therapy*, vol. 89, no. 1, pp. 38–47.

7. *Engineers Australia* 2009, 'Continuing professional development policy', viewed 8 August 2009, <http://www.engineersaustralia.org.au/>.

8. Hardwick, S & Jordan, S 2002, 'The impact of part-time post registration degrees on practice', *Journal of Advanced Nursing*, vol. 38, no. 5, pp. 524–35.

9. Hogston, R 1995, 'Nurses' perceptions of the impact of continuing professional education on the quality of nursing care', *Journal of Advanced Nursing*, vol. 22, pp. 586–93.

10. International Council of Nurses 2005, 'Regulation terminology', *International Council of Nurses*, viewed 5 October 2009, <http://www.icn.ch/Regulation_Terminology.pdf>.

11. Mansouri, M & Lockyer, J 2007, 'A meta-analysis of continuing medical education effectiveness', *Journal of Continuing Education in the Health Professions*, vol. 27, no. 1, pp. 6–15.

12. Nolan, M, Owens, RG & Nolan, J 1995, 'Continuing professional education: identifying the characteristics of an effective system', *Journal of Advanced Nursing*, vol. 21, pp. 551–60.

13. Paul, C 1988, 'The New Zealand cervical cancer study: could it happen again?', *BMJ*, vol. 297, pp. 533–9.

14. Pearson, A, Fitzgerald, M, Walsh, K & Borbasi, S 2002, 'Continuing competence and the regulation of nursing practice', *Journal of Nursing Management*, vol. 10, pp. 357–64.

15. Perry, L 1995, 'Continuing professional education: luxury or necessity?', *Journal of Advanced Nursing*, vol. 21, pp. 766–71.

16. Prystowsky, JB & Bordage, G 2001, 'An outcomes research perspective on medical education: the predominance of trainee assessment and satisfaction', *Medical Education*, vol. 35, pp. 331–6.

17. Queensland College of Teachers 2008, 'Policy: Continuing Professional Development Framework', *Queensland College of Teachers*, viewed 8 August 2009, <http://www.qct.edu.au>.

18. Queensland Nursing Forum 1998, 'A focus on continuing competence', *Queensland Nursing Council*, vol. 6, no. 1, pp. 3–4, viewed 8 August 2009, <http://www.qnc.qld.gov.au>.

19. The Royal Australian College of General Practitioners 2008, 'Introducing the 2008–2010 RACGP QA&CPD Program', *The Royal Australian College of General Practitioners*, viewed 5 October 2009, <http://www.racgp.org.au>.

20. Thomson O'Brien, MA, Oxman, AD, Davis, DA, Haynes, RB, Freemantle, N & Harvey, EL 2001, 'Educational outreach visits: effects on professional practice and health care outcomes (Cochrane Review)', *The Journal of Continuing Education in the Health Professions*, vol. 22, pp. 121–4.

21. Yuen, F 1991, 'Continuing nursing education: some issues', *Journal of Advanced Nursing*, vol. 16, pp. 1233–7.

Chapter twenty

Leadership

by Anne McMurray

Overview

This chapter examines the potential of leadership development in practice nursing as well as the advantages of leadership for building personal and professional capacity. The resulting improvement in patient outcomes is also considered. The distinction is made between leadership and management and the discussion outlines the synergies between the two. The foundation of clinical leadership is explained and implications for practice addressed, particularly in the context of collaborative practice. The chapter ends with a discussion of mentorship and the importance of networking and mentoring programs for the ongoing development of practice nursing.

Objectives

At the completion of this chapter you should be able to:

- describe the characteristics of good leaders;

- compare the differences between leadership and management;

- explain your leadership strengths (and weaknesses) in practice and their impact on client outcomes;

- identify the leadership role of practice nurses in collaboration and teamwork; and

- describe the advantages of mentorship, the qualities of leadership mentors and strategies for developing mentoring programs.

Leadership

Leadership has been described as 'the capacity of a human community to shape its future' (Senge 2002, p. 13). This is based on the notion that leadership creates an avenue for influencing the way members of a community develop and sustain their common goals. Good leaders help develop this capacity by combining their innate skills and abilities with considerable hard work to challenge, inspire, empower and act as a role model for others. For some, this is embellished with artistic flair and charisma. For others it is a deliberate, conscientious and committed progression towards excellence achieved through rational planning and hard work. The best leaders are able to balance both sides of the coin (or the brain) sometimes simultaneously, sometimes sequentially. A charismatic personality which draws on personal charm can be helpful but it must be accompanied by the substance of strategic thinking, change management skills, personal strength, confidence, negotiation skills, knowledge management and willingness to form strategic alliances (Jooste 2004).

Leadership is widely acknowledged as an essential foundation for nursing practice across the entire continuum, from basic nursing care to making decisions that affect systems, policies or professional regulation. Nurses in all settings need leadership skills that are responsive to people's health needs, appropriate in the social and regulatory context, and visionary in terms of balancing current workforce and professional needs with the demands of home and community life and planning for an uncertain future (Davidson, Elliott & Daly 2006). This is a big ask.

Leadership at the point of service, such as occurs in practice nursing, is challenging, but it can sometimes be more rewarding in that context than in other nursing settings. Patients in hospital often feel 'processed' rather than cared for, being moved through the system quickly, with a sense of urgency and little time to discuss their ongoing needs, especially for information. In general practice there is an opportunity to engage with people on a more meaningful level, making sure that their needs for treatment, guidance, information and follow-up are met. This is both an opportunity and a challenge. It requires leadership skills to oversee the smooth transitions involved in a person's care, to promote continuity of services, and to ensure that the practice clients are

Reflections

Is continuity of care a priority in your practice?
Do you use a particular strategy for maintaining continuity of care?
How does your practice documentation system affect continuity of care?

provided with safe, high quality care and appropriate advice on maintaining their health and preventing illness or injury. Leadership skills that enable these activities are cultivated in working with others and interacting across personal and professional settings.

To help shape 'the human community' of practice nursing the following definition of good leadership behaviours as described two decades ago by Kouzes and Posner (1988) remains the gold standard.

Good leaders:

- challenge process, learning from the past but living in the present;
- inspire a shared vision, creating a force that invents the future;
- enable others to act, by mentoring, turning followers into leaders;
- model the way by example, living the values and planning for their successors; and
- encourage the heart by celebrating the achievements of themselves and others.

(Kouzes & Posner 1988)

The ideal image of a good leader epitomises courage. Courageous leaders practise with their eye and their intellect on the big picture; however, they also create cycles of personal and professional affirmation and confidence that are fuelled by small, incremental successes. Courageous leaders become adept at articulating their contribution and that of their team, which makes visible their acceptance of the leadership role, attracts support from those around them, and inspires others to become leaders.

Good leaders go where there is no path and leave a trail. They embrace the change agent role willingly, understanding that managing change is the primary role of a leader, and that role modelling for others will help grow their own as well as others' strengths (Graetz 2000; Porter-O'Grady & Malloch 2003). When change is rapid and substantial they take time to reflect, creating a natural space for themselves and other members of the team in the new version of the workplace, so each of them can find a level of stability and renewal (Sullivan 1999). They live out of imagination, not history. They trust others. They flatten and reshape hierarchies by building alliances. This is extremely important in practice nursing, where, just as in rural areas, it takes a concerted effort to connect nurses who are geographically isolated. Networking is therefore a critical, fundamental element of good leadership (Borbasi & Gaston 2002).

Reflections

Identify the most useful networks you have either established or joined in practice nursing.
Which of these are within your geographic area, or which are personal?
Which are 'virtual' networks?
What are the strengths and weaknesses of personal versus virtual networks?

Good leaders also design opportunities for ideas to flourish with good timing and good judgment. This creates mutual respect and an environment wherein 'difference, diversity and ambiguity' are not just tolerated; they are celebrated (Porter-O'Grady & Malloch 2003). As individuals, good leaders are self-regulating, stretching their capacity, rather than their ego, recognising their prejudices and shortcomings as well as their talents (Kouzes & Posner 1988). In nursing practice, they understand the 'bi-cultural' nature of professional leadership, retaining professional values on one level while recognising and influencing the wider social and policy context of health care on the other (Antrobus & Kitson 1999). They are confident in their own skills but not rigid. And they know that when leadership becomes an obligation rather than an opportunity for change, it's time to bail out (Drucker 1999; Kotter 1990; Porter-O'Grady & Malloch 2003).

Accepting a leadership role does not always come easily to nurses, especially when their practice experience has been predominantly in a rigid, hierarchical environment such as a hospital or other institution. This type of organisational culture often prohibits self-development and creative thinking, although this is beginning to change with the pressure to increases nurses' satisfaction to promote greater retention of the workforce. Another barrier to the development of leadership behaviours lies within nurses themselves. The motivation to develop leadership capacity can sometimes be sabotaged by nurses' propensity to bypass, downplay or devalue their work. This creates misunderstandings about the importance of nursing where it is most vital, that is, at the point of service, and perpetuates the myth that practising nurses are virtuous, meek and self-sacrificing (Miller et al. 2008). This couldn't be further from the reality of contemporary nursing practice, especially in the context of today's significant financial constraints and the pressure to manage effectively and efficiently.

Reflections

How do you convey the scope of your practice role to others in the practice?
How do you gain acceptance within the practice for your leadership skills?
To what extent do the financial aspects of the practice affect your leadership role?

Leadership and management

Because leadership and management are often confused as similar processes, it is helpful to look at the distinctive and complementary elements of both. Kotter, a well-known Harvard professor of business, contends that too many workplaces are over-managed and under-led. In his view, what our turbulent and rapidly changing workplaces need is active recruitment of people with leadership potential, who can then be exposed to capacity-building career experiences (Kotter 2001). He explains leadership as something that is designed to create change. It is a strategic endeavour, focused on promoting the aspirations of the group. Leaders establish direction, aligning people by helping empower them, and motivating and inspiring them to achieve the vision. Management is about controlling complexity to bring order and consistency to the work. It revolves around planning, budgeting, organising, staffing and problem solving (Kotter 1990). So although both leaders and managers may play a part in decision making and planning, management is primarily concerned with operational activities such as coordination and resource allocation, which are intended to meet organisational goals (Leach 2008). Table 20.1 below illustrates these differences.

Table 20.1 Comparison of management and leadership tasks

	Managers	**Leaders**
Create an agenda	plan and budget	set direction
Develop a human network	organise and staff	align people, groups
Execute the agenda	control, solve problems	motivate, inspire
Impact	**Create order**	**Produce change**

Source: Kotter 1990

Practice nursing requires a management skill set that is developed over time and on the job. This is especially relevant for the skills required for negotiation, advocacy and lobbying (Halcomb, Davidson & Patterson 2008). Advocacy is a necessary part of good and best practice to ensure appropriate, effective, responsive and safe patient care (Watson 2008). Negotiations are a cornerstone of both leadership and management interactions, especially in managing information and communication. The fine art of lobbying ranges from requesting resources for self-development to those needed to service the breadth of clients attending the practice. At another level, lobbying also involves the politics of professional practice in lobbying the profession and the health care system for greater visibility in what practice nurses are doing, clarifying what is changing in the context of practice or education, and anticipating how and when change or the lack of change is affecting the health of people. It requires courage to hold practice, its knowledge base and its outcomes up to scrutiny, even when this causes reconsideration of a course of action.

Reflections

To what extent does your practice involve you in planning and budgeting? How would you go about gaining recognition for your problem-solving skills? What strategies would you develop to 'align people' to achieve the goals of the practice?

Clinical leadership

Clinical nursing leadership is typically described in terms of the leader's behaviours, the particular situation requiring leadership, or the needs of followers (Shaw 2007; Sullivan & Decker 2005). By far the most prevalent theory of nursing leadership is *transformational leadership*, which is based on the idea of the nurse as *facilitator*, working with others to inspire and empower others, and help build capacity (Burns 1978; Leach 2008; Porter-O'Grady & Malloch 2003). Transformational leaders are often charismatic and work towards engendering trust in those around them (Porter-O'Grady & Malloch 2003). Members of the work team tend to gravitate to them because they seem to understand themselves and their place in the scheme of things. This self-understanding and consistency between values, beliefs and actions complement other skills such as expertise, flexibility and the ability to articulate expectations for the future (Ward 2002). These characteristics embody what has been described as emotional competence (Malloch & Porter-O'Grady 2005). As these authors suggest, the emotionally competent leader understands that:

- leadership is all about relationships;
- leadership requires emotional balance;
- conflict is present in all relationships;
- communication skills are not optional;
- the leader never owns others' issues or resolves others' problems;
- accountability means that the leader sees that defined outcomes are attained;
- friendship is not a component of the role; and
- the leader keeps no secrets, in fact, favours disclosure.

(Malloch & Porter-O'Grady 2005)

Nurses gravitate to transformational leadership theory because it is visionary, dynamic and focuses on 'doing' rather than 'creating' (Stanley 2008). This fits well with practice nursing, where the nurse can influence others by being a good communicator, building relationships, being motivational and articulating their clinical and leadership competence and knowledge (Stanley 2008).

There is a view that in practice, leadership and management should coexist, with all clinical leaders having some managerial responsibility to ensure operational effectiveness (Christian 1998; Sullivan & Decker 2005). However, as Kotter (1990) cautions, care must be taken to ensure that in assigning responsibility for effectiveness or efficiency, the practice does not become 'over-managed' and 'under-led'.

Reflections

Which aspects of your practice tend to require too much management or too little leadership?
Are you able to control the flow of work to negotiate improvements in efficiency?
How do you know when your leadership is enhancing practice effectiveness?

Collaboration, teamwork and leadership

One of the most challenging leadership issues in practice nursing lies in fostering genuine collaboration among all members of the practice team. Whenever teamwork is required in a workplace there must be complementary skills, commitment to a common purpose and goals, and mutual accountability (Javellana-Anunciado 2007). Good teamwork has a number of advantages. These include organisational benefits, benefits to team members themselves and, for the patients, enhanced satisfaction, acceptance of treatment and improved health outcomes (Mickan 2005). Ideally, the practice team focus is on instances of parallel, independent care around patient needs (Phillips et al. 2008). Putting patients at the centre of care ahead of managerial throughput and professional gatekeeping is a major step towards collaborative thinking (Donaldson 2001; Patterson & McMurray 2003). This reflects today's inclusive approach where patients are seen as partners in care, capable of making informed but autonomous decisions and participating in their own care (Iedema et al. 2008; Kravitz & Melnikow 2001). Good leaders nurture this type of participation.

Practice collaboration is a term that is readily accepted, but the notion of autonomy is often misunderstood. Autonomy implies authority, freedom and discretion in making judgments (Wiggins 2008). In nursing, *clinical* autonomy applies these principles to the care of patients, whereas *work* autonomy involves freedom and discretion in scheduling work, initiating processes and procedures, goal setting and evaluation (Weston 2009). Neither clinical autonomy nor work autonomy means that a person acts exclusively or independent of others, especially in a situation such as practice nursing where all members of the practice are accountable for outcomes. In a well-functioning team a nurse can make independent decisions within a nursing sphere of practice, and interdependent decisions in those spheres where nursing overlaps with other disciplines (Kramer, Maguire & Schmalenberg 2006). Depending on how the practice is managed, this could involve making some autonomous decisions in relation to health maintenance, prevention, caring and disease management, and participating in shared decision making in diagnostic, prescriptive or curative decisions, or alternatively, deferring these to medical management. Clearly, there is no reason why autonomy and teamwork cannot coexist, and this has been substantiated by research demonstrating that the interaction between the two can create synergies rather than conflict (Rafferty, Ball & Aitken 2001; Waldman, Smith & Hood 2003).

Reflections

What leadership skills would be most important in developing this type of approach?

How would you build a business case for developing this type of system?

Some practice nurses have developed innovative ways of dealing with GP shortages and high practice demands in regional and rural areas by conducting home visits for clients with chronic conditions or intermittent needs that can readily be dealt with in the home. This has increased efficiency while maintaining safe, high-quality care. The system has helped maintain patient flow as well as patient and staff satisfaction, which is important in a practice with frequent changes of locum practitioners.

Successful team leaders are able to persuade all members of the team to collaborate in working toward shared goals, and to develop a shared language with which to communicate (Carroll & Quijada 2004). This includes genuine attempts to help transform apprehensions about the change in status and relationships, to accommodate one another's vested interests and to reframe relationships. Like all changes, it requires time, energy and a collegial environment that helps build inclusiveness and solidarity. As nurses we tend to come from diverse backgrounds with few opportunities to consolidate our views or share our needs, especially when we practise in isolation. Most medical practitioners do not experience the same communication barriers because of their background and education, which often results in them forming strong bonds that become reinforced over time (McPherson, Smith-Lovin & Cook 2001). Unfortunately, the reality of work pressures, the subjugation of roles to the dominance of medical practitioners and continuation of a hierarchical model of practice often interfere with collaborative relationships. Perpetuating an 'expert' hierarchical model of practice wherein each level of practice is under the direct control of the practitioner dilutes nurses' willingness or ability to articulate an expansion of roles or capacity to make judgments on the basis of individual cases (Brown, McWilliam & Ward-Griffin 2006; Carryer et al. 2007). It is also a barrier to teaching and creating partnerships with patients, especially in situations where nurses know intuitively how important the transfer of knowledge would be to them. Other barriers to practice collaboration include a lack of explicit, appropriate tasks and role definitions, an absence of clear leadership, insufficient time for team building, the 'us and them' effects of professional education and socialisation, and frustration from power and status differentials (Zwarenstein & Reeves 2006).

Mentorship

Like other professionals, nurses become socialised to the profession and its core values primarily through mentoring and modelling (Campbell, Dardis & Campbell 2003). A mentor is typically an experienced (and often wiser) person who guides, supports and nurtures a less experienced person (Sullivan & Decker 2005). Professional values are learned when significant individuals or 'champions' model desirable behaviours. This can be invaluable in helping to clarify the ambiguities and contradictions that sometimes arise when a nurse is isolated, such as in rural practice or when new to a role, and can be reassuring to those new to practice nursing (Heartfield & Gibson 2005; Mills, Lennon & Francis 2006).

Mentorship programs can be formalised or simply be the spontaneous bonding that occurs informally between mentors and mentees. Mentoring can also be enjoyable and a source of personal satisfaction and growth as well as an effective pathway to leadership development (Campbell, Dardis & Campbell 2003; Van Eps et al. 2006). Currently, the Australian General Practice Network (AGPN) has initiated a pilot project to inform development of a national structured mentoring program to support practice nurses in dealing with a range of challenges. Most of these have been identified in the Commonwealth review of practice nurses (AGPN 2009). They include fragmentation of the sector and variation in size and structure of practices; diversity of roles and cultures; a system of accreditation that does not link continuing education to registration; the need to share across settings; the need to integrate nurses' career plans with practice plans; the challenge of developing shared understandings between general practitioners and nurses; and funding for appropriate and sustainable mentoring programs (Heartfield & Gibson 2005). Expectations are that the AGPN mentorship program will help address at least some of these.

Mentoring programs vary to some degree, but there is widespread agreement on the fundamental characteristics of a mentor. These include the following:

- trust
- openness to new ideas
- valuing knowledge

- compassion
- presence—being able to 'walk' the journey
- mindfulness
- passionate optimism
- resilience
- balance
- impulse control and
- emotional competence.

Emotional competence allows the mentor to demonstrate optimism and emotional availability (Porter-O'Grady & Malloch 2003).

Being a mentor means showing a person how to access the appropriate clinical knowledge and tools, how to make accurate clinical judgments and when to refer on to secure the required expertise. As the mentee develops, the mentor takes on a role as the 'guide on the side' rather than the 'sage on the stage', helping build the toolkit rather than the outcomes. This is done with a commitment to walk a mile in the other's shoes, and a deep understanding of the vulnerabilities we all have as learners. The mentor then provides the impetus for mentees to stretch their capacity while preserving egos that are porous and receptive, not ones that become a casualty of the process. The opposite of this is toxic mentoring, where the mentor tries to transfer knowledge rather than building capacity. In this case, the mentor sets up a situation where they try to shape the mentee's development to mirror their own. This leads to failure to thrive. If people are being mentored toward emotional competence, they will embrace the *next* step in the journey, rather than the last, and rather than mimic the characteristics of the mentor, they will develop their own career openly and decisively (Porter-O'Grady & Malloch 2003). Of course, mentorship is also reciprocal: as a person fosters another's development they also build their own capacity, which has benefits for both individuals and helps strengthen the profession.

How can mentoring programs be developed?

Little research evidence is available to guide the development of mentoring programs, which makes best practice difficult to define (Smith, McAllister & Snype Crawford 2001). However, leadership programs can help, especially in women's leadership programs. It is difficult for some women to keep up with changes when they have career interruptions, and the longer span of work life adds a multiplier factor to their disadvantage. Goleman (2002) suggests we create a more tribal feel. Like others, he argues that becoming a good leader requires 'soul'; that is, using the emotion, identity and character that we all have in us, and using it to maximise our leadership potential (Goleman 2002; Shaw 2007). In Goleman's view, the tribal leader creates the table and invites others to sit down. This approach celebrates everyone's accomplishments, bringing to the team a sense of safety and encouragement for sharing ideas and working within their own style or comfort zone, which can help create a stronger professional identity.

The implication for change in practice nursing is that all change must begin with developing sensitivity to our own and others' capabilities and tendencies by fostering a culture of self-reflection and a place for the safe exchange of ideas and feedback (Caramanica, Cousino & Petersen 2003; Ray, Turkel & Marino 2002). This type of work culture is energising. Expectations are made explicit, reinforced, and are based on the knowledge that each action has some bearing on client outcomes (Davies, Nutley & Mannion 2000). In contrast, when disillusionment reigns, high levels of stress interfere with clarity of thinking and receptivity to change. The quality of communication suffers, leaving the work unit bathed in suspicion rather than anticipation of success. This creates stagnation rather than the empowerment to be persuasive and to consider new and innovative health care models, which runs counter to the Commonwealth Government's vision of the new wave in health care where practice nurses feature prominently. Linking personal affirmation with this type of political savvy is crucial to professional development (McKenna, Keeney & Bradley 2004).

At the organisational level there are some explicit steps that can be taken to make leadership more integral to professional practice. The first and most important of these revolves around making nursing work visible. Knowing and communicating the things that matter, how *you* made a difference, how this fits into the bigger picture, how your ideas and approaches to your work can be justified as strategies for another occasion, how your work helps advance the work of the team, how your mentorship helps pass knowledge and skills onto the next person. The second step involves our professional obligation to socialise successive generations of nurses into the profession and into our specialty areas which is not always guaranteed in our education programs (Aagaard & Hauer 2003). Empowerment, even the perception of empowerment, is contagious. Where the leadership is powerful and there is organisational support, others become empowered by association and everybody's job satisfaction increases.

The source of work satisfaction for most of us flows from making a difference, from questioning the possible, pondering the probable and choosing the preferred future (Miller, Maloney & Maloney 2008). Where this is valued, rewarded and modelled in the workplace it creates structural empowerment (Patrick & Spence Laschinger 2006).

Even the greatest leaders have moments of personal insecurity, uncertainty in practice judgments or strategies, and times when the busyness of work overrides their ability to act with tact and diplomacy. Yet these are the traits leaders aspire to achieve (Hyett 2003). Enabling 'ordinary people to produce

Reflections

1. Think of someone in your sphere of influence (either at work or in your personal network) with a charismatic personality. How does that person seem to influence decisions? To what extent do you think that person is perceived to be more knowledgeable than others? What lessons on leadership would you take from how that person handles themself in a group situation?

2. What would be some practical strategies for connecting practice nurses with one another? What persuasive arguments could be made for the practice to support your membership in the local and national practice nurse association or network?

3. It can be said that good leaders use their personal characteristics to best advantage. What are some of your personal leadership qualities? How are you able to use these qualities to influence others?

4. One of the most difficult leadership challenges is trying to help co-workers who do not understand their role in the workplace. In this type of situation how would you, as the leader, help build others' capacity to achieve team goals?

5. Consider the extent to which you have clinical autonomy and work autonomy. Is either or both sufficient for what you would like to achieve in your practice environment? If not, how would you go about securing a change? What obstacles or facilitating factors would you have to deal with to succeed?

6. What are some of the things that promote or enhance collaboration in your practice? What leadership strategies would promote collaboration or ensure its continuity?

7. Think of a mentor who has influenced your career. Describe that person's distinguishing features in rich detail, especially those you'd like to emulate.

extraordinary things in the face of challenge and change' creates inner leadership that can make a difference to people's lives, and the work of the team or the practice (Jooste 2004, p. 217). It is circumscribed within the simple act of watching over those entrusted to nursing care, knowing when and how to influence them, being prepared to celebrate your diversity and theirs, your knowledge and theirs, your needs and theirs. This is a partnership mindset. It is a prescription that cuts across all challenges, all settings and all nations. It begins with a clear vision, a willingness to share and a commitment to the work of the health care and practice team, its actions and outcomes. This builds capacity from within and without, perpetrating understanding and shared solutions to the breadth of problems that often seem insurmountable. With strong leadership these can be resolved one step at a time.

Conclusion

Practice nursing is increasingly recognised as a major element of our health care system. Leadership skills are crucial to ensuring the continuing development of this important specialised role. The main objectives of leadership development are to improve client outcomes, enhance practice effectiveness, and advance personal and professional goals. This requires teamwork, collaboration and excellent communication skills, all of which are fundamental characteristics of good leaders.

Judy Evans, president of Australian Practice Nurses Association, 2007–08
My experience of leadership and what it has taught me

Working as a sole nurse in a large practice challenged my skills as a leader and my ability to seek mentorship as I pursued a career as a practice nurse. To consolidate my place within the practice team I found I had to defend my decisions, argue my worth and demonstrate the preservation of the nursing process in the medical model of general practice. As I achieved goals, demonstrated my abilities and gained respect from my colleagues my confidence grew and I took on the challenge to understand what was required of a leader.

My first experience of leadership was in organising a local nursing network. Through this I learnt that leadership required clarity of vision, the ability to enthuse others to broaden their potential and to choose goals that were valued and balanced with expected outcomes. I also recognised the value of mentoring. The nursing network that I nurtured grew and when I chose to step aside there were others who had the confidence, skills and vision to become leaders and continue the work that I had started.

Within a few years I found myself as president of the Australian Practice Nurses Association. Between these two milestones I developed a clear understanding of my vision for practice nursing; belief in my abilities to lead, advocate for colleagues and negotiate our position. I sought relationships with others who had similar energy to me, but who had diverse expertise so that we could work together and learn from one another to get the job done. The key elements to building these relationships were reliable and honest communications and inclusivity when making decisions. This was a journey that included the influence of mentors and the privilege of engaging with nursing colleagues. A mentor provided me with a central point in which I could reflect on my achievements and disappointments. It provided me with a forum to build my opinions and the ability to defend and debate them.

My own experience of leadership taught me the worth of questioning and challenging the status quo, and that it is okay to be a lone voice in the discussion. To have independence in your opinion and a questioning mind can open opportunities for learning for yourself and for others. Leadership, I have learnt, is not about ownership of the agenda but about encouraging others to take some steps with you through what can be a perilous journey at times, to forge ahead despite setbacks, to inspire and motivate others to achieve their goals as well as your own.

The skill of being a good leader requires the time to reflect and build on your vision. Choose where to start, apply critical thinking and set goals that are achievable but also inspirational. When you are in the position of a nursing leader, whether it be in your practice or as leader of an organisation, others are watching and observing you. I feel that is it important that leadership be infectious; encouraging others to step into the arena. At all times maintain your enthusiasm for the job and create humour in the process.

By taking on the role of leader, diverse opportunities opened up that I would not have had the privilege to take and grow from.

Key messages

Leadership skills are essential for practice nurses.

Leadership skills can affect continuity of patient care and help maintain practice efficiency, effectiveness and quality.

Good leaders challenge process, inspire a shared vision, enable others to act, model the behaviours they expect of others and celebrate their achievements and those of others.

Leadership creates change, while management strives for order and consistency. Both require high-level communication skills.

Teamwork and collaboration are fundamental to practice nursing.

Mentoring and networking are essential for practice nurses to remain connected with one another and stretch their capacity for change.

References

1. Aagaard, E & Hauer, K 2003, 'A cross-sectional descriptive study of mentoring relationships formed by medical students', *Journal of General Internal Medicine*, vol. 18, pp. 298–302.

2. Antrobus, S & Kitson, A 1999, 'Nursing leadership: influencing and shaping health policy and nursing practice', *Journal of Advanced Nursing*, vol. 29, no. 3, pp. 746–53.

3. Australian General Practice Network (AGPN) 2009, *National mentoring pilot program for nursing in general practice*, viewed 18 May 2009, <http://www.generalpracticenursing.com.au/>.

4. Borbasi, S & Gaston, C 2002, 'Nursing and the 21st century: what's happened to leadership?', *Collegian*, vol. 19, no. 1, pp. 31–5.

5. Brown, D, McWilliam, C & Ward-Griffin, C 2006, 'Client-centred empowering partnership in nursing', *Journal of Advanced Nursing*, vol. 53, no. 2, pp. 160–8.

6. Burns, J 1978, *Leadership*, Harper & Row, New York.

7. Campbell, D, Dardis, G & Campbell, K 2003, 'Enhancing incremental influence: A focused approach to leadership development', *Journal of Leadership and Organizational Studies*, vol. 10, no. 1, pp. 29–44.

8. Caramanica, L, Cousino, J & Petersen, S 2003, 'Four elements of a successful quality program', *Nursing Administration Quarterly*, vol. 27, no. 4, pp. 336–43.

9. Carroll, J & Quijada, M 2004, 'Redirecting traditional professional values to support safety: changing organisational culture in health care', *Quality & Safety in Health Care*, vol. 13, suppl. 11, pp. ii16–ii21.

10. Carryer, J, Gardner, G, Dunn, S & Gardner, A 2007, 'The capability of nurse practitioners may be diminished by controlling protocols', *Australian Health Review*, vol. 31, no. 1, pp. 108–15.

11. Christian, S 1998, 'Clinical leadership in nursing development units', *Journal of Advanced Nursing*, vol. 27, p. 118–116.

12. Davidson, P, Elliott, D & Daly, J 2006, 'Clinical leadership in contemporary clinical practice: implications for nursing in Australia', *Journal of Nursing Management*, vol. 14, no. 3, pp. 180–7.

13. Davies, H, Nutley, S & Mannion, R 2000, 'Organisational culture and quality of health care', *Quality in Health Care*, vol. 9, pp. 111–119.

14. Donaldson, L 2001, 'Safe, high quality care: Investing in tomorrow's leaders', *Quality in Health Care*, vol. 10, suppl. 11, pp. ii8–ii12.

15. Drucker, P 1999, 'Managing oneself', *Harvard Business Review*, vol. 77, no. 2, pp. 65–74.

16. Goleman, D 2002, *The new leaders*, Little Brown, London.

17. Graetz, F 2000, 'Strategic change leadership', *Management Decision*, vol. 38, no. 8, pp. 550–62.

18. Halcomb, E, Davidson, P & Patterson, E 2008, 'Promoting leadership and management in Australian general practice nursing: what will it take?' *Journal of Nursing Management*, vol. 16, pp. 846–52.

19. Heartfield, M & Gibson, T 2005, 'Mentoring for nurses in general practice: national issues and challenges', *Collegian*, vol. 12, no. 2, pp. 17–21.

20. Hyett, E 2003, 'What blocks health visitors from taking on a leadership role?' *Journal of Nursing Management*, vol 11, pp. 229–33.

21. Iedema, R, Sorensen, R, Jorm, C & Piper, D 2008, 'Co-producing care', in R Sorensen & R Iedema (eds), *Managing clinical processes in health services'*, Elsevier, Sydney, pp. 105–20.

22. Javellana-Anunciado, C 2007, 'Effective team building', in P Kelly (ed), *Nursing leadership and management*, 2nd edn, Thomson Delmar Learning, Clifton Park NY, pp. 246–58.

23. Jooste, K 2004, 'Leadership: A new perspective'. *Journal of Nursing Management*, vol. 12, pp. 217–23.

24. Kotter, J 1990, *A force for change: How leadership differs from management*, The Free Press, New York.

25. Kotter, J 2001, 'What leaders actually do', *Harvard Business Review*, vol. 79, no. 11, pp. 85–97.

26. Kouzes, J & Posner, B 1988, *The leadership challenge*, Jossey-Bass, San Francisco.

27. Kramer, M, Maguire, P & Schmalenberg, C 2006, 'Excellence through evidence: the what, when, and where of clinical autonomy', *Journal of Nursing Management*, vol. 36, no. 10, pp. 479–91.

28. Kravitz, R & Melnikow, J 2001, 'Engaging patients in medical decision making' *British Medical Journal*, vol. 323, pp. 584–5.

29. Leach, L 2008, 'Nursing leadership and management', in P Kelly (ed), *Nursing leadership and management*, 2nd edn, Thomson Delmar Learning, Clifton Park NY, pp. 1–30.

30. Malloch, K & Porter-O'Grady, T 2005, *The quantum leader: applications for the new world of work*, Jones and Bartlett, New York.

31. McKenna, H, Keeney, S & Bradley, M 2004, 'Nurse leadership within primary care: the perceptions of community nurses, GP's policy makers and members of the public', *Journal of Nursing Management*, vol. 12, pp. 69–76.

32. McPherson, M, Smith-Lovin, L & Cook, J 2001, 'Birds of a feather: homophily in social networks', *Annual Review of Sociology*, vol. 27, pp. 415–44.

33. Mickan, S 2005, 'Evaluating the effectiveness of health care teams', *Australian Health Review*, vol. 29, no. 2, pp. 211–17.

34. Miller, T, Maloney, R & Maloney, P 2008, 'Power', in P Kelly (ed), *Nursing leadership and management*, 2nd edn, Thomson Delmar Learning, Clifton Park NY, pp. 259–68.

35. Mills, J, Lennon, D & Francis, K 2006, 'Mentoring matters: developing rural nurses knowledge and skills', *Collegian*, vol. 13, no. 3, pp. 33–6.

36. Patrick, A & Spence Laschinger, H 2006, 'The effect of structural empowerment and perceived organizational support on middle level nurse managers' role satisfaction', *Journal of Nursing Management*, vol. 14, no. 1, pp. 13–22.

37. Patterson, E & McMurray, A 2003, 'Collaborative practice between registered nurses and medical practitioners in Australian general practice: moving from rhetoric to reality', *Australian Journal of Advanced Nursing*, vol. 20, no. 4, pp. 43–8.

38. Phillips, C, Pearce, C, Dwan, K, Hall, S, Porritt, J, Yates, R, Kljakovic, M & Sibbald, B 2008, 'Charting new roles for Australian general practice nurses': *Abridged Report of the Australian General Practice Nurses Study*. Australian Primary Health Care Institute, Canberra.

39. Porter-O'Grady, T & Malloch, K 2003, *Quantum leadership: a textbook of new leadership*, Jones and Bartlett, Mississauga.

40. Rafferty, A, Ball, J & Aiken, L 2001, 'Are teamwork and professional autonomy compatible, and do they result in improved hospital care? *Quality in Health Care*, vol. 10, no. 4, pp. 32–8.

41. Ray, M, Turkel, M & Marino, F 2002, 'The transformative process for nursing in workforce redevelopment', *Nursing Administration Quarterly*, vol. 26, no. 2, pp. 1–14.

42. Senge, P 2002, 'Servant leadership: Afterword', in L Spears (ed) *Servant leadership*, [25th anniversary edn]: a journey into the nature of legitimate power and greatness', Paulist Press, New York, pp. 1–13.

43. Shaw, S 2007, *Nursing leadership*, International Council of Nurses and Blackwell Publishing, Oxford.

44. Smith, L, McAllister, L & Snype Crawford, C 2001, 'Mentoring benefits and issues for public health nurses', *Public Health Nursing*, vol. 18, no. 2, pp. 101–7.

45. Stanley, D 2008, 'Congruent leadership: values in action', *Journal of Nursing Management*, vol. 16, no. 5, pp. 519–24.

46. Sullivan, E & Decker, P 2005, *Effective leadership & management in nursing*, 6th edn, Pearson Education Inc, Upper Saddle River, NJ.

47. Sullivan, T 1999, 'Leading people in a chaotic world', *Journal of Educational Administration*, vol. 37, no. 5, pp. 408–23.

48. Van Eps, M, Cooke, M, Creedy, D & Walker, R 2006, 'Mentor evaluation of a year-long mentorship program: A quality improvement initiative', *Collegian*, vol. 13, no. 2, pp. 27–30.

49. Waldman, J, Smith, H & Hood, J 2003, 'Corporate culture: The missing piece of the healthcare puzzle', *Hospital Topics*, vol. 81, no. 1, pp. 5–14.

50. Ward, K 2002, 'A vision for tomorrow: Transformational nursing leaders', *Nursing Outlook*, vol. 50, pp. 121–6.

51. Watson, C 2008, 'Assessing leadership in nurse practitioner candidates', *Australian Journal of Advanced Nursing*, vol. 26, no. 1, pp. 67–76.

52. Weston, M 2009, 'Validity of instruments for measuring autonomy and control over nursing practice', *Journal of Nursing Scholarship*, vol. 41, no. 1, pp. 87–94.

53. Wiggins, M 2008, 'The partnership care delivery model: an examination of the core concept and the need for a new model of care', *Journal of Nursing Management*, vol. 16, no. 5, pp. 629–38.

54. Zwarenstein, M & Reeves, S 2006, 'Knowledge translation and interprofessional collaboration: where the rubber of evidence-based care hits the road of teamwork', *The Journal of Continuing Education in the Health Professions*, vol. 26, no. 1, pp. 46–54.

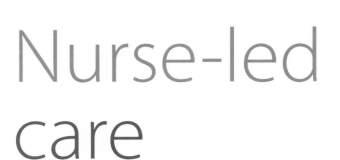

Chapter twenty-one

Nurse-led care

by Judy Evans, Lynne Walker
and Peter Larter

Overview

International and Australian literature provides the evidence that supports a change of orientation of nursing services and offers the opportunity for nurses to review how health care is delivered in general practice. Any change in health care delivery requires the development of new models of care and achieving this will require planning, development, implementation, evaluation and assessment of the sustainability of any new model (Davidson et al. 2005). These skills and processes will form crucial elements in the development of a new nursing care model. This chapter uses the Quality Framework for Australian General Practice developed by the Royal Australian College of General Practitioners (RACGP) to outline a systematic approach that can be used by nurses to develop and implement a nurse-led service. Innovation alone will not guarantee success and the development of a new nursing service will need to be supported by the formulation of a sound business proposal to the practice principals or funders of the service.

Objectives

At the completion of this chapter you should be able to:

- describe the elements of a quality framework;

- relate a quality framework to the establishment of nurse-led care; and

- formulate a business proposal to support the introduction of nurse-led care.

Introduction

The Australian health system is undergoing a reform process which is likely to see many opportunities for health care professionals to provide care in new ways. In response to the ageing of the population, the increasing burden and cost of chronic disease and a recognition of inequities in access to health care, government is looking for ways to fund services that have more of a focus on prevention and ongoing disease management while maintaining an emphasis on improving the safety, quality and equity of access to care (Jolly 2007). Over the past few years, the role of the practice nurse has expanded considerably and includes the shift from nurses performing task-orientated activities to more advanced, team-based clinically autonomous care to meet the needs of the broader community. As the need for redesigning care is recognised, health services will place *'nurses at the forefront with the aim of enabling patients to have greater choice, access and equity of service'* (Redsell & Cheater 2008, p. 69). For nurses to take up this opportunity, they will need to develop skills beyond those regarded as the traditional domain of nursing.

Background

The term 'nurse-led' has been described by Hatchett (2003, p. 5) as

> *a continuum of practice ranging from the nurse having delegated authority to make decisions regarding patient care at one end of the spectrum, to being responsible for all care provided including clinical assessment, treatment, and management of patients undifferentiated by need.*

This is a broad definition but one which encourages practice nurses with a range of skills and scope of practice to initiate a model of nurse-led care in their own health setting. Nurse-led care is patient-centred care founded on equality of opportunity and mutual respect among team members (Hatchett 2005).

There is growing evidence to support nurses being able to provide care within the primary care context that is equal to that provided by primary care doctors and that will achieve positive health outcomes for patients. Keleher et al. (2009) concluded that the evidence suggests that nurses can provide effective health care and that they are particularly effective in enhancing patient knowledge and patient compliance. Positive results have been reported in studies testing the feasibility and outcomes of nurse-run clinics. These include improved clinical outcomes, the feeling of being valued and increased satisfaction with services (Wong & Chung 2006). Sibbald, Laurant and Reeves (2006) state that extending the nursing role is a strategy that will improve service delivery and the evidence suggests that nurse-led chronic disease clinics offers as high-quality clinical care as that delivered by conventional medical practice. The following quote summarises the findings:

> *Not only have nurses been deemed as satisfactory alternative providers of primary health care, patient satisfaction has been found to be higher following nurse consultations for chronic disease and minor illness conditions.*

(Laurent et al. 2008, p. 2)

It can be seen, therefore, that there are many advantages to the health system in supporting nurses in planning, implementing and evaluating models of nursing care that meet both the needs of the community and the patient.

Models of care

A model of care describes the delivery of health care within the broad context of the health care system. Davidson et al. (2005) discusses the ambiguity in the literature in defining the meaning of a model of care, however, they reinforce that the development and evaluation of care delivery should be motivated by improved patient and organisational outcomes. Although part of a team, in this context we are referring to a model of care that is primarily coordinated by nursing staff with support from the general practice team. Nurse-led care focuses on health in the broader sense and has an emphasis on life management rather than diagnosis and intervention (Centre for Evidence-based Nursing South Australia 2007). Although the evidence may point to the effectiveness of alternative models of care, with innovation comes a certain level of uncertainty about whether the model will be safe, effective, sustainable and of high quality. The National Health and Hospitals Reform Commission (NHHRC) has suggested that new models of primary care should meet certain criteria (Chiarella 2008; NHHRC 2009) and Davidson and Elliott (2001) have added further points for inclusion. Together they suggest that models of care should:

- incorporate best practice and evolving evidence regarding health;
- facilitate evidence-based preventive care;
- lead to increased effectiveness, access and efficiency in health care delivery;
- be economically sustainable;
- streamline and strengthen the care for older people and those people with high level and complex care needs due to chronic and/or multisystem illness;holistically manage people close to home;
- holistically manage people close to home;

- be based on evidence wherever possible;
- be based upon assessment of patient and health provider needs;
- include consultation with key stakeholders;
- be considerate of the safety and wellbeing of nurses;
- involve a multidisciplinary approach wherever possible; and
- include interventions that are culturally sensitive and appropriate.

These factors need to be taken into consideration when addressing the challenges of fiscal constraints; the expectations of consumers and other health professionals; quality and safety; the ageing population; and the increasing burden of chronic disease. Although these challenges are well documented, there needs to be a balanced view that identifies the benefits to the patients, the nurse and the practice as to why a new nurse-led model of care deserves the necessary investment in planning, marketing and financial resources.

Benefits of nurse-led care

Benefits of nurse-led care to patients, nurses, practices and the health care system have been identified by Proudfoot et al. (2005) and Whitehorse Division of General Practice (2007) as listed below.

Benefits of nurse-led care to the **patients** include:

- improved access to health and community services;
- improved management of chronic diseases including self-management support;
- increased choice of health provider; and
- improved clinical outcomes.

Benefits of nurse-led care to the **nurses** include:

- increased recognition as a health care provider;
- increased responsibility for patient outcomes;
- further education and professional development;
- increased employment opportunities;
- improved job satisfaction;
- development of management skills; and
- empowerment.

Benefits of nurse-led care to the **practice** include:

- improved working relationships and a multidisciplinary approach;
- cohesive approach to patient care;

- decreased general practitioner (GP) workload;
- increased capacity of the practice;
- increased income;
- increased health promotion opportunities to patients;
- increased range of services offered by the practice;
- improved patient satisfaction; and
- improved recall and reminder systems.

Benefits of nurse-led care to the **health system** may include:

- better population health outcomes;
- lower hospital utilisation;
- better use of skilled health workforce through role redefinition; or
- cost efficiencies.

Reflections

What other benefits to nurse-led care can you add?

A quality framework

A quality framework is a structure that facilitates the systematic analysis of the core principles that underpin the delivery of high-quality care. The importance and relevance of applying a quality framework has been recognised by The Australian Commission on Safety and Quality in Health Care as a key component in ensuring high-quality care for all. Indeed, the commission has begun to develop a framework to improve and align safety and quality of health care delivered across the entire health sector. This framework is being designed for use as the basis of planning and improving all health services.

The Royal Australian College of General Practitioners (RACGP) has developed a quality framework (see Figure 21.1 overleaf) specifically for general practice. The RACGP describes this quality framework as 'a model, a reference, a plan, a source of ideas or a benchmark' (Booth, Snowdon & Lees 2005, p. 3). It can highlight achievements and gaps allowing needs to be targeted without duplication and can be a valuable tool to identify needs, inform decision making and evaluate progress of efforts to deliver health care (Booth & Snowdon 2007). Being adaptable to practices and communities with individual structures makes this a flexible tool in planning any new service.

This chapter will explore the use of these domains at the setting of care level and will be examined separately.

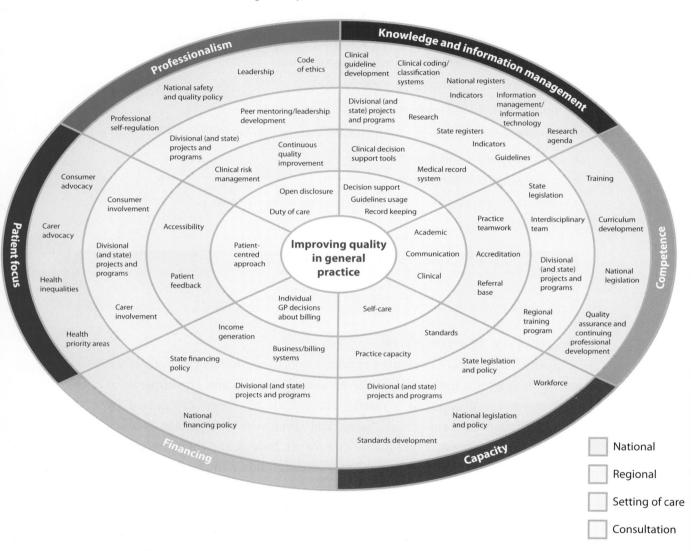

Figure 21.1 A quality framework for general practice
Source: Australian Family Physician 2007

Domains of quality

The RACGP quality framework has identified six interconnected domains to the framework. These domains can be used to systematically identify the quality and safety elements necessary to consider when designing, implementing and evaluating a nurse-led service in the workplace.

Patient focus

One of the six dimensions of quality identified by the Committee on Quality of Health Care in America (2001) was that a health service should be patient-centred and provide respectful and responsive care to individual patient preferences, needs and values. This means providing care in partnership between patients, their families, carers and other health care providers. Patient-centred care should be designed to optimise the patient experience. It is

> responsive to and respectful of the needs, values, differences, and preferences of the patient. It includes additional components: coordinating continuous and timely care; relieving pain and emotional suffering; listening and communicating; providing education and information; sharing decision making and management; preventing disease, disabilities, and impairments; and promoting wellness and healthy behaviour.

(Pruitt & Epping-Jordan 2009, p. 638).

Furthermore the Australian Charter of Healthcare Rights (Australian Commission on Safety and Quality in Health 2008) describes the rights of all people using the Australian health care system as:

1. *Access*—the right to health care
2. *Safety*—a right to safe and high-quality care
3. *Respect*—a right to be shown respect, dignity and consideration
4. *Communication*—a right to be informed about services, treatment, options and costs in a clear and open way
5. *Participation*—a right to be included in decisions and choices about care
6. *Privacy*—a right to privacy and confidentiality of provided information
7. *Comment*—a right to comment on care and having concerns addressed.

The efforts for quality improvement will be futile without a focus on patient involvement in their care as the health outcomes of patients will be influenced by their own engagement in their health care. New technologies are emerging to support patient-centred care and should be considered when new services are being established. These include the use of email, SMS messaging and practice websites to communicate with patients, and Web 2.0 applications (for example, Facebook, Twitter) to engage patients in their care, particularly for youth-orientated clinics.

Reflections

Questions to consider within the patient focus domain in planning a nurse-led service:

- *Is there a need or demand for this service?*
- *How will the patient benefit?*
- *How will it be ensured that patients will use the service?*
- *How will the background of the patient (for example, culture, gender, age) affect what they expect of the service?*
- *Will interpreting services be required?*
- *How will the participation of families and carers be incorporated?*
- *How will patient privacy and confidentiality be respected, and how will this be communicated?*
- *How will the service be evaluated to ensure it meets the patient's expectations?*
- *Does the practice collect patient data that can be used to identify patient needs? Sources include:*
  - *patient feedback, including surveys*
  - *patient complaints register*
  - *data aggregation software, for example, PEN Clinical Audit Tool.*

Example 21.1 Well women's clinic

Cervical screening rates in the geographical region were noted to be well below the national average. The practice nurse, Jane, conducted an audit of the appointments system and discovered that patients were waiting approximately four weeks for a routine Pap test. A patient survey was developed and implemented, and the results provided overwhelming support for the practice to initiate a Well Women's Service. Another finding was that some women indicated that they would only attend the clinic if they could be screened by another female. The service was thus designed to increase access to a female provider in a timely manner for cervical screening and other preventive activities. Jane undertook an accredited Pap test training course and the clinic was established. Marketing for the Well Women's Clinic was pursued through the local paper; a practice information sheet; a phone message on 'call waiting'; posters in the waiting room; and notification on practice recall letters. Patient education material was sourced to better inform patients and provide education on women's health. The clinic was assessed using a range of evaluation tools: written exit survey for all patients attending the clinic; audit of the demand and waiting times for appointments; and a review of the cervical screening rates for the region.

Competence

This domain requires the implementation of appropriate processes to ensure that all health care practitioners are appropriately trained, are actively engaged in ongoing professional development and have current registration to provide the stated service. Competence is discussed in detail in Chapters 3 and 19 but can be defined as:

> *the combination of skills, knowledge, attitudes, values and abilities that underpin effective and/or superior performance in a profession/occupational area.*

> (Australian Nursing and Midwifery Council 2005, p. 8)

Competence implies a specific skill set that can be demonstrated; that is, a proven ability to undertake certain tasks. It is important to be able to define and differentiate between **competence** and **confidence**. Competence in nursing requires reflective practice which enables nurses to develop clear self-knowledge of individual professional competence. Confidence alone may encourage a nurse to undertake a task or skill that they are not fully competent to do.

The level of service provided should be commensurate with the competence of the nurse providing the service. Nurses need to demonstrate competence in the area of clinic service that is being provided. Quality care is more than individual practitioner skills and knowledge. Systematic high-quality care requires competent delivery of clinical care by teams and individual professionals that are appropriately trained and skilled for the tasks.

Reflections

Questions to consider within the competence domain in planning for a nurse-led service:

- Who is going to run the service?
- What skill mix is necessary to provide the service?
  - Registered nurse (Division 1) and/or enrolled nurse (Division 2 nurse)?
  - nurses, administration and general practice staff?
- Will staff require additional training?
- Will staff be interested in this area of clinical work?
- What will be the referral pathway?
- How will you build workforce or human resources sustainability into the service?
- Are the roles and responsibilities for each person involved clearly delineated?

Example 21.2 Nurse-led weight loss clinic

Mary, a practice nurse in a busy rural clinic, identified from practice data that many patients recorded a body mass index (BMI) and waist circumference in excess of guidelines adopted by the practice, and would benefit from weight loss. Mary proposed that a nurse-led service could be offered to patients with a chronic illness as part of their management plans. Furthermore, the clinic would form an important component of the health checks for 45- to 49-year-old patients already at risk of developing a chronic disease. Mary attended nutrition training and a motivational interviewing course to ensure her competence to add weight loss counselling to her scope of practice. Mary became the lead in establishing this clinic and included in the team a GP with interest in this area and key reception staff. Evidence-based advice and information was offered and referral pathways were established to internal and external health care providers, including the dietician and exercise physiologist. An evaluation tool was developed to monitor the success of health outcomes for patients and patients' satisfaction with the service.

Capacity

This domain describes what is essential for sustainable, high-quality and accessible patient-care services. The general practice team cares for patients with a broad and diverse range of health concerns and requires a mixture of skills, equipment, resources, facilities and organisational infrastructure to be able to support the delivery of competent clinical care. Elements such as occupational health and safety, human resource management, infection control, and practice-specific processes and systems are included in this domain. Care is delivered across episodic presentations, planned prevention interventions and ongoing clinical management, and these require planned appointments, recall and reminder systems, rosters, practice management and strategic systems and processes.

Reflections

Questions to consider within the capacity domain in planning for a nurse-led service:

- Are there adequate resources within the practice to run this service? For example, is there:
  - room availability and appropriate equipment?
  - evidence to support the clinic?
- What are the occupational health and safety issues?
- Are practice policies and procedures in place and are they current?
- Who will absorb the additional workload in running the clinic?
- What actual services will be offered?
- Where will the service be delivered?
- Will the service be delivered:
  - in clinic hours or after hours?
  - weekdays, weekends or evenings?
- Will patient privacy be preserved?

Example 21.3 Nurse-led immunisation clinic

At a monthly team meeting The Wellness Medical Practice identified that the episodic management of immunisations was demanding and inefficient. It was agreed that the practice would benefit from a more structured approach. An electronic audit of the practice population identified that the percentage of patients in the practice demographic who were under the age of seven was increasing rapidly. Sue, a registered nurse (Division 1), expressed an interest in this area and the practice agreed to fund her initial and ongoing education

Continued >

Example 21.3 *continued*

to the level of nurse immuniser status. A room was allocated that provided privacy for the patient, space for a dedicated vaccine refrigerator and a couch for patients under observation. Reception staff coordinated the appointment sessions: three mornings per week and one Saturday morning per month. Established clinical guidelines were followed and a practice policy was written in consultation with all staff to ensure that roles and responsibilities of staff were clear. Immunisation rates were tracked over time to evaluate the impact of this quality improvement activity.

Knowledge and information management

General practice operates in an environment that is complex and changing. Maintaining awareness of new evidence, changing clinical management guidelines and new technologies can be difficult. Health information systems are emerging as essential tools within general practice for storing, analysing and acting on information as the profession moves from paper-based recording systems to electronic systems. There is evidence that the development of information management and information technology systems, practice management and business processes improve the capacity of practices to deliver high-quality care (Proudfoot et al. 2007). Computer software can be used to support knowledge and information management in many ways including decision support, accessing discharge summaries, case findings, accessing and storing clinical guidelines, performing clinical audits and managing recall/reminder systems. There are also other technologies that can be used to manage and utilise knowledge and information, including online learning applications for education; online service directories and referral tools; use of SMS messaging and email systems for patient reminders; and mobile devices for care delivered away from the practice. This domain challenges the clinical evidence for establishing the nurse-led clinic but also prompts nurses to investigate the resources, knowledge and information management systems that will help to facilitate the development of a highly effective service.

Reflections

Questions to consider within the knowledge and information management domain in planning for a nurse-led service:

- What evidence supports the assertion that clinical intervention will add value to patients' health outcomes?
- What evaluation tool will be used to measure success and achievements?
- What documentation will be required?
- What technology can be utilised in planning the service? Suggestions include:
  - clinical audit tools to identify health needs for the practice's population
  - online service directories to identify local providers with which to partner
  - websites with clinical guidelines and evidence repositories, for example, Cochrane Library.
- What technology can be utilised in the delivery of the service? Possibilities include:
  - computers, including desktops and mobile devices
  - medical software packages
  - clinical audit tools for ongoing evaluation
  - forms of communication such as email and SMS messaging
  - websites and web-based technologies, such as the practice's website, and information websites for patients, for example, Better Health Channel resources.
- What policies and procedures are in place for:
  - follow-up of results?
  - referral pathways?
  - recall and reminders?
  - use of information to evaluate the service?

Example 21.4 Nurse-led asthma clinic

Rod, a registered (Division I) practice nurse, used an audit tool to analyse patient health needs and identified a high number of asthmatics attending the practice. He had recently been concerned by an increase in the number of patients attending the practice requiring an emergency appointment to treat their episodic asthma.

Continued >

Example 21.4 *continued*

In reviewing the literature and evidence supported by the National Asthma Council, he identified that the implementation of an asthma action plan for patients with asthma would reduce episodic presentations to hospital emergency departments and general practice. Rod attended an accredited asthma course and established a dedicated clinic to manage patients in the practice population with the diagnosis of asthma. The practice purchased a spirometer that linked directly into the patient's electronic medical file. Patients with the diagnosis of asthma (identified through the practice's medical software program) were sent a recall letter to attend the clinic for review and education in the management of their asthma. A pre-questionnaire was developed to establish a baseline of their symptoms and management. An asthma action plan was developed for each patient as part of a Medicare Benefits Schedule (MBS) funded 'Asthma Cycle of Care' and a timely review entered into the recall system. Referral pathways were established both between the clinical team (nurse and GP) and external providers (respiratory physicians, physiotherapist and pharmacist). A bimonthly meeting was established with the GP for Rod to report on patient management, improved health outcomes and review patients whose condition remained unstable. Rod worked with the GPs to ensure that patient information held within the patient's electronic medical file was updated regularly and he worked closely with administrative staff to bill appropriately for the service.

Professionalism

The domain of professionalism has a broad reach. This domain includes reference to the behaviour of both the individual professionals and the organisation in which they work. Accountability is a primary consequence of being a professional nurse. This includes accountability for all decisions both within interdisciplinary and affiliate working relationships. This domain includes the values, ethics, leadership and culture of all who are involved in the delivery of care to patients.

The dimensions of quality used in the RACGP quality framework are themselves grounded in basic principles of ethics—avoid harm (safety); doing good (appropriateness and effectiveness); respect for autonomy (appropriateness and acceptability); and justice (accessibility and efficiency) (Flynn, Booth & Portelli 2007). There is also a particular focus on a commitment to continuous quality improvement in the delivery of services. This underscores the necessity that an evaluation framework be built into any nurse-led clinic from its inception to enable monitoring of its successes and to identify areas for improvement.

In summary, professionalism addresses the education and accountability of the professional; promotes good practice and high standards; endorses ethical conduct; and underpins cooperation with other health professionals in the provision of patient-centred care.

Reflections

Questions to consider within the professionalism domain in planning for a nurse-led service:

- Are the practice management and principal doctor(s) supportive of the new service?
- Does the practice have a culture of quality improvement?
- How will evidence be collected and used to identify opportunities for continuous improvement?
- How will risks, particularly clinical risks, be managed?
- Is there anyone who can assist you? Who can you identify to be a lead champion?
- Does this program align with identified national priority health areas?
- Does this fit within your personal and professional goals?
- Are there any medico-legal requirements?
- Do you have a mentor or preceptor who has had experience in this area?

Example 21.5 Smoking cessation clinic for Aboriginal and Torres Strait Islander people

Nicole had been working as a remote area nurse for many years but had recently moved to work in an urban general practice that primarily cares for Aboriginal and Torres Strait Islander people. The practice was very supportive of engaging in activities that would improve the management of chronic disease and had a robust system of monthly data collection to measure patient health outcomes. These data demonstrated a high use of tobacco within the practice's population. Nicole was aware that Aboriginal and Torres Strait

Continued >

Example 21.5 *continued*

Islander people experience a heavy burden of disease, particularly chronic disease. She reviewed the evidence behind the risk factors for development of chronic disease in Aboriginal and Torres Strait Islander communities and found that tobacco use contributed to 12% of the overall disease burden and 17% of the health gap between Indigenous and non-Indigenous Australians (NHHRC 2009). Nicole worked with a leading GP and established a dedicated clinic to encourage smoking cessation in the community. The clinic operates within the practice and also as an outreach clinic where Nicole consults with the elders of the community in developing health promotion activities in the schools. She also worked to ensure that smoking status was recorded in each patient's clinical record, and monitored changes to smoking status among the population over time as part of a strategy to evaluate the success of the clinic. Patient surveys were also implemented and she found that the patients were satisfied with the way the clinic operated.

Finance

Ideally, resources for financing the highest quality models of health care would be unlimited; however, resources are always scarce and financing is an important determinant of quality in its own right. The financial domain is concerned with the funding mechanisms that must be considered and detailed as part of a business case to establish a nurse-led model of care. Financing a nurse-led model of care involves two key tasks. First, the resources, systems and competencies that need to be financed in order to establish and then run the service must be identified and listed. Second, the financing for them must be secure to ensure that patient access to the service is not limited in any way by excessive out-of-pocket costs. It is important to keep in mind during this second step that funding mechanisms can either encourage or hinder high-quality care and can also either make health care affordable for patients or be a financial barrier to access (Booth, Portelli & Snowdon 2005).

The kinds of resources, systems and competencies required to establish a new model include:

- physical resources (for example, computers, clinical equipment);
- labour (for example, nurse, GP and external provider time, superannuation and insurance costs);

- human capital (for example, education and training, knowledge, teamwork, referral pathways);
- technological capital (for example, software programs, data interrogation tools); and
- organisational systems (for example, policies, procedures, recall/reminder systems, appointments systems).

Opportunities to finance these components may come from a range of sources. Government funding models determine what is possible to a large

Reflections

Questions to consider within the finance domain in planning for a nurse-led service:
- What are the costs in developing the nurse-led service?
- What are the costs in maintaining the nurse-led service?
- Is this service going to be a financial risk to the practice?
- Is it acceptable to the practice for the service to be delivered as cost-neutral?
- What income streams will support this service? Are they sustainable?
- Are patient co-payments necessary? If so, can they be applied to all patients or should they be applied selectively?

Example 21.6 Nurse-led diabetes clinic

Peta, a diabetes nurse educator, decided to investigate the financial feasibility of establishing a clinic aimed at targeting patients who are at risk of developing diabetes or who have a definitive diagnosis of diabetes. In building the business case, Peta balanced the costs of implementing the program against the income gained. She considered: labour costs relating to nursing time; training for reception staff; organisational time costs (establishing appointment systems and recall and reminder systems); costs related to data cleansing; and printing costs in relation to patient educational handouts and promotional flyers to advertise the clinic. Peta then documented potential forms of income which included: MBS item numbers; Service Incentive Payments; patient co-payments and private heath insurance. It was decided that there were sufficient funding sources to enable the service to be delivered.

degree and must be fully understood and harnessed if they are to be used to support quality care. These include MBS item numbers, incentive payments for quality (Practice Incentive Payments and Service Incentive Payments) and specific programs such as the Mental Health Nurse Incentive Program. Additional sources include patient co-payments, private health insurance rebates, grants and sponsorship arrangements.

The business proposal

Many good ideas never come to fruition because of a lack of planning and/ or poor strategies for change management. Using a structured method such as the RACGP quality framework for General Practice helps in the systematic consideration of all aspects needed to create a high-quality and sustainable service. Putting your ideas into a business proposal is recommended. This will ensure that you have a comprehensive plan and that you give others in the practice an opportunity to consider and reflect on your idea in some detail.

Writing a business proposal will enable you to:

- clarify your objectives, structure your ideas, and record all that needs to be done;
- demonstrate the rationale for a new service, based on evidence;
- demonstrate a commitment to, and foster, quality improvement in care;
- outline implementation, evaluation and sustainability plans;
- outline risks and develop a risk management plan; and
- identify 'gaps' in the model, and invite input from others in the practice.

A good proposal can be daunting to write. Often, health professionals can articulate their plan verbally but find it difficult to put it down on paper. This takes practice and becomes easier over time. Nurses may identify proposal writing as a specific skill they wish to develop professionally. Project management approaches provide useful tools for nurses to appraise the feasibility and implementation of novel care models (Davidson et al. 2005), and so a short course in project management may be considered.

This section, however, intends to equip a nurse with a basic plan for constructing a business proposal following consideration of the six domains of quality outlined. All of the 'questions to consider' in each of the six domains of quality listed earlier should be carefully considered prior to beginning writing the business plan, and your answers will provide guidance about what needs to go into the plan. A thorough proposal should contain the elements listed in Table 21.1 opposite.

Table 21.1 Elements of a business proposal

Section	Purpose	Description	Approximate length
Executive summary	Provide the reader with a 'snapshot' of the entire document so that they can easily conceptualise what is being proposed.	A very brief summary of the proposal, including the problem that the model is seeking to solve, what the model will look like, who will be involved, what resources are required, where the financing will come from and how it will be evaluated.	4 – 6 sentences
Introduction	Capture the reader's interest and encourage them to keep reading.	This section should – describe in more detail the problem that the model is seeking to address (a situation analysis) including any evidence gathered about problems identified or gaps in service – specifically outline how the proposed clinic will be an improvement on current practices – briefly outline how the clinic will be implemented, touching on the detail later in the proposal.	½ – 1 page
Rationale	Provide evidence to support the need for change.	The rationale should be squarely based on evidence, which can highlight gaps between best practice and current practice. Evidence can be sourced from: – within the practice (e.g. clinical audits, patient surveys) – academic literature searches – treatment guidelines – government or peak body publications and journals.	½ – 1 page
Objectives	Clearly state what you are aiming to achieve.	Outline the objectives of the clinic—what, when, where and how it will actually deliver the services required, and how you will know whether these objectives are being achieved over time. The rationale for these objectives should already be clear to the reader.	½ page

Continued >

Table 21.1 *continued*

Section	Purpose	Description	Approximate length
Scope	Outline what you are seeking to change and what will not be changed.	Some clinics may seek to completely change current practice in the clinic, while others will simply add to current practice. It is important to provide clarity to the reader in this section if necessary (e.g. a cervical screening clinic may be an addition to current screening by GPs or a replacement of that screening).	½ page
Implementation plan	Outline the steps that will need to be taken to begin operating the clinic.	This is the heart of the business proposal. Each step should be outlined and a timeline for completion of the step documented. Important elements of the implementation plan include outlining: – changes needed to the roles of people within the practice – new staff that may need to be employed/ engaged – whether policies and procedures need to be created and/or amended – resources needed to run the clinic—both existing resources and those that need to be purchased – education and training required to ensure competence in service delivery – medico-legal issues that may arise – occupational health and safety issues that may arise – how information will be managed – technology that will be utilised – how patient privacy will be protected – systems for patient feedback and complaints – how equity of access to the service for different kinds of patients will be ensured – referral pathways to be used – how the model will be financed—where the income will come from and how costs will be met – how the model will be marketed.	1– 4 pages

Section	Purpose	Description	Approximate length
Evaluation plan	Assure the reader that the clinic will be subject to ongoing evaluation and show how the clinic will be evaluated over time.	This section should show the reader how evidence will be collected, analysed and presented to others in the clinic in order to identify opportunities for continuous quality improvement. Wherever possible, evidence should be collected to analyse whether the clinic's objectives are being met over time.	½ – 1 page
Risk identification and control	Show that risks and potential pitfalls have been anticipated and have either been mitigated entirely, or that a plan exists to address them if and when they arise.	Any change involves risks. These risks need to be clearly outlined and their likelihood of occurring and the potential consequences should they occur also detailed. For each risk, a short statement of how the consequence will be addressed should follow. Risks may include clinical risks, business and financial risks, personnel risks (e.g. OH&S, morale, workload), and legal risks.	½ – 1 page
Conclusion	Outline the 'next steps' following the presentation of the business proposal.	After everyone in the practice who needs to read the proposal has done so, a process for incorporating their feedback and making a final decision about whether or not you should proceed with the clinic needs to be outlined.	

Conclusion

The changing environment of general practice presents barriers and opportunities to the advancement of the nursing role and the development of nurse-led care. Nurses can be instrumental in taking the lead to develop new and diverse models of care. Phillips and colleagues (2008, p. 25) suggest that 'nurses have a role in enhancing organisational resilience and assisting in the orientation to change'. Adapting a quality framework may work towards alleviating the fatigue of driving change while, in turn, further develop interprofessional collaboration within the practice team. The business case for the employment of nurses is well established for the traditional nursing role, but the innovation of more advanced nursing care models requires creativity, planning and evaluation.

Key messages

Thorough planning is required before implementing nurse-led care.

Consultation for establishing a nurse-led service involves the entire practice team, including the patients.

An understanding of available funding opportunities is essential when planning a new service.

Useful resources

AGPN business case models
   http://www.agpn.com.au

National Quality Framework for General Practice
   http://www.racgp.org.au/qualityframework

Haydon, R 2007, *The shredder test—the Australian guide to writing winning proposals*, Monterey Press, Melbourne.

References

1. Australian Commission on Safety and Quality in Health (ACSQHC) 2008, Australian Charter of Health Care Rights, viewed 24 October 2009, <http://www.health.gov.au/internet/safety/publishing.nsf/Content/52533CE922D6F58BCA2573AF007BC6F9/$File/17537-charter.pdf>.

2. Australian Family Physician 2007, *A quality framework for Australian general practice*, The Royal Australian College of General Practitioners, January/February, vol. 36, no. 1–2.

3. Australian Nursing and Midwifery Council 2005, *National Competency Standards for Registered Nurses*, viewed 24 October 2009, <http://www.anmc.org.au/userfiles/file/competency_standards/Competency_standards_RN.pdf>.

4. Booth, B, Portelli, R & Snowdon, T 2005, *A quality framework for Australian general practice*, The Royal Australian College of General Practitioners, Melbourne, viewed 19 September 2009, <http://www.racgp.org.au/>.

5. Booth, B & Snowdon, T 2007, 'A quality framework for Australian general practice', *Australian Family Physician*, vol. 36, no. 1–2, pp. 8–11.

6. Booth, B, Snowdon, T & Lees, C 2005, *A quality framework for Australian general practice*, The Royal Australian College of General Practitioners, Melbourne, viewed 19 September 2009, <http://www.racgp.org.au/>.

7. Centre for Evidence-based Nursing South Australia 2007, 'Nurse-led cardiac clinics for adults with coronary heart disease', *Australian Nursing Journal*, vol. 14, no. 6, pp. 25–8.

8. Chiarella, M 2008, *Discussion Paper: New and emerging nurse-led models of primary health care*, Australian Government Health and Hospitals Reform Commission, viewed 24 October 2009, <http://www.health.gov.au/>.

9. Committee on Quality of Health Care in America 2001, *Crossing the quality chasm: a new health system for the 21st century*, viewed 26 March 2010, <http://www.nap.edu/catalog/10027.html>.

10. Davidson, P & Elliott, D 2001, 'Managing approaches to nursing care delivery, in E Chang & J Daly (eds), *Preparing for Professional Nursing Practice*, MacLennan & Petty, Sydney.

11. Davidson, P, Halcomb, E, Hickman, L, Philips, J & Graham, B 2005, 'Beyond the rhetoric: what do we mean by a model of care?', *Australian Journal of Advanced Nursing*, vol. 23, no. 3, pp. 47–55.

12. Flynn, J, Booth, B & Portelli, R 2007, 'Professionalism and the quality framework', *Australian Family Physician*, vol. 36, no. 1–2, pp. 16–18.

13. Hatchett, R 2003, 'Nurse-led Clinics Practice Issues', Routledge, London.

14. Hatchett, R 2005, 'Key issues in setting up and running a nurse-led-cardiology clinic', *Nursing Standard*, vol. 20, no. 14–16, pp. 49–53.

15. Institute of Medicine 2001, '*Crossing the quality chasm: a new health system for the 21st century*', National Academy Press, Washington DC, viewed October 2009, <http://www.nap.edu/html/quality_chasm/reportbrief.pdf>.

16. Jolly, R 2007, *Practice Nursing in Australia*, Parliament of Australia, Department of Parliamentary Services, Canberra.

17. Keleher, H, Parker, R, Abdulwadud, O & Francis, K 2009, 'Systematic review of the effectiveness of primary care nursing', *International Journal of Nursing Practice*, vol. 15, no. 1, pp. 16–24.

18. Laurent, M, Reeves, D, Hermens, R, Braspenning, J, Grol, R & Sibbald, B 2008, 'Substitution of doctors by nurses in primary care', *The Cochrane Library*, issue 4, John Wiley and Sons.

19. National Health and Hospital Reform Commission (NHHRC) 2009, *A Healthier Future For All Australians—Final Report of the National Health and Hospitals Reform Commission*, Commonwealth of Australia, Canberra.

20. Phillips, C, Pearce, C, Dwan, K, Hall, S, Porritt, J, Yates, R, Kljakovic, M & Sibbald, B 2008, *Charting new roles for Australian general practice nurses*, Australian Primary Health Care Research Institute, Canberra.

21. Proudfoot, J, Infante, F, Holton, C, Powell-Davies, G, Bubner, T, Beilby, J & Harris, M 2007, 'Organisational capacity and chronic care—an Australian general practice perspective', *Australian Family Physician*, vol. 36, no. 3, pp. 286–8, viewed 1 December 2009, <http://www.racgp.org.au/afp/200704/200704proudfoot.pdf>.

22. Pruitt, S & Epping-Jordan, J 2005, 'Learning in practice: preparing the 21st century global healthcare workforce', *British Medical Journal*, vol. 330, pp. 637–9, viewed October 2009, <http://www.bmj.com/cgi/content/full/330/7492/637>.

23. Redsell, S & Cheater, F 2008, 'Nurses' roles in primary care: developments and future prospects', *Quality Primary Care*, vol. 16, no. 2, pp. 69–71.

24. Sibbald, B, Laurant, M & Reeves, L 2006, 'Advanced nurses role in UK primary care', *Medical Journal of Australia*, vol. 185, no. 1, pp. 10–12.

25. Whitehorse Division of General Practice 2007, *Nurse-led clinics—chronic disease management in general practice*, viewed 24 October 2009, <http://www.gpv.org.au/>.

26. Wong, F & Chung, L 2006, 'Establishing a definition for a nurse-led clinic: structure, process, and outcome', *Journal of Advanced Nursing*, vol. 53, no. 3, pp. 358–69.

Glossary

Glossary terms appear as bolded orange text

Anaphylactic reaction An immediate severe hypersenstivity reaction.

Antisocial personality disorder Personality disorder where a pervasive pattern of disregard for or violation of the rights of others begins in early life and continues into adulthood.

Aseptic technique Work practices used during clinical procedures to minimise the risk of introducing infection.

Australian Childhood Immunisation Register National register that records details of vaccinations in children aged under seven years who live in Australia.

Australasian Triage Scale A five-tier urgency scale that is used for categorising clinical urgency in emergency department settings.

Autolytic debridement Employs natural processes of macrophage and endogenous proteolytic activity resulting in selective liquefacation, separation and digestion of wound debris.

Autonomy Involves the authority of the individual providers to independently make decisions and carry out the treatment plan.

Biosurgical debridement Uses scavengers to digest necrotic tissues of the wound.

Borderline personality disorder Personality disorder with a prolonged disturbance of personality function in an adult, characterised by depth and variability of moods.

Chronic care model A holistic framework for transforming health care so that patients receive coordinated care from an interdisciplinary team that includes a planned follow-up.

Clinical justice Speed of intervention that is required to achieve an optimal outcome.

Cognitive behaviour therapy Cognitive therapy is a structured psychological therapy that is based on the idea that the way we think affects the way we feel.

Cold chain monitoring System of transporting and storing vaccines within their safe temperature range.

Cost-effectiveness of intervention A form of economic analysis that compares the relative costs and outcomes (effects) of two or more courses of action.

Collaborative practice An inter-professional process for communication and decision making that enables the separate and shared knowledge and skills of care providers to synergistically influence the client or patient care provided.

Competence The ability to perform tasks and duties to the standard expected in employment.

Continuing professional development The ongoing, systematic learning process that nurses and midwives undertake to maintain their competence to practise and enhance their professional and personal skills and knowledge.

Determinants of health Conditions under which people live which determine their health.

Decision-making framework A national framework to assist nurses and midwives in decision making about their scope of practice.

Enzymatic debridement Application of topical exogenous enzymes to remove debris of the wound.

E-health The organisation and delivery of health services and information using the internet and related technologies.

Empathy Identification with and understanding of another's situation, feelings and emotions.

Evidence-based medicine The conscientious use of current best evidence in making decisions about the health care of patients.

Evidence-based practice The systematic interconnecting of scientifically generated evidence with the tacit knowledge of the expert practitioner to achieve a change in a particular practice for the benefit of a well-defined client/patient group.

Flinders model Structured self-management assessment, goal setting and care plan for chronic diseases.

Glasgow Coma Score A standardised system used to assess the degree of brain impairment and identify the seriousness of injury in relation to outcome.

Health education Strategies to improve health literacy, improve knowledge about health and healthy lifestyles for the community and the individual.

Home medicines reviews A strategy that promotes **Quality use of medicines** by incorporating inputs from accredited pharmacists in a primary health care team.

Incidence A measure of the risk of developing some new condition within a specified period of time.

Mechanical debridement Physical removal of debris from the wound.

Medication adherence Extent to which patients conform to agreed timing, dosage and frequency of medication taking.

Medication reconciliation Process for comparing the patient's current medications with those ordered for the patient while under the care of another organisation (e.g. hospital).

National Medicines Policy A national policy that aims to ensure the availability of essential affordable medications of acceptable quality, safety and efficacy.

Negligence Failure to exercise reasonable care and skill.

Newly emerging infection An infectious disease whose incidence has increased in the past 20 years or threatens to increase in the near future.

Parents' Evaluation of Developmental Status Screening tool used by parents to assess a child's development through a number of specific tasks observed in a brief period of time.

Personal protective equipment Use of gloves, water impermeable aprons or gowns, masks, protective goggles or face shields, and appropriate footwear to minimise direct unprotected contact between staff and the patient.

Pervasive development disorders A group of disorders characterised by delays in the development of socialisation and communication.

Practice nurse A registered nurse or an enrolled nurse who is employed by, or whose services are otherwise retained by, a general practice.

Primary prevention Avoiding disease by reducing susceptibility or controlling risk factors in an otherwise well population.

Prevalence Total number of cases of the disease in the population at a given time.

Primary health care Care that can be accessed directly by individuals and communities.

Primary medical care A form of primary care that provides continuing, comprehensive health care for the individual and family across all ages, sexes, diseases and parts of the body, in the context of the family and the community, emphasising disease prevention and health promotion.

Quality of life An evaluation of the general wellbeing of individuals and societies in a wide range of contexts.

Quality use of medicines An objective of National Medicines Policy which aims to promote wise selection of management options and suitable medicines, and safe and effective use of medicines.

Readiness to change model Categorises change of behaviour in five stages: pre-contemplation, contemplation, preparation, action and maintenance.

Regulation All of those legitimate and appropriate means—governmental, professional, private and individual—whereby order, identity, consistency and control are brought to the nursing profession.

Screening A procedure performed to detect the presence of a specific disease.

Secondary prevention Avoiding irreversible damage through early

detection of disease before it becomes symptomatic.

STAR skin tear classification tool Assesses the skin and any remnant flap for haematoma and ischaemia which could affect tissue viability.

Strive for 5 Australian Government Department of Health and Ageing guidelines for safe vaccine storage.

Scope of practice Practice for which nurses and midwives are educated, competent and authorised to perform.

Teamwork Coordinated action carried out by two or more individuals jointly, concurrently or sequentially. It implies common agreed goals, clear awareness of, and respect for others' roles and functions.

Tertiary prevention Avoiding complications, disability or dependence in irreversible states of the disease.

Tissue assessment tools An evaluation on the wound based on its characteristics (e.g. **TIME/CDE**).

Transtheoretical model of behaviour change A health psychology theory involving the progression through a series of six stages (see **Readiness to change model**) to explain or predict a person's success or failure in achieving a proposed behavioural change.

Triage Triage is the rapid systematic process that is used in health care services to determine a person's level of urgency at point-of-entry to the service.

Index